Conversations between AIDS counsellors and their clients bring delicate and potentially threatening issues into play. In this study Anssi Peräkylä applies the principles of conversation analysis to his exploration of AIDS counselling, using data from video-recorded counselling sessions in a London teaching hospital. He meticulously analyses this data to show how various questioning techniques – in this case arising from the Milan School Family Systems Theory – operate in these situations, and how counsellors attempt through the design and placement of their questions to achieve the co-operation of their clients, with varying success. His conclusions provide a timely and illuminating insight into the management of a sensitive topic through various techniques of indirectness.

W0055292

Studies in Interactional Sociolinguistics 11

General editor: *John J. Gumperz*
Advisory editors: *Charles Briggs*
                      Paul Drew
                      Deborah Schiffrin

AIDS counselling

Studies in Interactional Sociolinguistics

AIDS counselling
Institutional interaction and clinical practice

Anssi Peräkylä

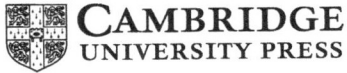
CAMBRIDGE
UNIVERSITY PRESS

CAMBRIDGE UNIVERSITY PRESS
Cambridge, New York, Melbourne, Madrid, Cape Town, Singapore, São Paulo

Cambridge University Press
The Edinburgh Building, Cambridge CB2 2RU, UK

Published in the United States of America by Cambridge University Press, New York

www.cambridge.org
Information on this title: www.cambridge.org/9780521454636

First published 1995
This digitally printed first paperback version 2005

A catalogue record for this publication is available from the British Library

Library of Congress Cataloguing in Publication data

Peräkylä, Anssi
    AIDS counselling: institutional interaction and clinical practice
    Anssi Peräkylä.
        p.   cm. – (Studies in interactional sociolinguistics: 11)
    Includes bibliographical references and index.
    ISBN 0 521 45463 8 (hardback)
    1. AIDS (Disease) – Patients – Counselling of. I. Title.
    II. Series.
    RC607.A26P449 1995
    616.97′92 – dc20   95-38246   CIP

ISBN-13 978-0-521-45463-6 hardback
ISBN-10 0-521-45463-8 hardback

ISBN-13 978-0-521-02288-0 paperback
ISBN-10 0-521-02288-6 paperback

Ja Oravalle

But when one comes in contact with social phenomena, one is, on the contrary, surprised by the astonishing regularity with which they occur under the same circumstances. Even the most minute and the most trivial practices recur with the most astonishing uniformity.

E. Durkheim *The Rules of Sociological Method.*
New York: Free Press, 1964, p. 94.

A quite specific *astonishment* stands at the beginning of every theological perception, inquiry and thought, in the fact at the root of every theological word. This astonishment is indispensable if theology is to exist and be perpetually renewed as a modest, free, critical, and happy science.

K. Barth *Evangelical Theology: An Introduction.*
New York: Holt, Rinehart and Winston, 1963, p. 62.

CONTENTS

Preface

This study has been made possible by the solidarity, help and sympathy of a number of people, all of whom I want to thank. For three years (1989–1991) I was privileged to work with Professor David Silverman as Glaxo Research Fellow at Goldsmiths' College, London. The intellectual environment of my work was created by him; and throughout the three years, he patiently gave invaluable advice and encouragement. An earlier version of this book was prepared as a Ph.D. dissertation supervised by Professor Silverman.

Christian Heath gave his advice during the crucial times of the first year of the project. David Greatbatch commented upon many of the data analyses presented here, and made available his experience of the analysis of institutional interaction. While preparing the book, I was given an opportunity to stay twice for a month at UCLA, where John Heritage gave me insightful suggestions and encouragement. On various occasions during the research project, Paul Drew gave most helpful advice. Towards the end of the project, Marja-Leena Sorjonen commented upon the data analyses related to several chapters.

During my research project, I also had an opportunity to discuss the work with experienced AIDS counsellors at the Royal Free Hospital, London. Riva Miller, Eleanor Goldman and Robert Bor gave invaluable advice. Their writing on AIDS counselling based on Family Systems Theory was a crucial source of insight for me.

Financially, my work has been supported by Glaxo Holdings plc, University of Tampere, and the Academy of Finland. I gratefully acknowledge the permission of Mouton de Gruyter to use materials that have earlier appeared in TEXT, in the articles 'Owning experience' (co-authored with David Silverman, in TEXT 11-3) and 'Invoking a hostile world' (in TEXT 13-2).

In revising the typescript, Judith Ayling of Cambridge University Press gave her most valuable support, which I gratefully acknowledge.

I am particularly grateful to the clients and the counsellors participating in the sessions that I have used as my data. By giving their consent to the use of the video recordings for research they have made my work possible. I am painfully aware that a sociological analysis like this falls short of fully understanding the suffering, uncertainty and hope with which the people I have been observing live. Many sessions that I have analysed have touched me personally; and I am sure that they will touch everybody who reads this study.

Finally, I want to thank my wife, Outi Paloposki. She gave her appreciation and sympathetic criticism of my work and also helped with the English language. But most importantly, through her presence she has created the *milieu* for living, in which it is possible to love and to work; and I am always grateful for that.

Anssi Peräkylä
University of Helsinki

Transcription conventions

Symbols

[	C:	Quite a [while.	Left square brackets:

[C: Quite a [while.   Left square brackets:
    P: [Yeah.   the point at which a current speaker's talk is overlapped by another's talk. The point at which the overlapping talk stops may be marked with a right-hand bracket.

    C: Q[uite a while.   Spaced-out letters are sometimes used to indicate the approximate duration of the overlap of two speakers' talk.
    P: [Y e s I know

=   W: I'm aware of =   Equal signs, one at the end of a line and one at the beginning of the next line: no gap between the two lines.
    C: =Yes. Would you confirm that?

(.4)   Yes (.2) yeah   Numbers in parentheses: elapsed time in silence in tenths of a second.

(.)   to get (.) treatment   A dot in parentheses: a tiny gap, probably no more than one-tenth of a second.

___	What's <u>up</u>?	Underlining: some form of stress, via pitch and/or amplitude.
: :	O:<u>kay</u>?	Colons: prolongation of the immediately prior sound. The more colons, the longer the prolongation.
WORD	I've got ENOUGH TO WORRY ABOUT	Capitals, except at the beginnings of lines: especially loud sounds relative to the surrounding talk.
.hhhh	I feel that (.2) .hhh	A row of hs prefixed by a dot: an inbreath; without a dot, an outbreath. The more hs, the longer the in- or outbreath.
( )	future risks and ( ) and life ( )	Empty parentheses: the transcriber's inability to hear what was said.
(word)	Would you see (there) anything positive	Parenthesized words: possible hearings.
(( ))	confirm that ((continues))	Double parentheses: author's descriptions, not transcriptions.
*	*no*	Asterisks on both sides of a word: it is uttered at a low volume in contrast to the surrounding talk.
.,?	uhu?	Punctuation marks are used to indicate intonations: full stop indicates falling intonation; question mark rising intonation, and comma slightly rising intonation.

>>	but (.) >>can I	Two 'greater than' signs: a hurried beginning.
> <	>I would like< to	The section of talk surrounded by 'greater than' and 'smaller than' symbols is spoken at a quicker pace than surrounding talk.
-	I would li-	A dash at the end of a word indicates a 'cut-off'.

Speaker designations

In the extracts, the participants' institutional identities are abbreviated as follows.

C = Counsellor
C1 = Principal counsellor in two-counsellor sessions
C2 = Co-counsellor in two-counsellor sessions
P = Patient
O = Observer

There are also other abbreviations, which are explained in each individual case. If the transcriber has not been quite sure about a speaker's identity, the speaker designation is in brackets, thus, (P).

In the extracts, all clients' and counsellors' proper names have been changed. In the text, the term 'Client' includes the patient and whoever accompanies him or her in the counselling session.

Numbering of extracts

The extracts are numbered separately in each chapter, starting always with number 1 (the first number at the top of each extract). The second set of numbers indicates the location of the segment in the data base. Thus (2) (E4-20) identifies the second extract in a chapter; the location of which in the data base is 'E4-20'.

Transcription of the postural orientation

The presentation of postural orientation is made by using two different systems. In the excerpts where several participants' postural orientation is indicated, arrows and explanatory texts are used. An example is shown below. Note that the length of a silence (at the end of C's talk) is indicated by a broken line, where each dash indicates a tenth of a second. In the segment below, C's utterance is followed by 0.6 sec. silence, during which P shifts his orientation from C to M.

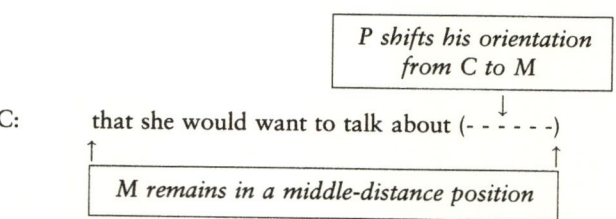

```
                          ┌─────────────────────────┐
                          │   P shifts his orientation │
                          │      from C to M          │
                          └─────────────────────────┘
                                           ↓
C:        that she would want to talk about (- - - - - -)
          ↑                                            ↑
          ┌─────────────────────────────────────────┐
          │  M remains in a middle-distance position │
          └─────────────────────────────────────────┘
```

When only one participant's postural orientation is indicated, or when the system above would have been insufficient, a more complex notation developed by Goodwin (1981) and Heath (1986) is applied. In this notation, a person's orientation towards another person is indicated by different types of lines. At the beginning of each line, the person whom the subject orients to is indicated by letters in brackets.

A row of commas (,,,) indicates a process where the person disorients from somebody to whom he/she was oriented to; and a row of full stops (. . .) indicates a process where a person is turning towards somebody. The letters 'md' are sometimes used to indicate a middle-distance orientation, where a person is not oriented to anybody, but nevertheless is gazing up. The more complicated system is exemplified below. In this segment, the postural orientation of C2 and C1 is presented: C2 is stably oriented to W, whereas C1's postural orientation alternates between W and C2.

```
C2:   (w) - - - - - - - - - - - - - - - - - - - - - - - - - - - - - -
C2:   or not because [(      ) later.
C1:   (w) - - - - - - - -,,,,...**(c2)**********,,..(w) - - - - - -
W:                         [Oh I would want to know.=[Rather
P:                                                    [yes
```

Ad hoc symbols have been used to indicate other forms of bodily expression. They are explained separately in connection with each transcript where they appear.

1

Introduction

This book is about verbal interaction in AIDS counselling sessions at a London teaching hospital. In the first place, then, it is a study about structures of interaction in a social setting called 'AIDS counselling'. More specifically, it is a study about the particular structures of interaction which arise when such counselling is informed by a certain kind of theoretical thinking, namely the Milan School Family Systems Theory.

The book also seeks to be an application of Conversation Analysis. This by now well-established method of interaction research will here be used in the examination of a specific type of professional–client intercourse: one where the professionals have a strong theoretical consciousness which informs their activity. Therefore, the study reported in this book is also an experiment demonstrating the applicability of Conversation Analysis in the research of theory-based interaction.

This is not a study of AIDS, nor is it about the experiences of people living with AIDS. It is not a study of AIDS counselling in terms of the development and distribution of the counselling services, or in terms of the professionals' understanding about what they should be doing, or in terms of the clients' needs for counselling or their satisfaction with what they have received. Moreover, it is not about Family Systems Theory *per se*. It is an empirical study about face-to-face interaction.

In the Introduction I wish to give the reader the necessary background information which will make it easier to understand the analysis of actual interactional data to be presented later. Three topics will be introduced: first, AIDS counselling as a newly emerged professional practice will be discussed. Thereafter, some key concepts and methods related to the Milan School Family Systems Theory will be presented; and finally, Conversation Analysis, which will give the methodological tools for the data analysis, will be introduced.

AIDS counselling

Apart from human suffering, the AIDS epidemic has brought with it reorganization in many segments of contemporary social life. This concerns such varied spheres of life as conduct in intimate sexual relations, needle-sharing, administration and content of health education, ranking of medical sub-specialities, and funding of social research. The professional activity of counselling is one of the spheres affected.

One of the social responses to the HIV epidemic has been the setting-up of counselling services for the people whose lives have been touched by HIV and AIDS. In the UK, the (former) Department of Health and Social Security recommended that such counselling be given to anyone having an HIV antibody test. Counselling is also offered in clinics giving medical treatment to patients diagnosed as HIV-positive or as having AIDS (Chester 1987).

A World Health Organization definition describes HIV counselling in the following way:

HIV counselling is an on-going dialogue and relationship between client or patient and counsellor with the aims of preventing HIV transmission and providing psychosocial support for those affected, directly and indirectly, by HIV.   (cit. in Carballo and Miller 1989: 117)

Two leading experts in HIV counselling interpret this as meaning that HIV counselling has a two-fold aim. On the one hand, it seeks to prevent the transmission of the HIV virus through addressing both non-infected and infected groups. On the other, it seeks to provide psychosocial support for those affected by HIV, either carriers of the virus or their family members, friends and relatives. In doing this, it seeks to encourage and enhance the self-determination and self-confidence of the people concerned, and to improve family and community relationships (Carballo and Miller 1989).

In practice, HIV counselling in the UK is undertaken by several professional groups: social workers, health advisers, clinical psychologists, and medical doctors. The organizational and theoretical frameworks vary (Silverman 1990; Burnard 1992).

Chester (1987: 7) points out that what is generally called 'HIV counselling' can consist of three different types of activity. *Advice* involves delivery of information, explanation and guidance. *Support* involves encouragement, enhancement of morale and maintenance of sociability; and *personal counselling* is 'the skilled and principled use of relationship to facilitate self-knowledge, emotional acceptance and growth, and the optimal development of personal resource'. Moreover, activities like *health education* and *training of staff* working with HIV-positive patients are sometimes included in HIV counselling (see D. Miller 1987a); but they take place outside AIDS counselling sessions and therefore are not part of the activity that is to be analysed in this book.

Advice and support are self-explanatory terms that need no further clarification here. However, the third component of HIV counselling, personal counselling, deserves a further comment. By this term Chester refers to the professional activity of counselling in a more limited sense of the word. The British Association of Counselling defines counselling in this more narrow sense as follows:

People become engaged in counselling when a person, occupying regularly or temporarily the role of counsellor, offers or agrees explicitly to offer time, attention and respect to another person or persons temporarily in the role of client.   (cit. in Chester 1987: 60)

The counsellors exercise the professional skills acquired through training to facilitate personal change (such as alleviation of distress or activation of personal resources for coping with difficulties) in the client. Other key aspects of counselling interaction are that it is confined to certain places and times, it is based on a mutual contract, and it operates mainly through verbal exchange between the client and the professional.

All this makes counselling rather similar to what is usually called 'psychotherapy'. There is no general agreement on what actually constitutes the difference between these two (Chester 1987: 62).

Nelson-Jones (1982) suggests that counselling focuses on 'less disturbed' clients in non-medical settings, whereas psychotherapy deals with more severe cases. However, this is disputable, given the long tradition (beginning with Freud) of psychotherapeutic treatment of people suffering from mild neuroses within the context of private practice. Miller and Bor (1988) say that psychotherapy focuses exclusively on mental health, whereas counselling is more pragmatic and associated with a range of activities such as education, marriage guidance and pastoral and medical care.

However, when it comes to understanding what AIDS counselling is, it is sufficient at this stage to say that AIDS counselling contains elements of advice-giving, delivery of information and support, and elements that are more closely associated with 'counselling' as a psychosocially oriented helping profession.

Counselling at the different stages of HIV infection

In terms of the stages of HIV infection, there are three typical environments for AIDS counselling. *Pre-test counselling* takes place before the HIV antibody test. It aims at ensuring that the patient's consent to testing is genuinely informed and that the patient understands the result of the test (e.g. not a test for AIDS). The time of last risk is discussed so that the meaning of the test result can be understood. The practical and psychosocial consequences of being identified as seropositive are also addressed (Miller and Bor 1988; McCreaner 1989).

Post-test counselling involves giving the test result and addressing its implications for the person and others who may be connected with him or her. In the case of a positive test result, this means ensuring again that the patient understands the meaning of 'being HIV-positive', identifying the patient's immediate concerns, and helping him or her to plan (possibly in the very short term) what to do next (Miller and Bor 1988).

Counselling with HIV-positive patients aims to enhance the medical, social and emotional management of the illness. In particular, being HIV-positive may be a catalyst for many anxieties and relationship problems to emerge. The patient's fears concerning his or her future (illness, disfigurement, and death) are addressed (Bor and Miller 1988; George 1989). When counselling HIV-positive persons, the emphasis may gradually shift from 'advice' elements more towards 'support' and 'personal counselling' (Chester 1987: 8); and in addition to the HIV-positive patient, his or her family members, friends or other associates may become increasingly engaged as clients of the counsellor (Miller 1987b).

The bulk of the data analysed in this book is from counselling with HIV-positive patients. I have examined no post-test sessions, and data from pre-test sessions has been used only to a very limited degree. Consequently, the interactions analysed here involve more 'support' and 'personal counselling' types of activity than only advice-giving and information. Therefore, all the observations made here may not be directly applicable to a pre- or a post-test setting.

HIV-positive haemophiliacs

Apart from the patient's stage of HIV infection, the way he or she became infected may influence the focus of counselling. In Western countries, diagnosed HIV infection has thus far most severely affected three specific population groups: homosexual men, intra-venous (IV) drug-users, and haemophiliacs. Most of the data used here is from counselling with haemophilic men.

Haemophilia is a hereditary illness involving a tendency for the patient to suffer internal haemorrhages through failure of the blood to clot normally. The genetic disorder causing haemophilia is carried by mothers, but the illness affects only males. During the first half of the 1980s more than 1,000 British haemophiliacs contracted HIV infection through contaminated blood products used for their treatment. Since 1985 it has been made virtually sure that all the blood products used are safe.

In the UK, HIV-positive haemophiliacs are offered counselling in all Haemophilia Centres, that is, in the out-patient clinics which are responsible for the treatment of haemophilia. Consequently, counselling is given on the same premises where the patients were treated prior to HIV infection, and most likely by staff members who already know them. Chester (1987: 21) talks about the 'distinctiveness of the haemophilic group in respect of HIV counselling', probably referring to the fact that the counselling services for HIV-positive haemophiliacs are well funded and organized.

Counselling services for haemophiliacs were largely already established *before* HIV infection, both because haemophilic families receive genetic counselling and chronic illness affects the whole family. It is also likely that counselling (as well as medical treatment) related to HIV/AIDS is much less stigmatizing in the context of haemophilia centres than in the context of sexually transmitted disease and genito-urinary medicine clinics.

Family Systems Theory

Counsellors working in different fields – including AIDS counsellors – have variable training and theoretical orientation. Family Systems Theory is one of the theories that has been applied in counselling. The data presented in this book comes solely from the practice of counsellors who identify themselves with this 'school' and, therefore, it is necessary for the reader to have some background knowledge about Family Systems Theory, as follows.

During the last decade, the Milan School Family Systems Theory[1] has been applied increasingly in various fields of therapy, counselling and social work in Britain and elsewhere (for an overview of recent developments in different settings, see Campbell and Draper 1985). This movement, now very influential, had its beginnings only some twenty years ago. It was initiated in a private clinic in Milan, Italy, when Mara Selvini Palazzoli, a child psychiatrist, together with her colleagues started 'The institute for family study' (in 1967) and then 'The centre for the study of family' (in 1971).

Selvini Palazzoli and her colleagues were initially treating anorectic and schizophrenic patients. Disillusioned by the ineffectiveness of psychoanalytic therapy, Selvini Palazzoli became interested in the family therapeutic and cybernetic ideas developed by Gregory Bateson and his co-workers in the US (Hoffman 1981). Instead of

---

[1] The systemic view in family therapy has been parallelly developed in various clinics and research institutions, both in the US and in Europe. The Milan Group was one of the most influential contributors to this. Because the counsellors whose work will be analysed in this book use the Milan approach, I will concentrate on this specific theory and technique also in my introductory notes presented here. In the text, the term 'Family Systems Theory' will therefore refer specifically to the Milan school of thought. For an overview of the different systemic perspectives in family therapy, see Hoffman (1981) and Sluzki (1983).

considering the behavioural symptoms as indications of the intra-psychic conflicts of the individuals involved, the Milan associates started to view the manifest problems as parts of the unacknow-ledged 'games' that the families were playing.

In these games, the 'symptoms' served as ways of coping with something that the families otherwise felt as threatening. In other words, individual symptoms were seen as a part of a 'system' com-prising the whole family. Since then, the Milan associates have widened their view further, now locating any 'problems' not only in the context of the family, but of other social and political institu-tions, including the therapy itself (Selvini Palazzoli *et al.* 1978; Boscolo *et al.* 1986; Hoffman 1988).

Given this new psychopathological understanding, the aim of the therapy is to make families aware of their games and of the func-tions which the behaviour labelled as 'problem' serves. The game is interrupted, and the family is helped to acknowledge the systemic functions of their problems (Hoffman 1981). Borrowing an analogy from biology, the Milan School associates began to view the thera-pists' task as inflicting a *perturbation* on to a system (which they themselves are part of), so that the system will react and find new (and possibly less problematic) ways of operating (Boscolo *et al.* 1986: 18). The interruption, or perturbation, is achieved by the therapists using specific interactive techniques.

The precondition of the use of the therapeutic techniques based on Family Systems Theory is that whole families, instead of indivi-dual clients, participate in the sessions, and that the therapists work in teams. The three most innovative new techniques involve 'circular questioning', 'live supervision', and concluding 'interventions'.

As a theoretical idea, 'circularity' emphasizes that knowledge is always gained through looking at difference. The therapists' activ-ity, therefore, consists of soliciting information in such a manner that differences between the family members' perspectives and experiences, as well as each individual's perceptions about the dif-ferences between the other family members, are brought into focus (Selvini Palazzoli *et al.* 1980). The theoretical idea of 'circularity' is translated into a specific technique called 'circular questioning' (Penn 1982; Fleuridas *et al.* 1986; Feinberg 1990; Mauksch and Roesler 1990). Following this technique, the therapist typically asks one member of the family to comment on the relationship of two others in their presence. The questions are preferably so constructed that they focus on differences, e.g. 'Who is closer to father, your daughter or your son?' Sometimes the circular questions are asked in a hypothetical manner, e.g. 'If you had not been born, what do you think your parents' marriage would be like now?' (Hoffman 1981). This kind of questioning is efficient in engaging the family in talk, and helps family members to realize how the problem of one member affects all the others, i.e. the 'systemic' character of their problems.

In 'live supervision' one (or sometimes two) of the therapists converses with the family members, while the rest of the team follow the session behind a one-way mirror. The team can communicate with the therapist during breaks in the session, or, in some cases, by telephone. This means that the functioning of the family and that of the family-plus-therapist is noted and discussed by the whole team. As the team members behind the screen are not actively involved in the interaction, their perspective is different from that of the therapist. This enables the team to see and discuss the family and the process of the interview more productively (Speed *et al.* 1982; Burnham and Harris 1985; Cade and Cornwell 1985; Selvini and Selvini Palazzoli 1991).

In the Family Systems approach, the term 'intervention' refers to the concluding stage of the session. After the therapist(s) have talked with the family there is a break, during which the team meets for discussion. The results of this discussion are then communicated to the family by the therapist(s) who conducted the session. Typically, the family is either given a message from the whole team, or a ritual task. In the message, a 'positive connotation' is created, whereby the team emphasizes that the problem is 'logical and meaningful in its context' (Boscolo *et al.* 1986: 4). The ritual task is an order for the family to behave in a certain way regularly at certain times. The ritual will demonstrate the systemic function of the symptoms. For example, other family members can be asked to regularly tell the bed-wetter how she helps them all by her bed-wetting, e.g. by making laundry for the mother to keep her busy.

In this book, the AIDS counsellors' use of 'circular questioning' and 'live supervision' will be studied in detail. The AIDS counsellors also use the technique of 'interventions' but unfortunately the space available will not allow us to study that in any detail.

Family Systems Theory in AIDS counselling

The Milan School Family Systems Theory was developed in the context of the psychiatric treatment of severely disturbed patients. There is a big difference between a private clinic treating anorectic and schizophrenic patients and a hospital based outpatient clinic treating haemophiliacs. Accordingly, the logic of activities based on Family Systems Theory cannot be exactly the same.

The counsellors whose work will be studied in this book are leading practitioners developing the methods of Family Systems Theory to AIDS counselling. Therefore, their writings will help us to see what is considered as relevant in this theory in the context of this particular counselling.

The systemic view concerning the 'problems' and what can be done with them is central. HIV/AIDS-related issues may be problematic in different ways for different individuals associated with the patient. For example, the worsening of the patient's condition may be a source of anxiety for him or herself, but also a problem for the physician who feels unable to give bad news (Bor *et al.* 1989). An HIV crisis may highlight any difficulties that the patient has had previously in his or her relationships with those close to them. Moreover, in order to deal with the problems change may be needed not only in the patient as an individual, but in the way that the different 'systems' involved operate (Miller and Bor 1988).

Along with the general systemic thinking, AIDS counsellors using the Family Systems Theory emphasize the same principles and techniques in conducting a session as their colleagues in other fields. The management of these techniques will be the primary research object in this study.

'Circular questioning' is consistently used in AIDS counselling to highlight the clients' different perspectives on their problems. Key aspects of this will be analysed in chapter 3. In particular, AIDS counsellors use *hypothetical questions*, which usually are *future-oriented* (Miller and Bor 1988). In such questions, counsellors ask clients to describe their life and relationships in a hypothetical future situation. They may ask, e.g. 'If you had to be admitted to

hospital as an in-patient, and had not told your boyfriend about your positive antibody test, what might be the effect of this on your relationship?' (Miller and Bor 1988: 17). This type of questioning makes it possible to address issues that the clients might be afraid to talk about (loss, disfigurement, death and dying) in a manageable way. Hypothetical future-oriented questioning will be analysed in chapters 6 and 7.

'*Live supervision*' is also used by AIDS counsellors. However, because in the clinic that we are studying the counsellors do not have available two adjacent rooms with a one-way screen, they have had to develop their own variation of this technique. There is an observing team member present in the same room where the counselling takes place. For this type of situation, a particular questioning practice has been developed: the observing team member can feed in questions, targeted to the clients but nominally addressed to the counsellor who is conducting the interview. The management of this questioning technique will be studied in chapters 4 and 5.

The setting

The bulk of the data used in this research is from AIDS counselling sessions in the Haemophilia Centre of the Royal Free Hospital, London. In addition to this, a smaller amount of data has been received from a clinic specializing in HIV and AIDS, and also operating in the Royal Free Hospital.

In the Haemophilia Centre sessions, there are three professionals who in turn work as principal counsellors at the interviews. One of them is a social worker and two are medical doctors. The social worker – Mrs Riva Miller – and one of the doctors – Dr. Eleanor Goldman – have received formal training in Family Systems Theory, and they were in charge of most of the sessions.[2] At the HIV/AIDS clinic there were two counsellors (both psychologists)

---

[2] All the proper names appearing in the transcripts shown in the book are pseudonyms. After the preparation of the transcripts, however, the two counsellors who most often appear on the tapes expressed their preference for disclosing their identities. Therefore, it might be relevant to indicate that 'Mrs Heller' is the pseudonym for Mrs Riva Miller, and 'Dr Kaufman' for Dr Eleanor Goldman.

who conducted sessions. One of them – Dr Robert Bor – had formal training in Family Systems Theory.

As already indicated above, the professionals whose counselling practice will be observed in this book are working in the forefront of the development of AIDS counselling based on the Family Systems Theory. They have written numerous influential publications, and are regularly in demand as consultants and teachers, not only in the UK, but worldwide. This active contribution to the Family Systems Theory by the subjects of this research adds an important aspect to the *theory-based* nature of the interaction studied here.

Tape-recordings of 32 counselling sessions were used as data. These included 26 sessions with HIV-positive haemophiliacs taking place at the Haemophilia Centre, and 5 pre-test sessions and 1 session with a newly diagnosed HIV-positive patient at the HIV/ AIDS clinic. All patients, except one at the HIV/AIDS clinic, were male (which is the reason for the subsequent use of the pronoun 'he' for the patients in the text.) The data base is described in detail in the appendix. In what follows, I describe briefly the setting for these counselling sessions and the general course of events during them.

The pre-counselling sessions at the HIV/AIDS clinic are linked with HIV testing. Most patients volunteer for a test, or alternatively they may be referred to the clinic by doctors from other units of the hospital where it has been thought that a test would be useful. In the data used in this study one pre-test session was with a patient referred by another unit of the hospital. Before blood is taken for the test, the patients are counselled. The only case not directly linked to testing at the HIV/AIDS clinic was of a patient who had come to that clinic for follow-up treatment shortly after having been diagnosed as HIV-positive in a small private clinic.

At the Haemophilia Centre, HIV-positive patients are counselled with intervals varying from a few weeks to more than a year. The initiative for a counselling session comes sometimes from a client and sometimes from the staff of the clinic. Clients may contact counsellors and ask for an appointment. In the majority of cases, however, counselling is linked with the patients' regular medical visits to the Centre. The usual reason for a visit is a medical review, either routine or one focused on a particular complaint. Along with the medical review, a counselling session can be arranged. The appointment is offered for the patient either by the administrative staff organizing the time of the medical visit or at the end of the previous counselling session.

The combination of the people present at the sessions varies. All 5 pre-test sessions at the HIV/AIDS clinic were one-to-one counselling. Sometimes there is only one counsellor with the patient at the Haemophilia Centre, too. However, the counsellors at the Haemophilia Centre prefer to work in pairs when pressure of work allows. One is the principal counsellor and the other adopts the role of the co-counsellor, who only occasionally takes part in the talk (this arrangement is analysed in detail in chapters 4 and 5).

Apart from one or two counsellors, there may be an indefinite number of observers present: doctors, nurses and other staff, who remain silent unless the counsellor conducting the session invites them to comment. Usually the principal counsellor asks at the end of the session if observers wish to comment upon what they have heard; their contributions may also be solicited if a matter arises in which they have a special competence (normally related to medicine or nursing). The rationale for the presence of observers is to teach them counselling, and to keep them aware of issues related to the patient which may be relevant in their own interactions with him.

The counsellors at the Haemophilia Centre repeatedly encourage patients to bring their 'significant others', usually spouses, family members or girlfriends, to the sessions. With adolescent patients, mothers or fathers are present in most interviews, and with other patients 'significant others' are present in about half of the sessions. When this is the case the counsellors treat all clients present on an equal footing, i.e. they address their questions and commentaries not only to the patient, but also to his 'significant others'.

The counselling sessions take place in ordinary office rooms, usually at the office of the practitioner who is conducting the interview. As previously mentioned, all professionals are in the same space with the clients during the session.

There is no standard agenda for the sessions. What the participants talk about varies according to the patients' situations. However, some themes are brought up recurrently. Especially if the doctor responsible for the patient's medical treatment is present, some time in the counselling session can be used to elicit information about his recent medical condition from the patient. This information is not treated as it would be in a purely medical interview: examinations, diagnoses and treatment decisions do not follow. Rather, the participants are setting up a 'list' of concerns that will be addressed further when the doctor examines the patient.

Issues related to the transmission of HIV recur in many sessions. The counsellors evaluate the patients' knowledge through their questions, and offer information and correct misconceptions when needed. With younger clients especially, birth control and family planning are discussed along with the transmission of the virus. Questions related to medication and drug trials are also often discussed. The patients' level of awareness is explored and further information offered when necessary. Socio-economic issues are always given some attention. Counsellors discuss practical matters such as housing, income, transport and education. Letters and medical reports are provided in support of social service benefits and housing.

Sensitive issues relating to the patients' fears concerning the future come up very often during counselling sessions. Counsellors encourage patients and their families to prepare themselves and to plan ahead of time, taking into account the possibility of distressing events in the future.

In general, the topics covered in the interviews are usually elicited from the patients. In other words, counsellors do not say 'Let's talk about safe sex / your housing / your fears of the future', but rather they ask the patients and the others present at the session to name what they want to talk about. This is not to say, however, that counsellors do not influence what is discussed during the sessions (much of the book concerns that kind of influence), but, at least nominally, they avoid imposing their agendas on the patients.

The length of the sessions varies. Some last less than half an hour, most are around 50 minutes, and some much longer than an hour. When HIV counselling was started at the clinic, the counsellors used to have a break during the course of the session if there were two of them present. During the break they consulted one another and then concluded the session with a summary and commentary on what was seen and heard in relation to how the clients were coping. Through pressure of work, however, time to discuss the concluding intervention has often been lacking, and most of the sessions examined in this book proceeded without a break. However, at the end of the sessions the counsellors still regularly summarize what they have heard and comment upon the clients' coping. If there is more than one practitioner present, the summary and commentary are often so arranged that the professionals talk to one another. To avoid diffusing the power of the conclusion, further discussion is discouraged.

The general aim of the study

Thus far, I hope to have offered the reader some essential background information for understanding the data analyses to be presented later. Apart from knowledge about the hospital and about AIDS counselling in general, it is important to remember that the counsellors whose work will be studied are informed by the Milan School Family Systems Theory: many features of the sessions are inspired by this particular model of thinking about therapy and family life.

Now we are in a position where we can formulate, in a preliminary fashion, the purpose of this study. It is to examine *how the tasks of AIDS counselling and the ideas of Family Systems Theory are translated into the practice of verbal interaction.* In other words, we want to study how, in the details of their talk, the counsellors (and their clients) work through their AIDS-related counselling agenda and their specific counselling theory.

As my brief introductory notes have already shown, the textbooks and articles arising from Family Systems Theory and the AIDS counselling manuals describe the activities involved in AIDS counselling based on Family Systems Theory. This book does not seek to be, and cannot be, any substitute for them. However, the counselling textbooks and manuals usually operate on a rather general level of specification: for example, different questioning techniques are presented in the form of paraphrased examples (such as the example 'hypothetical future-oriented question' cited above on pages 9–10). Needless to say, paraphrased examples work perfectly well in their context, which is to explicate counselling theory or to give advice to beginners.

In this study, however, we are concerned with another level of precision. We will seek to show, in the most minute detail, *how* the counselling agenda and the different techniques involved are worked through. This means we will study how the counsellors maintain their footing as questioners in the first place, how they design and deliver their questions arising from the various Family Systems techniques, and how the clients respond to these questions.

Our general purpose, therefore, will be to explicate the interactional competencies that the counsellors and the clients mobilize while operating in a Family Systems Theory framework in the context of AIDS counselling. As the data analyses will show, there is a vast array of such skills, most of which are normally activated by the participants in a semi-automatic, unreflective manner. As the data analyses will also show, the *clients'* interactional competencies and practices are as important as those of the counsellors: the functioning of Family Systems Theory is dependent on both. Unravelling the participants' competencies and skills will be one of the main contributions of this book.

In order to achieve the aim of this study, we need other theoretical and methodological tools than those that Family Systems Theory can provide. The focus of Family Systems Theory is primarily on understanding family relationships. As far as this theory is interested in the dynamics of counselling or therapy sessions, it is always primarily concerned with how things that happen during the sessions are linked with changes in family relations, which of course occur primarily outside the sessions.

In this book our sphere of interest is narrower. We want to concentrate exclusively on what is happening during the counselling session. We will not try to say anything about the effects of these interactions on the clients' relations to others outside the sessions. Nor have we tried to study any change in the clients as could possibly be seen by comparing consecutive sessions with the same clients. What we want to do is to study the interactional practices that *any* AIDS counselling sessions based on Family Systems Theory are assembled from – regardless of whether these sessions are effective in changing the clients or their family relations. The conceptual apparatus of Conversation Analysis provides the theoretical and methodological tools for this.[3]

---

[3] Gale (1991) points out that there is a close affinity between the systemic epistemology of Family Therapy, and the reflexive research methodology of Conversation Analysis. His review of recent literature shows that in Family

Therefore, in this book a practice which is in itself theory-based (on Family Systems Theory) will be analysed using the tools of another theory and method (Conversation Analysis). A brief introduction to Conversation Analysis and its application to research of client–professional encounters will be given in what follows.

A research programme on language use

During the last two decades, a new approach to research of spoken interaction, called Conversation Analysis (CA), has been established and has spread rapidly to a number of academic departments of sociology, linguistics and communications in various universities in the Western world. The original impetus for this school of research was given in the lectures and writings of the late Harvey Sacks (e.g. Sacks 1972; 1974; 1992a; 1992b) at the University of California, in the intellectual environment shaped by Harold Garfinkel's (1967) ethnomethodology. Sacks' most important co-worker was Emanuel Schegloff (e.g. 1968; 1979; 1981; 1992a) and his most influential student Gail Jefferson (e.g. 1974; 1984a; 1984b; 1985a); both currently carry on the research programme.

The growing interest in Conversation Analysis has been paralleled by the growth of other sub-disciplines of anthropology, linguistics, philosophy and sociology interested in spoken or written discourse, such as ethnography of speaking (Hymes 1974; Gumperz 1982; Duranti 1988), speech-act theory (Austin 1962; Searle 1969 and 1976; Labov and Fanshel 1977) and numerous variants of discourse analysis (Sinclair and Coulthard 1975; Brown and Yule 1983; Stubbs 1983; van Dijk 1985; Tannen 1990). Although conversation analysts are not, therefore, alone in their interest in language use in naturally occurring situations, their approach has a number of distinct features which will be outlined below.

Therapy research, 'methodologies have been sought that are contextually sensitive, incorporate systemic and cybernetic concepts, develop behaviorally focussed microtheory and provide clinicians with information relevant to their practices' (pp. 99–100). These challenges, Gale argues, are best met by Conversation Analysis, which provides for a 'methodology capable of yielding such a mixture of information'.

The point of departure for the following summary of the central principles of CA[4] is provided by a quotation from Schegloff , who characterizes the CA enterprise as follows:

[T]he target of its inquiries stands where talk amounts to action, where action projects consequences in a structure and texture of interaction which the talk is itself progressively embodying and realizing, and where the particulars of talk inform what actions are being done and what sort of social scene is being constituted.   (1991: 46)

Three central points involved in CA research appear to be encapsulated here. First, talk amounts to action. Second, actions accomplished through talk are structurally organized, and third, through the particulars of their talk the interactants create an intersubjective understanding about what they are doing. Each of these points will be elaborated below.

Talk amounts to action

For somebody reading Conversation Analytical research reports for the first time it might come as a surprise (if it were suggested) that this is research on social action. The technical details of CA (such as the concern with pauses, hesitations, small words like 'uh-hum' and overlapping talk) may easily overshadow the primary, initial, interest which nevertheless lies in understanding social action. Thus Schegloff (1986: 111) suggests: 'First, we must remember, in any examination of talk-in-interaction we are studying social action, and we are doing so by looking at actual determinate, singular social actions or acts.'

The study of social action, when exercised in CA, involves first and foremost an effort to lay bare the methods that people use in everyday life to accomplish whatever they are doing. In other words, conversation analysts are asking questions concerning the very constitution of social life: what makes it possible for us to do the ordinary things we routinely do, such as inviting, agreeing,

---

[4] The organization of this introduction of Conversation Analysis is in debt to some earlier key articles, such as Heritage and Atkinson (1984); Lee (1987); Zimmerman (1988); and Heritage (1989). Overviews of CA have also been given in Levinson (1983, chapter 6); Heritage (1984, chapter 8); Silverman (1993, chapter 6).

disagreeing, complaining, telling a story, opening a conversation, etc.

In its clearest way this approach was formulated by Sacks in his early lectures. In his first recorded lecture he invited the students to 'look to see how it is that persons go about producing what they do produce' (Sacks 1992a: 11). Or in a more complicated formula: 'What we want then to find out is, can we first of all construct the objects that get used to make up ranges of activities, and then see how it is those objects do get used' (ibid.).

The objects that Sacks probably had in mind are different kinds of turns or components of turns, located in specific slots in conversation, which then get a certain type of response from the co-interactants. In his first recorded lectures he analysed gambits like introducing oneself as a means of eliciting the co-interactant's name, and formulating the topic of an ongoing conversation as a way of inviting a newcomer to join in.

Schegloff (1992c) points out how this kind of an approach involved turning upside down some of the traditional premises of micro-sociology. Until Sacks, talk had been examined as 'a screen on which are projected other processes, whether Balesian system problems, or Schutzian interpretative strategies, or Garfinkelian common-sense methods'[5] (p. xviii). Talk was considered as a gateway to various spheres and aspects of social life which in themselves were essentially something else than talk. But in Sacks' work talk itself, in its own right, was brought into focus and thereby 'it seemed possible to give quite well-defined, quite precise accounts of how what was getting done was getting done – methodical accounts of action' (p.xviii).

Structural organization of action

The action as seen in CA is not of a voluntary character, or taking place in a social vacuum. What CA is primarily concerned with, then, are not singular acts carried out through singular utterances (such as the speech-acts studied by Austin and Searle), but the

---

[5] Placing Garfinkel among the scholars who view talk in this way is, however, open to dispute. Garfinkel's critique of the 'documentary method of interpretation' (1967) can be seen as a development in the same direction as that taken by Sacks.

patterns and structures of interaction built up in conversation or other verbal exchanges among two or more participants. This has been pointed out by Heritage: '[A]ll aspects of social action and interaction can be examined in terms of conventionalized or institutionalized structural organizations which analysably inform their production' (1989: 22).

These structural organizations have at least the following key features: (1) they operate through sequences of talk; (2) they are oriented to by the participants as normative standards; and (3) such structures are pervasively present in all interaction.

The structures of interaction operate through sequences of talk. This means that the structures concern primarily the relations of successive utterances. The type of a given utterance, i.e., what is done in it, is tied in a number of ways to the type of the preceding utterance, and will in turn create constraints on what will be done in the next utterance.

Sacks (1992a: 113-25) once provoked 'ethnomethodological wonder' (Pollner 1987) among his students by drawing their attention to the obvious fact that by knowing some parts of a sequence of actions we can easily infer others which we initially don't know. E.g. if we see the police come and take away someone from the house next door, we can infer that somebody has informed the police about a possible crime, that interrogation of the suspect is going to follow, etc. CA research has shown that a similar kind of sequencing operates in the very minute details of talk-in-interaction. Things that happen successively in talk 'are in some before and after relationship, have some organization as between them' (Sacks 1987: 54).

One of the technical terms which describe this relation is 'sequential implicativeness', suggested originally by Schegloff and Sacks (1973). There is sequential implication between two turns when 'the current turn projects some range of possibilities for next turn (...) and in next turn, one of these is done' (Schegloff 1979: 267). The strongest case of such relation can be seen in 'adjacency pairs', where the first utterance by a speaker creates a specific relevance (called 'conditional relevance') for a given type of response by the co-participant (Schegloff 1972). For example, a greeting makes relevant a greeting by the other party, a question invites an answer as its response, an invitation makes relevant its acceptance or rejection, etc. If the conditionally relevant second does not occur, it is noticeably and accountably absent, which means among other things that the one who failed to produce it is held accountable for the missing response.

It has been suggested by Heritage and Atkinson (1984: 6) that the structure of sequential implicativeness covers almost all the talk. '[T]he vast majority of utterances occur as selections from a field of possibilities made relevant by some prior utterance, and in their turn project a range of possible "nexts".' In other words, apart from conversational openings, what we say is always said with reference to the preceding utterance (unless some other prior utterance is marked as our point of reference: Sacks, Schegloff and Jefferson 1974: 728); and, equally, what we say creates a frame of reference where the following utterance will be located by its speaker and by the recipients (unless otherwise marked).

The structures of interaction are oriented to by the participants as normative standards of their conduct (Heritage 1984; Heritage and Atkinson 1984; Drew 1990). The structures operate only by virtue of the interactants persistently shaping their action with reference to them, and allowing them to inform their inferences of the others' action.[6]

The orientation to structures as normative standards can be seen very clearly in the case of adjacency pairs, such as questions and answers. At the most basic level, of course, evidence for the participants' orientation to the adjacency-pair structure is supplied by all the people who answer after they have been asked questions. But apart from this regularity of conduct, there are also more subtle indications of the orientation. Following Merritt (1976: 329; Atkinson and Drew 1979: 52–7) the following recurrent phenomena indicate the participants' orientation to the adjacency-pair structure as a normative standard.

First, if the second pair part (e.g. an answer) fails to appear, the first pair part regularly gets repeated. Secondly, if a silence occurs between the first pair part and the second, other co-present parties

---

[6] It needs to be emphasized that the understanding of the nature of 'norms' in CA is akin to that in Garfinkel's (1967) ethnomethodology, thus departing from Parsons' (1937; 1951) conception of 'norms'. In other words, norms in CA are not primarily understood as internalized motivating forces, but rather as something that the people themselves orient to and respond to, in an active fashion.

regularly do not begin to talk before the party selected as the next speaker by the producer of the first pair part has produced the second. Thirdly, the absence of the second pair part is treated as inferentially implicative, i.e. complaints can be made and there is an expectation of a 'reason for' the absence. Fourthly, where some other activity is inserted between the first and second pair part (i.e. the answerer-to-be first requests clarification of the question), the completion of the initial adjacency pair is likely to follow the completion of the 'insertion sequence'. And fifthly, the producers of the first pair part (e.g. questioners) regularly tend to treat anything that follows their turn as doing the work of the second pair part, even if the turn, when taken in isolation, could be heard otherwise.

CA researchers also claim that normatively based sequential structures of action are pervasively present in all talk. This means that such structures are not only occasionally and voluntarily invoked by the participants (say, by asking a question every now and then), but that all interaction inevitably is penetrated by them. There are no liberated zones and no time out from these constraints of social life.

Sacks argued programmatically that social life is highly organized through its smallest particulars. He criticized traditional sociology for treating small-scale phenomena as irrelevant or contingent, something beyond social determination and sociological analysis (Jefferson 1985b: 25–6). Against traditional sociology's disregard for small phenomena, CA has made a presupposition about 'order at all points' (Jefferson 1984c), assuming that 'no scale of detail, however fine, is exempt from interactional organization, and hence must be presumed to be orderly' (Zimmerman 1988: 415).

The claim about 'order at all points' is, however, the backbone of a research programme rather than a proven theoretical proposition. Thus Heritage (1989: 23) writes that 'no order of detail in interaction can be dismissed a prior as insignificant'. Nobody claims that all the structures penetrating small-scale interaction have already been laid bare by conversation analysts. But the 'order at all points' hypothesis has thus far been successful, leading to the identification of numerous 'generic forms of organization' (Drew 1990), such as the organization of turn-taking (Sacks, Schegloff and Jefferson

1974), the organization of repair (Schegloff 1979 and 1992a), the organization of adjacency pairs (Schegloff 1972), or the preference organization related to agreement and disagreement (Pomerantz 1984). These generic forms of organization are working wherever there is talk-in-interaction,[7] and they also inform the production and reception of the smallest particulars of talk, such as 'uh-hum's, pauses, inhalations or hesitations.

CA's emphasis on the structured character of interaction may give to some readers the false impression that the world of talk-in-interaction is a closed, mechanically determined system. CA, however, points out the *openness* of the structures of talk-in-inter-action. This openness arises from the fact that even though the structural constraints are inevitably *relevant* for interaction, they nevertheless do not *determine* it. In and through their interaction, people define their own position *vis-à-vis* the structures; in doing this, they may even make choices between the individual structural constraints that they orient to.

As was pointed out earlier, the structures of interaction concern primarily the relations of successive utterances and the actions of which these utterances are vehicles. What action(s) a given utter-ance performs is, however, a matter to be *interactionally defined*. The syntactic form and semantic content of an utterance are only partial factors determining this. What an utterance does is to be defined during the course of the interaction between the speaker and the hearer(s).

The recipients of any utterance *treat* the talk that they have heard as certain action or actions. In the last analysis, therefore, an utter-ance becomes a vehicle of a certain action only by virtue of having been treated as one. Let us consider talking about troubles as an example.[8] The recipient can treat a trouble-expressing utterance either as request for help (by offering help or advice) or as 'disclosure' of one's inner predicament (by offering sympathy). These two different ways of responding to a trouble-expressing utterance constitute two different interpretations of the current state of talk and of the local participant roles, and thereby make

---

[7] Note, however, that in certain forms of institutional talk, the generic practices are transformed (see e.g. the discussion on turn-taking in chapter 2).
[8] This is freely adapted from Jefferson and Lee (1981).

relevant different kinds of trajectory for the talk to follow. Thus, as Sacks (1992a: 20) has stated, 'others can, by virtue of their return, cast your activity into something other than it was produced to be'.

However, the first speaker has in the 'third turn position' an opportunity to try and correct the recipients' first interpretation (Schegloff 1992a). The person who talked about his or her troubles and was offered help can, e.g., say that he or she doesn't need help, but just wanted to speak the problem aloud. In sum, what utterances 'do' is a result of an ongoing negotiation between the interlocutors.

Intersubjective understanding

It is a standard critique of CA that it disregards the 'meaning' involved in speaking, and has therefore distanced itself from its origins in 'interpretative' sociology (Garfinkel's ethnomethodology) (e.g. Taylor and Cameron 1987: 99–107; Alexander 1988: 243). Within CA research, formulations that easily raise that kind of objection do occur; for example, Sharrock and Anderson (1987: 246) write: '[C]onversation analysis necessarily disattends to what actors may see as the business of their talk, in favour of the activities which actors engage in solely by virtue of their character as operators of a speech exchange system.' A critic can hear Sharrock and Anderson arguing that in CA the actors are necessarily treated merely as 'cogs in the wheels' in the machinery of conversation, rather than actors engaged in a meaningful activity.

However, at the root of Conversation Analytical research there is another kind of current. Conversation is understood as a major site – possibly the major site – for the creation and maintenance of intersubjective understanding. This has been pointed out by Heritage and Atkinson, among others, who write that 'a context of publicly displayed and continuously updated intersubjective understandings is systematically sustained' through the talk (1984: 11). In other words, the conversationalists operating within the organization of talk are not treated as mechanical automata, but as rational (analysing and inferring) subject actors.

In analytical terms, four different layers of intersubjective understanding can be distinguished, which are all systematically sustained in and through conversation. The first of them – and it may be the precondition for the other three – is the understanding of the prior turn. Each turn displays an analysis and an understanding of the prior utterance (or the utterance that it is marked as targeting at). The action that is performed through an utterance can often be understood in various ways; through selecting his or her response, the next speaker inevitably also brings forward his or her analysis of the preceding turn.

Atkinson and Drew (1979: 48) pointed out how the first speaker's action in (1) can be heard in many different ways: it is packaged as a question, but is also potentially hearable as an invitation. Moreover, the first turn also could be heard as a complaint.[9]

(1)   (Atkinson and Drew 1979)
       A: Why don't you come and <u>see</u> me some[times
       B: [I would like to

By producing an acceptance, B displays an understanding of A's turn as an invitation.

There is no 'time out' from this kind of display of understanding of the prior turn. Whatever action we take, it will be heard in connection with the prior turn. Adjacency pairs may again be the most illustrative case, but any other consequent utterances have the same features. For example, in (2) below, by responding with a mere 'mmh:' to W's answer in line 10, and by allowing a gap of 1.5 sec to emerge thereafter (arrows numbered 1), the counsellor displays an analysis of W's prior talk as not yet complete (cf. Schegloff 1981). The counsellor's 'mmh' and the ensuing silence make relevant a continuation of W's answer, thereby providing W, for example, with the possibility of answering in more detail. Moreover, by expanding her statement (arrow 2), W in turn displays an analysis of C's preceding 'mmh:' and the silence as phenomena which allow her to continue the description of her concerns.

---

[9] If the second speaker's turn was not completed by the end of 'I would like to', it could also be heard as the beginning of an account for B not having come to see A. (E.g. 'I would like to but I've been so busy lately and I'll still be busy for two weeks.')

```
(2)   (E4-12)
      (C = Counsellor, P = Patient, W = patient's wife)
 1    C:          ↑Can I just ask you what are your greatest
 2                conce:rns:: (.) Liz.
 3    P:          [Liza
 4    C:          [Liza: I ca:n't get it [(        )
 5    W:                                 [((coughing))
 6    C:          Liza about- .hh (.4) at this mo:ment in ti:me.
 7                (.)  can you s:ay alou:d.
 8                (3.0)
 9    W:          Erm:: (.) the uncertainty[:?
10    C:  (1) ->                           [mmh:
11        (1) ->  (1.5)
12    W:  (2) ->  obviously:? (.6) an::d (3.0) trying to get John
13                to cope with it (.2) an:d- (.3) lead as normal
14                a life as possible? (.) I'd (.) I don't see
15                .hhh (1.0) I don't really see any f::easible
16                r:ealistic alterna:tive.
```

The second turns are followed by third turns, which allow the first speaker a chance to correct a possible misunderstanding by the second speaker (on third position repair, see Schegloff 1992a). In question–answer sequences, for example, the answer displays an understanding of the question; and in the third turn position, the first speaker can correct a possible misunderstanding. In any third turn position, the producer of the initial action can resist the interpretation made about it in the second turn.

Apart from an understanding of the talk and action involved in the preceding turn, the speakers reach an intersubjective understanding about the 'state of talk' (Heritage and Atkinson 1984) in a broader sense. For example, Heritage and Atkinson point out, 'when a speaker initiates a new topic or direction for talk that is disjoined from what precedes it, the speaker exhibits an analysis that "then and there" is an appropriate place for something new to be raised' (1984: 10). Initiating a new topic displays an understanding that here is an appropriate slot to begin something fresh and new.

The third layer of intersubjective understandings relates to the 'context' of talk. (On the 'context' of talk, see articles in Duranti and Goodwin 1992.) By designing their utterances in specific ways, speakers can display their understanding that the current talk is taking place under the auspices of some specific context, such as 'professional–client interaction', 'press conference' or 'cross-examination'. Displaying an understanding of the context is closely linked with displaying the identities of the speakers: the participants may talk in a specific manner so as to portray one another as 'doctor' and 'patient', 'counsel' and 'witness', etc. We will return to this issue below, when talking about institutional contexts.

The fourth layer of intersubjective understanding is rather different from the others, because it primarily concerns the 'content' of the talk, i.e. what the interlocutors *talk about*. In Conversation Analysis, this aspect of intersubjectivity has not been explicated as systematically as have the other aspects, even though the work on topic organization (see e.g. Jefferson 1984a; Button and Casey 1984 and 1985; Sacks 1987; Sacks 1992a: 752–63; Sacks 1992b: 254–5 and 561–9) has produced many relevant findings. Because intersubjectivity concerning the topic is nevertheless of primary importance for this particular study, something needs to be said about it here.

To be engaged in conversation or other talk-in-interaction does *not* require that the participants share a common world-view or general social norms. It does, however, require that they share a *focus of attention* (cf. Goffman 1967: 113-14). The shared attention on some objects in the world is maintained turn-by-turn and word-by-word; and it is momentarily changing and still continuous.

Turns of talk invoke images of the world and its objects (past, present and future; real and imaginary; close and remote). The principle of sequential implicativeness (see above) is also concerned with these worlds, called forth by the turns of talk (Moerman 1988). If a speaker has focused the interlocutors' shared attention on something, the next speaker is inevitably in the position of speaking 'after such-and-such was mentioned'. He or she is indeed free to maintain the focus or to shift the attention elsewhere; but in any case, his or her turn will be hearable in connection to what was mentioned just before.[10]

This may be illustrated by two examples. In the question–answer sequence in (3) below, the participants focus their shared attention, step by step, beginning from 'concerns' via 'depression' to 'bike accident'. Each turn builds upon the earlier one, so that the participants progress from general descriptions towards specific ones.

---

[10] The 'state of talk' documented in the previous turn of course creates specific constraints for the speaker's choice.

```
(3)    (E4-65)
1      C: (1) ->   So if I was to ask what's your main concern
2                  today Mike what is it.
3                  (1.0)
4      P: (2) ->   Uh::m: (1.0) Nothing really. (0.2) I'm feeling
5                  a bit depressed lately but
6      C:          About what.=
7      P: (3) ->   =Uh:m Over that bike accident I had.
```

In (4) below, however, the progression is not as seamless as in (3). Through the counsellor's enquiries and the client's answers, the participants' attention moves first from 'main concern' to 'house settling' (arrows 1 and 2). Thereafter, the counsellor (instead of inviting some elaboration of the first concern, as in (3)) asks the client to name another concern ('what comes after that'). As the client produces 'good news of Bonnie' (arrow 4), the counsellor responds only minimally; probably prompted by the minimal response, the client finally produces[11] still another object of attention, his 'little job' (arrow 5), which the counsellor topicalizes through her follow-up question (arrow 6).

```
(4)    (E3-20)
1      C1: (1) ->   If [I was to ask you Mr Wood=
2      P:              [( )-
3                    (.)
4      C1:          =[sort of what is your main concern=
5      P:            [Mm hm
6      C1:          =at the moment what would that be.
7                    (1.0)
8      P:   (2) ->   Well I suppose the main concer:n er: w- w-
9                    would be the house settling.
10                   (.)
11     C1: (3) ->   [So getting out of the [house:.=And=
12     P:           [(set)- (set)-          [Yes:.
13     C1:          =what comes after that.
14                   (1.0)
15     P:           Uh:m hhh
16                   (0.5)
17     P:   (4) ->   Well of course as er as (Anna er says) the-
```

---

[11] As Marja-Leena Sorjonen has pointed out to me, P's 'I suppose really: er that-that's the main thing:,' (lines 24–5) seems to close the talk about 'concerns'. P's ensuing description of his job appears to open up a new kind of talk where P constructs his life as 'ordinary' (cf. Sacks 1984b).

```
18                     the- the good news of er Bonnie.=She's all right.
19      C1:            Mm:
20                     (.)
21      P:             [Uh:m
22      C1:            [( )
23                     (1.4)
24      P:             I suppose really: er that- that's the main
25          (5) ->     thing:.=I'm settled down with the little
26                     job that I ha:ve,=
27      C1: (6) ->     =What is the lit[tle job you've got.
28      P:                             [and that is in-
29                     in: in (Woki:ng),
```

As a summary, then, it can be suggested that the fourth layer of intersubjective understanding systematically sustained in conversation involves the participants achieving a shared focus of attention. This focusing is in itself sequentially organized, and it is embedded in the whole range of other sequentially organized activities (such as turn-taking and questions and answers) taking place in and through conversation. The focus of attention is maintained on a moment-by-moment basis and is continuously subject to change as a result of the unfolding of the interaction.

The participants' and the analyst's perspectives

After having outlined the four layers of intersubjective understanding, a further comment is due concerning the participants' and the analyst's perspectives on them. It was pointed out by Sacks, Schegloff and Jefferson (1974) that whatever understanding the speakers display in their talk, concerning the prior talk, these displays are available for the co-interactants and the analysts alike.

It is an intrinsic feature of conversational interaction that its participants exhibit continuously their understanding of one another's conduct. Any claims in CA studies about the participants' understanding in conversation are based on what the participants themselves publicly do during the course of talk. The participants' understanding about each other's activities is displayed in their own activities. According to Sacks, Schegloff and Jefferson, this 'affords both a resource for the analysis of prior turns and a proof procedure for professional analyses of prior turns – resources intrinsic to the data themselves' (1974: 729). The availability of this resource makes it possible for the CA researcher to remain 'agnostic' (Heritage and Atkinson 1984) concerning the 'inner' motivations and experience of the participants. Understanding is displayed publicly for co-interactants, and professional analysts can confine themselves to examining these.

Gaze and talk

In studying social interaction, 'it is necessary to have available as much information as possible about what people actually do when they communicate' (Erickson and Shultz 1982: 49). A large part of Conversation Analytical research has used tape-recorded *telephone conversations* as data. In examining telephone conversations, the analyst obviously cannot pay attention to gaze and body posture as these are not publicly available to the participants. In face-to-face interaction – such as counselling – gaze and body posture *are* available, and therefore the analysis has to take them into account.

Research on social interaction has recurrently demonstrated that gaze and body movement have most important parts to play in the organization of social intercourse (see e.g. Pike 1967, Scheflen 1973; Kendon 1990). In Conversation Analysis, the work of Goodwin (1981 and 1984) and Heath (1986) has been trail-blazing: they have analysed in detail the interrelationship between talk and the organization of gaze and body posture of the speakers and hearers.

In this study of AIDS counselling interaction, the analysis of gaze and body posture has a subsidiary role. The counselling sessions were video recorded. During the research process, the visual aspects of interaction were given attention along with the vocal ones. In the presentation of the data analyses in this book, however, our primary focus will be on the talk of the participants. The analysis of the non-vocal aspects of interaction will be presented only in those cases where the analysis of talk would remain incomplete otherwise.

In the data analyses presented here, two basic functions of gaze are central. One is to *demonstrate hearership*: through gazing at the speaker, a non-speaking party can indicate that he or she is acting as a hearer. The other function of gaze is related to *address-ship*: 'A speaker can use gaze to indicate that the party being gazed at is an addressee of his utterance' (Goodwin 1981: 9). Some other aspects of gaze will be discussed along with the presentation of the empirical results.

Features of institutional talk

Initially, most Conversation Analytical studies concerned 'ordinary conversation' – i.e. informal everyday talk between friends, acquaintances or family members – or alternatively, when the data were from professional–client settings, the studies did not differentiate between 'ordinary conversation' and the particular setting from which the data were collected. The aim of these studies was, and still is, to unravel more or less *universal, generic* structures and practices of talk-in-interaction. Research on ordinary conversation remains in the central focus of Conversation Analysis.

During the 1980s, however, there has risen a growing interest within CA in a phenomenon labelled 'institutional interaction' (e.g. Atkinson and Drew 1979; Boden and Zimmerman 1991; Drew and Heritage 1992). This kind of interaction most typically takes place between professionals and clients, e.g. in a doctor's surgery, a classroom, or in a legal setting. The intention of CA studies on institutional interaction is to find out the *particular* and *specific* structures and practices of talk-in-interaction which emerge in *specific institutional settings*. The general assumption guiding these studies is that the institutional context – i.e. the ways in which the interlocutors are related to one another as incumbents of their institutional roles – is in some way related to the structures and practices that can be observed in the verbal interaction within that setting. The challenge of these studies is to explicate in detail what kind of relation there is.

This book continues the rapidly expanding tradition of CA studies on institutional interaction. Therefore, in what follows, we will outline briefly some of the key characteristics of the CA research on institutional interaction.

How 'institutional context' is understood in CA

CA research into institutional interaction involves, in the first place, an analysis of the bearing of different institutional contexts on the organization of talk-in-interaction. Such a research interest was once formulated by Sacks (1971: 8)[12] as 'The idea then, it to try to connect where someone is in the world, relevant to the interaction, to how they deal with whoever they deal with . . . '. People may deal with one another in interaction in a particular way because they stand in a specific relation with one another within an institutional context.

A fundamental premise in CA research into the interaction within institutional contexts is the *primacy of ordinary conversation*. Ordinary conversation is taken as the basic form of talk-in-interaction, and the institutional types of talk are seen as transformations of it (Sacks, Schegloff and Jefferson 1974: 230; Heritage 1989: 33–4; Drew and Heritage 1992: 19).[13] This argument has both ontological and methodological aspects. In ontological terms, it is assumed that the variety of different conversational practices is 'full blown' in ordinary conversation, and the institutional interaction involves selective reduction and concentration on fewer practices (Heritage 1984: 239–40). In methodological terms it is assumed that ordinary conversation is used as a 'bench-mark' (Heritage 1989: 33) against which the other forms of interaction are recognized. This methodical use of ordinary conversation is basically the same for conversationalists making sense of the interactive settings in which they are participating, and the professional analyst trying to pin down the specific characteristics of any recorded data.

Most importantly, the selective reduction and concentration of conversational practices involved in institutional interaction is not understood as a result of the context unilaterally 'affecting' the conduct of interaction.[14] On the contrary, the institutional context is assumed to be an achievement, brought about by the participants through their very activities. In other words, by selectively reducing the scope of conversational practices, by concentrating on some practices, the participants can activate a certain institutional

---

[12] This citation is from an earlier, mimeographed edition of Sacks' lecture of 10 May 1971. I have not found it in the later, published edition (1992b: 391–5).

[13] The original argument by Sacks, Schegloff and Jefferson concerned the primacy of the *turn-taking system* of ordinary conversation as compared to other 'speech exchange systems'. Later, Heritage and others expanded the scope of the argument to include 'conversational practices' in general.

[14] According to Maynard (1988), this is where CA differs from 'ethnography of speaking'. In the ethnographic approach, the context is understood as affecting

context. The interaction can be rightly analysed as 'institutional interaction' insofar as the participants, through the linguistic detail of their conduct, render their talk observably (for one another and by virtue of that, for the professional analyst) 'talk-within-a-particular-setting' (Schegloff 1987, 1991 and 1992b; Heritage and Greatbatch 1991; Goodwin and Duranti 1992).[15]

Now it could be argued that conversation analysts in effect deny the existence of large-scale social institutions. Do they think that the institutions are created *ex nihilo* if and only if the people involved in interaction so decide? This is not the case: the CA programme does not presuppose that legal arrangements, bureaucracies, occupational roles, gender stereotypes, social classes, relations of authority and power, traditions, etc. are non-existent if you and I choose to ignore them. What the programme does presuppose, however, is that these institutional arrangements may or may not be present in particular interactions; and they may or may not be present at particular *moments* in these particular interactions. If they are present, then their presence is observable for the participants and the analyst alike.

Schegloff (1991 and 1992b) has formulated this as *the problem of relevance* of categorization. There are many aspects of context potentially available for any interaction: we may categorize one another on the basis of gender, age, social class, education, occupation, income, race, etc., and we may understand the setting of our interaction accordingly. In the momentary unfolding of interaction, Schegloff elsewhere argues, 'the parties, singly and together, select and display in their conduct which of the indefinitely many aspects of context they are making relevant, or are invoking, for the immediate moment' (1987: 219).

---

the language use in ways which may not be available for observation in the talk itself. E.g. the different conceptions that the patients and doctors have about disease may affect the way they talk about it, and (mis)understand each other's words.

[15] As an antecedent of later CA studies, Silverman's early paper 'Interview talk' already spelled out this kind of understanding of 'context' more than twenty years ago: '[T]he resources for the contexting of talk which the sociologist shares with the lay members themselves constitute a central research topic.' He recommended, thus, that rather than trading off their members' knowledge about contexts of talk, sociologists should try the explicate the 'managed accomplishment of a "knowable" context' (1973: 46).

Awareness of this 'problem of relevance' requires the professional analyst to proceed with caution. There is a danger of 'importing' context to data. The professional analyst may be tempted to assume, without going into the details of data, that this or that feature of talk is an indication of a particular context having affected the interaction. Such stipulation for context may, Schegloff (1991: 24–5) argues, result in the analysis being terminated prematurely, so that the inherent organization within the talk is not thoroughly understood. Phenomena which in the beginning may appear as indications of the workings of a 'context', may in a more thorough examination turn out to be primarily connected to the organization and dynamics of talk which can be even better understood without reference to the 'context'.

Another key issue addressed by Schegloff (1991 and 1992b) involves what he calls *procedural consequentiality of context*. He argues that it is not sufficient to say that a particular context is oriented to 'in general' by the participants in interaction, but instead it has to be shown how specifiable aspects of the context are consequential for specifiable aspects of the interaction. The goal is to make 'a direct "procedural" connection between the context . . . and what actually happens in the talk' (Schegloff 1991: 17). What is said, when it is said, and how, and by whom, and to whom, may invoke the context; and the goal of the CA research is to explicate exactly how the things said bring forward the context. Rather than trying to deny the existence of any large-scale institution, then, the CA programme is trying to find ways of specifying how these can be present in interaction.

In an important text, Drew and Heritage (1992: 22–5) have suggested that the participants' orientation to institutional context can involve three different types of phenomena. First, institutional talk is normally informed by *goal orientation*. At least one of the participants is oriented to some institutionally relevant goal. As Drew and Heritage point out (1992: 23), however, this orientation can take varying forms: it may be clear or less clear (especially for the non-professional participants); and the different participants' goals may be shared or conflicting. In this book, all the empirical chapters will in various ways deal with the goal-oriented character of AIDS counselling interaction, especially from the point of view of the counsellors' goals.

Second, Drew and Heritage (1992) argue that institutional inter-action often involves *special and particular constraints* on what each participant is allowed to contribute. Restrictions on turn-tak-ing (to be discussed in chapter 2) are perhaps the most typical form of institutionally specific constraints. Finally, institutional talk may also be associated with specific *inferential frameworks*. Inference refers to the process of interpretation 'by which participants in an exchange retrieve relevant background knowledge and assess others' communicative intentions' (Gumperz 1992a: 306; see also Gumperz 1992b). In institutional settings, this may have a special institutional character. In this book, institutionally specific inferen-tial frameworks are dealt with particularly in chapters 5 and 6.

As a summary, it can be said that in the CA perspective the institutional context of interaction is a joint achievement of the participants; brought about through the details of their talk, on a momentary basis. This is the point of departure of this study, too. In the data analyses that will follow, we are going demonstrate how the participants of AIDS counselling sessions, in various ways, invoke Family Systems Theory as the context of their talk. In doing this, they repeatedly make relevant the categories of 'client' and 'counsellor' as the coordinates of their action.

Detailed research tasks

Earlier in this chapter, the general purpose of this study was for-mulated as follows: to examine how the tasks of AIDS counselling and the ideas of Family Systems Theory are translated into the practice of verbal interaction. Seen from the point of view of CA research on institutional interaction, this involves explicating *how AIDS counselling based on the context of Family Systems Theory is brought out in and through the details of the counsellors' and their clients' conduct.*[16]

This is a very broad research task, and therefore it has to be specified and narrowed down. In one study it is impossible to exam-ine all the aspects of interaction which might contribute to invoking

---

[16] Buttny (1990) and Gale (1991) were among the first to adopt Conversation Analysis in research of Family Therapy. In their work, as well as in this book, Conversation Analysis makes visible the detailed practices by which the therapeu-tic agenda is worked through.

the context of counselling. I have narrowed down the phenomena to be explored very simply, by concentrating on those activities in counselling which have as their vehicle *questions* and *answers*. This means that I have *not* studied in any great detail information and advice-giving (which are a central part of any AIDS counselling; but see Silverman *et al.* 1992), nor the counsellors' concluding 'interventions' (which are an essential aspect of the Family Systems technique).

The question–answer-based activities that I have chosen as the objects of this study are as follows. Almost directly from Family Systems Theory arises *circular questioning*, which will be studied in chapter 3. The AIDS counsellors' application of the practice of live supervision based on Family Systems Theory, which can be called *live open supervision*, also operates largely on the question–answer format, and it will be studied in chapters 4 and 5. In chapters 6 and 7, the object of research is a central task of any AIDS counselling, namely *talking about the clients' fears concerning the future*. As we will see, a particular type of query arising from Family Systems Theory, *hypothetical future-oriented questions*, constitute a central tool in this and they will be analysed in detail.

The analyses of these different question–answer-based activities require each some specific Conversation Analytical tools and concepts. The analysis of 'circular questioning' and 'live open supervision' is largely based on the notion of *participation framework*; it will be introduced in the beginning of chapter 3. The examination of the talk about the future and of the 'hypothetical future-oriented questions' will require some other Conversation Analytical concepts related to *turn design and sequence organization*; these will be introduced at the beginning of chapter 6.

However, before analysing in detail the different question–answer-based AIDS counselling activities, some possibly even more primary data analysis has to be conducted. This involves examining *how the counsellors maintain their footing as questioners* in the first place. Any of the activities to be analysed in the later chapters will presuppose that the counsellors ask questions and the clients answer these. Most importantly, the question–answer pairs are often *chained*, so that clients' answers are followed by new questions by the counsellors (this is the case particularly in circular questioning analysed in chapter 3, and in the talk about the clients' fears concerning the future, analysed in chapters 6 and 7). The ways in which the counsellors maintain their footing as questioners will be analysed in chapter 2. The central Conversation Analytical concept that will be used in this chapter is *the organization of turn-taking*.

2

Quasi-conversational turn-taking

Counsellors of the Royal Free Hospital once described the method of AIDS counselling based on Family Systems Theory as follows: 'questions are used in order to explore different perceptions and views of relationships' (Bor and Miller 1988: 400).

As the quotation above indicates, a central feature of this method of AIDS counselling is its extensive reliance on *questions* and *answers*. Counsellors help clients to deal with the social and psychological strains caused by the illness, and prepare them mentally for possible worsening of their condition at some future time. This is done in the first place by asking the clients questions. The counsellors at the Royal Free Hospital also believe that AIDS-related problems are embedded in a complex system of relations and perceptions; and that making the clients aware of these can be helpful for them. Invoking this kind of awareness is also done through questions.

Asking questions is not, however, the only thing that the counsellors do during the sessions. There are many issues that the clients have to be *informed and advised* about. These include the details of the transmission of the virus and of safer sex, and medical issues related to the meaning of different symptoms and to various drug trials that take place at the clinic. Counsellors also have knowledge about the different social services that are available for HIV-positive patients; many clients need to be told about these, too.

Therefore, on a general level, it can be said that the tasks of the counsellors are accomplished through two types of turns of talk: (1) *questions* and (2) *informative and advisory statements*. Accordingly, during the counselling sessions, the clients spend most of their time either *answering* the counsellors' questions, or *listening to* the counsellors' advice and information.[1]

Consequently, the interaction in the AIDS counselling sessions is very uniform and asymmetric. For most of the time, one party asks questions and proffers statements, whereas the other answers and listens. This asymmetric uniformity could in principle be demonstrated and measured using quantitative techniques (such as the 'initiative–response analysis' developed by Linell *et al.* 1988); but I trust that it is visible enough for the reader in almost all the extracts that will be given throughout this book.

The topic of this chapter will be the asymmetric distribution of questions, answers and statements among the participants of the AIDS counselling sessions. However, we are not going to describe this asymmetry *per se.* Instead, we are going ask *how the distributive asymmetry is achieved.* This will involve an examination of *turn-taking practices* in AIDS counselling sessions.

There is something very paradoxical in the asymmetric distribution of questions, answers and statements in AIDS counselling sessions. The paradox is this: there are no norms or rules that would prescribe that only the counsellors may ask questions and give statements during the counselling sessions. In other words, no norms or rules forbid or disapprove the clients' questions, statements, or other 'ordinary' conversational activities. In spite of this lack of normative regulation, the participants of the counselling sessions end up producing scenes of interaction that are striking in their asymmetric uniformity.

In this chapter, the details of this paradox will be explored. It will be argued that asymmetric uniformity of counselling interaction is achieved in a very different way from the asymmetric uniformity in many other institutional settings, such as news interviews or cross-examinations. The asymmetric uniformity of interaction in news interviews and cross-examination *is* a result of the participants' orientation to sanctionable social norms that prescribe the types of turns (such as questions, answers and statements) that each par-

---

[1] See Erickson and Shultz (1982) for the description of educational counselling. Also in that kind of setting, activities are predominantly carried out through either the counsellors' questions and the clients' answers, or through the counsellors' statements (ibid., esp. pp. 22–3).

ticipant is entitled to. In contrast AIDS counselling, as it was just pointed out, is not regulated by such social norms.

In AIDS counselling, the asymmetry of interaction is achieved in a different way. It will be argued that the participants' orientation to *their tasks* and and to the various *activities* taking place during the session is the key issue here (see Drew and Heritage 1992: 27–9). The counsellors' task is to explore the clients' feelings, beliefs and perceptions; and to give them advice and information. Performing these kinds of tasks is made possible by the counsellors asking questions and proffering statements, over and over again. Moreover, the activities taking place in AIDS counselling – exploration of relations, beliefs and perceptions, and information and advice – are such that they predominantly presuppose that the clients adopt both a passive and a responsive footing. So the clients end up answering questions and listening to the counsellors' statements.

The empirical analysis that will shortly be presented seeks to demonstrate the character of AIDS counselling as an informal institutional setting. However, before examining the data, some Conversation Analytical concepts related to turn-taking have to be introduced.[2]

Turn-taking in ordinary conversation

In CA research, turn-taking is considered an aspect of primary importance in the structural organization of talk-in-interaction. The system of turn-taking is pervasively present as a regulator of oppportunities of action in any interaction (Heritage 1984).

[2]Chapter 2 will be different from the rest of the book in one respect: the phenomena that we will examine in this chapter have *not* been addressed to any larger extent in the Family Systems Theory literature. In the chapters to come later, we will analyse questioning techniques and practices that the counsellors' own theory has dealt with extensively. In those later chapters, therefore, we will apply Conversation Analysis to phenomena that have already been recognized and studied in Family Systems Theory. The turn-taking practices *per se* – i.e. the subject-matter of chapter 2 – are, however, something that Family Systems Theory has *not* discussed.

The reader who is primarily interested in the analysis of the interaction techniques of Family Systems Theory is advised to only glance through chapter 2. Those readers who are more generally interested in the analysis of institutional interaction, however, might find this chapter more rewarding.

Whatever the participants do in interaction, their conduct is regulated by the turn-taking system.

As was hinted above, turn-taking is different in ordinary conversation if compared with many forms of institutional talk. Because the organization of ordinary conversation is considered as the 'bedrock' of all forms of talk-in-interaction, the conversational turn-taking practices will here be presented first, whereafter we will examine some institutional modifications.

In ordinary conversation a number of features, normally taken for granted, can be seen as achievements brought about by participants orienting to a specific regulatory structure. According to Sacks, Schegloff and Jefferson (1974: 699–701), among those features are the following: (1) For most of the time, only one party speaks at a time. (2) The speakership changes recurrently, so that one speaker follows another; (3) the speaker change occurs in an orderly manner, so that the gaps and overlaps are minimal; (4) the length of any individual turn is not specified in advance, and (5) the number of people participating in conversation may vary. Sacks, Schegloff and Jefferson (1974) have outlined a formal model of organization of turn-taking which accounts for these and other related features.

This structural organization was crystallized into simple rules. The rules, however, presuppose some technical concepts. A *turn constructional unit* is the smallest amount of talk which, in its sequential context, counts as a turn. It may be a single word (e.g. 'Yes', or 'No'), or it may be a full sentence. A speaker is initially entitled to one unit only. At the completion of any turn constructional unit, therefore, there emerges a *transition relevance place*, where the speaker change may occur. Moreover, the rules presuppose a distinction between two basic *techniques of turn-allocation*. A current speaker may select the next speaker (most commonly, by addressing the first pair part of an adjacency pair to one of the other participants), or the next speaker may self-select (by volunteering his or her talk).

The rules regulating the change of speakership in conversation are the following (see Sacks, Schegloff and Jefferson 1974: 704). A current speaker may select the next, which gives the following turn to the party thus selected. If the current speaker does not select the next, then anybody present can self-select when the current speaker's turn for the first time can be heard as completed. In the case of self-selection, the one who starts talking first is entitled to the next turn. If the current speaker has not selected the next, and if no one self-selects when the turn is first hearably completed, the current speaker may (but need not) continue; and the change of the speakership may occur, following the same procedure, in the first following slot where the speaker's turn can be heard as completed.

It was pointed out by Sacks, Schegloff and Jefferson (1974), and has thereafter been emphasized by Atkinson and Drew (1979), that the above-outlined system of turn-taking allows for an *interactional and local management* of various aspects of conversation. The timing of the change of speakership, who takes the next turn, and what kind of activity is accomplished in any turn: matters like these are settled between the speakers on a turn-by-turn basis. This appears to be one of the reasons that Sacks, Schegloff and Jefferson (1974: 699–700) characterize the machinery of turn-taking sketched above as combining the twin features of being context-free and capable of context sensitivity: it is context-free because it operates in any conversation, and it is context-sensitive because it allows several aspects of conversation to vary on a local basis.

Institutional variations of the turn-taking rules

The rules outlined by Sacks, Schegloff and Jefferson (1974) are primarily meant to be a description of turn-taking in *ordinary conversation*. There are forms of institutional talk (taking place in what Drew and Heritage (1992) call *formal* settings) where the participants observably orient to sanctionable turn-taking rules other than those above. As it was already pointed out earlier in this chapter, AIDS counselling is *not* among these formal settings; but in order to better understand the special character of AIDS counselling, we need first to examine some features of the formal settings.

The possibility of 'non-conversational' turn-taking was first suggested by Sacks, Schegloff and Jefferson (1974: 729–31). They proposed that there may be an array of different 'speech exchange systems', which all have in common the fact that one party talks at a time and speaker change recurs. The other speech exchange systems differ from conversation (and from one another) in terms of other turn-taking parameters, i.e. they all have different system of turn-taking providing for the speaker change. Sacks *et al.* in effect

suggested a research programme involving 'comparative investigation of the speech-exchange systems available to members of a
single society' (1974: 729). Since the publication of their seminal
paper, considerable advance has been made in this field.

Atkinson and Drew (1979: 61–81) analysed *cross-examination*.
They pointed out that the specific character of the turn-taking system in that setting, compared to ordinary conversation, involves
two parameters: *turn type* and *turn order*. The turn types are pre-
specified so that the talk in examination is organized into a series of
question-and-answer pairs. Whatever the participants do in cross-
examination, it is done through questions and answers. Turn order
pre-specification means that the party conducting the examination
(generally the counsellor) has the right to ask questions, and consequently the examined party's utterances occupy 'the sequential
position of post-question' (1979: 62) and will thus be normally
treated as responses to the questions asked.

Greatbatch (1988) and Heritage and Greatbatch (1991) have
analysed the turn-taking system of television and radio news interviews. Their work can be seen as a continuation of that of Atkinson
and Drew: news interview and cross-examination have much in
common, and the core part of the analytical apparatus therefore
can be the same.

Just as in cross-examination, in news interviews there are con-
straining provisions concerning the turn types and the turn order.
The interaction in news interviews proceeds as a sequence of
Interviewer's (IR's) questions and Interviewee's (IE's) answers.
Consequently, the turn order is confined to the pattern IR:Q >
IE:A > IR:Q > IE:A etc., regardless of the number of participants.
This means that even if there is more than one Interviewee, the next
turn after each single answer is usually the Interviewer's question;[3]
and in the case of many Interviewers, each answer is followed by a
question from one of them.

It is interesting to note that the most thoroughly examined turn-
taking systems different from conversation involve extensive use of

---

[3] With the exception of questions which are not specifically addressed to one of the
interviewees. More than one interviewee can respond to such 'undirected' questions, without the interviewer intervening (Greatbatch 1988).

questions and answers.[4] It was suggested by Atkinson (1982), as a preliminary hypothesis, that reliance upon a multiple question–answer sequence (with the professional as the questioner) is, indeed, a characteristic feature of professional–client encounters in our society. Empirical work in many settings remains to be done. But the existing evidence for the use of questions and answers in some settings already suggests the functionality of such arrangements. The pre-specification of turn types and turn order modifies radically the actions involved in talking, and it also relates to the broader social environment of the action.[5]

Quasi-conversational turn-taking practices

However, the turn-taking perspective also has its limits. Even in those environments which are doubtlessly characterized by turn type and turn order pre-specification, many aspects of the talk

[4] For description of institutional turn-taking systems in classroom interaction, operating predominantly through questions and answers, see Mehan (1979 and 1985) and McHoul (1978). Frankel (1990), West (1983) and Schegloff (1987), among others, also describe turn-taking practices where questions and answers are extensively used.

[5] As was noted by Sacks already in his early lectures (1992a: 49–56), the organization of turn-taking strongly affects the shape and character of the action sequences accomplished through the talk. For example, in presidential press conferences each journalist is entitled to one question only: therefore, the president can easily turn down a question by giving a minimal answer, knowing the initial questioner cannot ask a follow-up question. Schegloff (1987) adds that this arrangement generally leads to topics not being thoroughly elaborated in the conferences, because each new questioner usually opens up a new issue.

Greatbatch (1992: 273) suggests that 'essentially simple modifications of the conversational turn-taking system can have radical implications for the management of other interactional activities'. The organization of *disagreement* in news interviews constitutes an example. Delays – which in ordinary conversation are associated with disagreeing turns – do not apply to disagreements in news interviews. This is because, Greatbatch argues, the disagreeing turns are usually produced as answers to the Interviewer's questions, and in this sequential position, a delay would do another kind of work than a delay of e.g. 'second assessment' (Pomerantz 1984) does.

A distinct organization of turn-taking can also be *functional* in relation to the macro-institutional environment of talk. Heritage and Greatbatch point out that the turn-taking organization of news interviews 'is pervasively associated with a central task and a core exogenous constraint of the news interview' (1991: 130): the structure based on the Interviewer's questions and the Interviewee's answers is apt to produce talk for an overhearing audience, and it makes it possible for the Interviewer to maintain at least a nominally neutral position.

can remain interactionally managed. In cross-examination, for example, the action sequences related to blaming are managed on a turn-by-turn basis (Atkinson and Drew 1979). The understanding of these can be helped by understanding the turn-taking procedures; but they need to be analysed 'in their own right', too.

Moreover, along with the accumulation of new studies on institutional interaction in the 1980s, it has transpired that not all institutional talk necessarily involves a distinct modification of the turn-taking system (Dingwall 1980; Zimmerman 1988; Drew 1990; Heritage and Greatbatch 1991). In a number of institutional environments the turn-taking may be managed on a local basis, just as in conversation. Drew and Heritage (1992) call these environments *informal*, as opposed to the *formal* environments where turn-taking rules are distinctively different. Tentatively, they describe as informal many forms of medical interaction, various business environments and interaction within social services, where, they assume, the turn-taking is conversational or 'quasi-conversational'. As it has already been pointed out, AIDS counselling is best characterized as an informal institutional setting.

The interaction in informal institutional settings may look quite different from mundane conversation. There may be aggregative asymmetries in the types of action between the participants – such as the uneven distribution of questions and answers (cf. West 1983; Frankel 1990). Long question–answer sequences may make interaction in some informal settings appear very similar to interaction in formal settings. But Drew and Heritage (1992) point out that in informal settings such asymmetries are not the result of a modification of the turn-taking system (see also Schegloff 1987; Heritage and Greatbatch 1991). Orientation to the *institutionally ascribed tasks* may result in one party predominantly asking the questions and the other answering them. Therefore, Schegloff's (1987 and 1991) warning concerning premature stipulation of context apply, among other things, to the unwarranted use of the turn-taking concepts.

AIDS counselling is best characterized as an informal institutional setting, without specific, institutional turn-taking rules. The absence of such rules does not, however, make the turn-taking in AIDS counselling (or in other informal institutional settings) an uninteresting phenomenon.

Thus far the Conversation Analytical studies on turn-taking have largely concentrated either on mundane conversation, or on formal institutional settings. Because AIDS counselling belongs to the 'grey' area between these two, it is of greatest analytical importance to study in detail the turn-taking practices in this environment. That will be done in the following. What we aim at is a description of something that might be called, using Drew and Heritage's (1992) phrase, 'quasi-conversational' turn-taking practices. It will be shown how the participants of the AIDS counselling sessions continuously orient to the conversational rules of turn-taking, even when they produce scenes which in their uniformity appear very unlike ordinary conversation.

Uniform turn-taking practices in AIDS counselling

Interaction in AIDS counselling, for most of the time in the sessions, follows a relatively uniform pattern. In this pattern, the counsellors do two things: they either ask questions of the clients, or proffer statements conveying information, advice or comments. The clients do only one thing, which is to answer the counsellors' questions. As will be argued throughout this chapter, this uniform pattern is a result of the participants' orientation to their tasks and the different activities arising from these tasks.

This pattern can be observed in the following extracts. We will begin with two extracts where the participants confine their actions to questions and answers. In extract (1), there is only one client present in the session. The counsellor (C1) explores his perception of his health and HIV. The elicitation of the client's perception is made through a series of questions and answers.

```
(1)    (E4-48)
 1    C1: (1) ->    But what about your health apart from
 2                  haemophilia,
 3    P:   (2) ->   Well it's just been fine. (.2) ( [  )
 4    C1: (1) ->                                     [Been fine
 5                  [in what way.
 6    P:            [( )
 7                  (0.7)
 8    P:   (2) ->   Well hhh fine in like the sort of same as it
 9                  has been [really it's
10    C1:                    [Mm:
```

```
11   C1: (1) ->    Ha[ve you any concerns about that?
12   P:               [(    )
13                  (0.5)
14   P:   (2) ->    (I don't know) (.2) not really.
15                  (0.6)
16   C1: (1) ->    And what about (.3) you (.2) mentioned the
17                  blee:ds and you mentioned your (.5) concern
18                  about transport and things .hhh uhm (.2) how
19                  about the HIV: (.) business.
20   P:   (2) ->    I mean that's (0.7) (                              )
21                  (0.5) further from my memory than- sort of mind
22                  at the moment really.=I'm more concerned (of my
23                  leg) my joints for example it's
24                  not [something I can
25   C1:                [Mm:
26                  (1.0)
27   C1: (1) ->    Is there anything (.3) that if you were to
28                  bring in to your mi:nd, you'd want to ask about
29                  that.
30                  (2.6)
31   P:   (2) ->    Not that I can see (    ) at the moment.=[(I am)
32   C1: (1)- >                                              [What
33                  do you understand about meeting Doctor Smith
34                  after this.
35                  (0.8)
36   P:   (2) ->    er I've actually got his letter so hhh and
37                  there are changes and it's uh:m (.) we're on
38                  AZT I believe (or something like that).
```

In extract (1), the interaction unfolds as a string of the counsellor's questions and the patient's answers. Questions are marked with arrows numbered 1 and the answers with arrows numbered 2. The only moment where a possibility of another kind of organization surfaces is in lines 27–31, where the counsellor indirectly offers the patient an opportunity to ask a question about HIV. This would reverse the roles of the participants. Even this offer is packaged as a question; and by answering that there isn't anything, P indirectly declines it. So the string of C's questions continues uninterrupted.

Extract (2) is from a session where there are three clients present. The HIV-positive patient is Richard, an adolescent boy, and he is accompanied by his mother (Mo) and Penny, his younger sister (S). In this segment, the counsellor explores the clients' perceptions of the patient's health, and their beliefs concerning one another's

perception.[6] Just as in extract (1), the interaction unfolds exclusively as questions and answers.

```
(2)    (E4-37)
 1     C1:   (1) -> Do you think Richard ever thinks of he might
 2                  get sick?
 3                  (4.5)
 4     Mo:   (2 )-> I think he- (0.3) basically doesn't.=no.
 5     C1:   (1) -> Umh:: (.) [And what about Penny. Do you think=
 6     ( ):                   [(     )
 7     C1:          =she thinks about Richard getting sick ever?
 8                  (.5)
 9     Mo:   (2) -> hhh (.2) heh I k(h)n(h)o(h)w i(h)t heh I
10                  d(h)o(h)n't heh thi(h)nk she .hhh rea(h)l(h)ly
11                  t(h)hi(h)nks [heh .hhh (        ), I don't=
12     P:                        [*heh*
13     Mo:          =think she really thinks about it,
14     C1:   (1) -> Do you Penny, is Mum right?=Do you never think
15                  abo[ut it.
16     S:    (2) ->    [*No*
17                  (.2)
18     S:           *No*
19     C1:   (1) -> Have you ever thought of Richard getting sick.
20                  (0.8)
21     S:    (2) -> N:o. hh
22     C1:          No.
23                  (4.0)
24     C1:   (1) -> Do you think of getting sick (.) (Richard)=
25     P:    (2) -> =No.
26     C1:          No.
27     P:           No
28                  (1.8)
29     C1:   (1) -> Can you help me a little bit Richard.=Because
30                  ((continues, leading to another question))
```

In (2), the questions and answers are marked with arrows numbered 1 and 2 respectively. The counsellor addresses each individual
question to one of the clients, and after each answer (and the possible receipt actions like repeating the answer in lines 22 and 26),
she produces another individually addressed question. The individually addressed questions create a strong conditional relevance for

---

[6] The technique of circular questioning, applied in this segment, will be analysed in
detail in chapter 3.

the addressed person to produce the answer in the next turn. Accordingly, the clients withhold activities other than answering the questions that were addressed to him or her.

Counsellors' statements

Apart from eliciting clients' feelings, beliefs and perceptions, counsellors also have to give information and advice to them. This requires other types of turns than questions: information and advice are delivered through statements. Statements can also be used as a vehicle for the counsellors' general comments upon the clients' situation.

In terms of the sequence organization, a key feature of such statements is that they are independent 'first acts', which do not create a strong conditional relevancy for a particular type of 'next' to appear.[7] By virtue of being fresh first acts, the statements are distinguishable from 'third turn responses', such as evaluations or corrections, which the counsellors occasionally produce after the clients' answers.[8]

Extract (3) illustrates advice-giving. The third participant here is M, the mother of P who is an adolescent boy. The counsellor's questions are again marked with arrows numbered 1, and the clients' answers with arrows numbered 2. The beginning of the advisory statement is marked with arrow numbered 3.

```
(3)    (SS/2/28)
1    C:    (1) -> Right. (0.6) But who do you fee:l m- (0.6) m-
2                 ought to: you would want to te:ll that you:
3                 (0.5) had met the virus in the past that you're
4                 antibody positive.
5                 (1.0)
6    C:    (1) -> Is there anyone you think (.3) you ought to
7                 te:ll or want to tell?
8                 (0.6)
9    P:    (2) -> Not really,
```

[7] This is not to say, however, that the delivery of the statements would not create the relevancy for the patient to align himself as a recipient, and to display this alignment by withholding talk and by producing 'response tokens' and other related acts.

[8] Such third-turn responses are closely connected to the question–answer sequence: they expand the adjacency pair with a third member. We will return to these later in the chapter.

```
10   C:        No.
11             (2.0)
12   C:    (1) -> Do you agree with him?
13   M:    (2) -> Mm::: I told the doctor to use gloves when he-
14             (.4) she was going to cut his toe:.
15   C:        Mm=
16   M:        =Or (.) look at his toe:.
17   (?):      Mm:
18             (.)
19   C:        But that would be:: whether he was antibody
20             positive or not because one doesn't
21             rea[lly know:.
22   M:            [(This is) why I tol[d him to.
23   C:                                [Right.
24             (1.2)
25   M:        To use glo:ves. .hhhh
26             (1.6)
27   C:    (3) -> .hh I mean (.3) if you: (0.5) take (.2) the
28             necessary precautions in your li:fe (0.5) then
29             (.2) I would agree with you, (.3) nobody needs
30             to know.
31             (1.1)
32   C:        Except if you develop a very strong
33             relationship with someone, .hh which a lot of
34             our boys do:, .hh (.3) then: (0.5) it's just
35             (.2) you would have to find way:s, over time,
36             of telling someone (1.6) if you were actually
37             going- (0.5) we:ll (.) that (.2) would be one
38             of the issue- (.) one of the people who you
39             might want to tell.
40             (2.0)
41   C:        But otherwise
42             (3.2)
43   C:    (1) -> Any questions you'd want to a:sk at this point.
44             (3.5)
45   P:    (2) -> No:.
46             (2.3)
47   C:    (1) -> You think what you've heard today is going to
48             make any difference to how you carry on?
49             (2.0)
50   P:    (2) -> I can't help it can I? (1.4) I can't help what
51             (0.8) what might happen or (0.2) can happen.
```

In the first part of the extract, the participants are aligned as questioner and answerer. In line 19, the counsellor does not ask a new question after the completion of M's preceding answer, but instead comments on the answer at the 'third position'. M responds to this commentary with an expansion of her preceding answer (lines 22, 25). After this exchange, the counsellor produces a multi-unit turn, in which she delivers advice to the patient (lines 27–41). This statement is followed by the reinstatement of the Q–A sequence. The counsellor's first question (line 43) is an indirect offer for P to ask something; as P declines this offer, the counsellor continues with another question.

In (3), the counsellor's advisory statement was relatively short. In extract (4), however, we have much longer statements, successively produced by two counsellors. The clients here are an HIV-positive man and his wife (W). Questions and answers are marked with arrows 1 and 2 respectively, and statements withs arrows numbered 3. These statements convey information and advice about the risk of transmission of the HI-virus, especially after childbirth.

```
(4)    (SS/2/30)
  1    C1:   (1) ->   And then you just- er when you got
  2                   pregnant did you have to try a lot of
  3                   times?=[or
  4    W:    (2) ->            [No:. [Just at first
  5    P:                            [No.
  6                   (0.2)
  7    C1:            Well that was (quite [clever wasn't i(h)t).
  8    W:                                  [hheh heh heh heh
  9    C1:            .hh[hh
 10    C2:   (1) ->      [Well I understood- (0.5) from last time
 11                   that we talked that (0.4) you used precautions
 12                   till about May last [year.
 13    W:    (2) ->                       [Yeah=
 14    P:             =Yeah.
 15    W:             And then we (.3) [stopped it and then
 16    C2:                             [Mm
 17    C2:            Mm
 18                   (0.6)
 19    W:             That was (in May) (.3) (      [    ) last=
 20    C2:                                          [I mean-
 21    W:             =year.
 22    C2:   (3) ->   Doctor Jay this isn't really the time because
 23                   the baby's going to be born but I- (1.6) I mean
 24                   (.) I think it's important to (0.2) uhm (.)
 25                   think about (0.3) the degree of risk you are
 26                   prepared to take [now: and in the fut[ure.
```

```
27  (W):                        [(Mm)              [
28  C1:   (3') ->                                  [Yeah I
29              think- I mean I think one of the things:: (.2)
30              that we should stress to you: .hh *eh-eh* I
31              mean we have to be honest and say that a lot
32              our information about (.3) intercourse and
33              pregnancy and having babies .hh uh:m that (.2)
34              knowledge is limited.
35              (.3)
36  C1:         .hh (.) But one of the things that has happened
37              in our: (.) small experience here .hh is that
38              (.3) one (.) mother (1.4) probably got (.3)
39              infected (1.0) very soon after the birth of her
40              chi:ld. (0.4) Her first child. I mean her
41              first [chi:ld was negative, .hhh=
42  W:               [Mm
43  C1:         =uhm: (0.5) her husband was positive, .hh and
44              then she came along and she (.3) she was found
45              to be (.2) positive. (0.2) .hhhh So (.2) I
46              think it is (0.5) very important (.2) that
47              after you have the baby (0.6) that you are
48              very very careful.
49  P:          Mm hm
50  C1:         And [I think I would=
51  (W):            [Yes.
52  C1:         =actually: (0.4) say: (.2) that (.) you
53              probably should avoid penetrative sex (1.6) for
54              (.2) I would say at least two months.
55              (2.2)
56  C1:         Because (0.4) (if) the inside of your: (.) your
57              womb=
58  W:          =M[m
59  C1:           [is all raw:.
60              (0.4)
61  C1:         And it- (.2) you know you know that you bleed
62              after [you have your baby.
63  W:                [Mm
64              (0.9)
65  C1:         So that is a very easy wa:y for infection to
66              get i:n.
67              (1.8)
68  C1:         Uh:m
69              (0.4)
70  C1:         So I- (.2) I- (.) I think (.3) that would be a
71              sensible thing for you to do:.
72              (0.4)
```

```
73   C1:              Uhm (0.2) In any event I think (0.8) we: (1.6)
74                    the advice we would give you (.3) is- (.) is
75                    that you really should always take
76                    precautions.=
77   P:               =Mm hm=
78   C1:              =If you have penetrative sex.
79   (W):             Mm=
80   C1:              =Uhm (0.8) And I mean the other: (.2) things to
81                    think about which is what we talk about (.3)
82                    with a lot of our patients now is that .hh
83                    (0.2) that isn't necessarily the only wa:y. You
84                    know you can have (.2) sexual fulfilment (0.4)
85                    without actually doing that.
86                    (.2)
87   C1:              Sometimes.
88                    (.)
89   P:               Mm
90   C1:              But I (0.4) do be careful (.2) after y- (.2)
91                    you've- (.) you've had the baby.
92                    (0.5)
93   C1:              Now the other thing is:=
94   C2:    (3″) ->   =Doctor Jay while we're on it you might have
95                    been getting to talk about it.=But I think this
96                    we'll talk about after the baby but really-
97                    .hhhh when I was talking about degree of risk
98                    (.3) Doctor Jay's right (.) if you want no risk
99                    you don't have sex. .hhh If you want to take
100                   the maximum (0.7) care: .hh then you should
101                   think about using a diaphragm or a cap, (1.0)
102                   [and a condom,
103  P:               [Ye:s.
104                   (.)
105  W:               M[m hm
106  C2:                [and crea:m.
107                   (1.2)
108  C2:              And then (0.4) at least it (.2) preserves a
109                   little bit. I don't kn[ow what the degree [is=
110  (W):                                   [mhm               [
111  P:                                                        [Yes.
112  C2:              =so .hhhh (.2) *but* (0.2) anything less than
113                   that (.2) condoms alo:ne (.) is not sufficient.
114  P:               Mm:
115                   (1.8)
116  C1:    (1) ->    Now (.3) the: (2.0) pregnancy and having the
117                   baby: (.2) uh have you (.) any idea (on) what
118                   kind of (.) tests and things we might (0.4)
```

```
119                      want to do when you've- (.) you've got your
120                      baby?
121                      (1.2)
122   W:    (2) ->       *No:*
123                      (1.3)
124   C1:   (1) ->       Have- [can you h[elp you[r wife.
125   P:                       [(    )  [(    ) [(    )
126   P:    (2) ->       They'll be similar tests to the ones (.) that I
127                      have.
```

In this extract, the participants are first aligned as questioners and answerers. But unlike the preceding extracts, here both counsellors (in a two-counsellor session) are asking questions of the clients.

The first statement, produced by C2, is marked with arrow 3. The first part of the turn is addressed to the main counsellor (C2 uses the address term 'Doctor Jay') and the latter part to the clients (C2 uses the second person pronoun when talking about risks). Given this dual addressing, C2's statement seems to do a double work: apart from asserting the importance of thinking about the risks, C2 also invites the main counsellor to elaborate the issue further.

There follows a very long statement by the main counsellor. The beginning of that is marked with arrow 3'. This turn – or rather a string of successive turns – includes a story about a woman having got infected in a similar kind of situation where W is now, leading to strongly emphasized advice to avoid having sex after the birth of the baby. Thereafter C1 moves on to give an explanation of the reasons for increased risk after childbirth, and advice about seeking sexual fulfilment not only through penetrative sex.

Arrow 3'' marks the beginning of the co-counsellor's long statement, conveying information about different means of protection to the clients. Again, the address of her statement changes during its course: C2 begins by addressing C1 (thus recognizing her as the conductor of the session),[9] but soon thereafter she shifts to address the clients with the information (and thereby indirect advice) about different means of protection.

Finally, the re-emergence of arrows numbered 1 and 2 indicates where the participants return to the question–answer format. Here

---

[9] Issues of different participant roles are touched upon more thoroughly in chapters 3–5.

the main counsellor begins to ask questions about the client's knowledge about the tests done after the birth of the child.

In extract (4) the co-counsellor addressed her statements to both clients and the main counsellor. Often in these sessions, counsellors' statements are addressed entirely to other professionals, not to the clients. The main counsellor may interrupt the flow of her questions and instead address a statement to the co-counsellor; or the co-counsellor may intervene and address one to the main counsellor. Statements like this operate as indirect commentaries upon the clients' situation, and sometimes upon their conduct in the session. They are regularly produced at the end of sessions as a 'concluding intervention' (see p. 8); sometimes they are used as a device for managing difficult situations during the session. Extract (5) provides an example of a co-counsellor commenting upon the client's situation. The co-counsellor's statement is addressed to the main counsellor, and it serves as a way of managing an apparently difficult junction. Apart from the two counsellors (C1 and C2) and the patient, there are present two medical doctors as observers (one of whom participates in the talk), and the patient's brother Philip.

```
(5)    (E4-72)
 1    C1:   (1) ->   ((...)) Now let's leave that question, and let's
 2                   (0.5) get back to Doctor Jay's question.=she
 3                   said .hhh that you said the worst thing about
 4                   being in hospital was to be bore:d.
 5    O:             And foll[owing that up-
 6    C1:                    [What stops you being bored at home
 7                   that you couldn't bring here[:.=To stop=
 8    O:                                        [(            )
 9    C1:            =you being bored here.
10                   (0.2)
11    O:             (                    )=
12    P:    (2) ->   =Well I just don't like the idea- >Ever since I
13                   had my operation in 1979. .hh
14                   for that le:g (0.5) I thought that would be
15                   (the end of) the hospital.
16                   (0.4)
17    P:             And then (0.4) better than (        ) come in
18                   again as a patient (0.3) never.
19                   (0.7)
20    C1:            Well that's fi:ne.=We understand tha:t.
21                   [.hh But things have cha:nged
22    P:             [(Presume that)-
23                   (0.3)
```

```
24   P:              I ha[d a lot of problems,
25   C1:                  [And it's NO GOOD DIScussing what you
26                   feel like.
27                   (0.5)
28   C1:   (1) ->    We have to discuss (.2) what i:s. And what is
29                   is that we have a chest infection.=If you think
30                   you'll be er bored in hospital can (.) someone
31                   bring your video here for you?
32                   (.)
33   P:    (2) ->    No.
34                   (0.5)
35   C2:   (3) ->    It seems to me Doctor Kaufman (.2) the decision
36                   (.) I don't know.=I'm [just talking to you=
37   P:                                  [Mm
38   C2:              =now:.
39                   (0.4)
40   C2:             But it seems to me (0.8) that we've heard
41                   several things here toda:y (0.2) that Philip if
42                   he was in Doug's position would be: (0.5) .hh
43                   s- very scared.=I've for- I've forgotten the
44                   words he used.
45   C1:             Shit [(scared)-
46   C2:                  [Shit scared.
47   O:                   [Shit scar(h)ed hh .hhh heh .hhh
48                   hh [.hh h
49   C2:                 [Doug[:
50   H:                       [Excuse [me.
51   O:                               [.hh [hh
52   C2:                                    [is (0.5) has the idea
53                   that this could be the beginning of AIDS.
54                   (2.0)
55   C2:             He: (.3) has the choice (0.9) whether he
56                   allo:ws the medical team here (.3) to have a
57                   chance to treat it and go (out) like we've we
58                   done (.2) for many other patients, (1.3) or he
59                   might deci:de (.) he doesn't want to treat
60                   anything and he just goes home .hh and (.3) his
61                   mother gets more worried, and Philip gets more
62                   worried, and Laura gets more worried,
63   C1:             And he gets [more sick.
64   C2:                         [and he gets more sick to the stage
65                   when (he) can't make decisions for himself.=At
66                   the moment he's able to .hh decide what to do:.
67                   And there is a chance he might get better very
68                   quickly.
69                   (0.5)
```

```
70    C1:    (1) -> If you: (0.2) reach the stage Doug where you
71                     couldn't make decisions anymore who would have
72                     to make them for you.=You heard what Mrs
73                     Walker said.=At the moment you can sit here
74                     saying that you don't want to come into hospi-
75                     tal.=but supposing (0.4) you went home and
76                     instead of getting better this infection got wor:se
77                     (0.5) Who would then make th[e decision about=
78    P:                                          [((coughs))
79    C1:            =whether you had to come in or [not.
80    P:     (2) ->                                 [My mum.
81                     (0.8)
82    C1:    (1) ->  So if your mum were here now to make the
83                     decision when you're not that bad what would
84                     she ((continues))
```

At the beginning of extract (5), the main counsellor (C1) is asking questions of the patient. The questions are again marked with arrows numbered 1 and the answers with arrows numbered 2. The counsellors are in the process of trying to persuade the reluctant patient to remain in hospital for the treatment of his current infection, probably pneumonia.

The arrow numbered 3 indicates the co-counsellor's (C2) ensuing intervention with a long turn, addressed to the main counsellor. Apart from the use of personal pronouns and names, the address is set up by the formulation 'I'm just talking to you now:.' at the beginning of C2's turn (lines 36 and 38). She thereby marks her talk as something not primarily meant for the clients.[10] The clients (the patient and his brother Philip) align correspondingly by withholding any activity, except Doug's 'Mm:' in the beginning of C2's turn, and Philip's apology (line 50) after the term 'shit scared' he had used earlier in the session is reiterated.[11]

---

[10] The patient, however, is apparently meant to be the indirect target of this talk; but we leave aside the analysis of the details of the participation framework here.

[11] The co-counsellor's turn addressed to the main counsellor appears to be an ultimate device in the counsellors' efforts to persuade the patient to remain in hospital. Its use is apparently triggered off by the difficulties that C1 has in persuading the patient through her questions. By addressing her turn in this way, the co-counsellor creates a 'protected' space for herself and the main counsellor to assert and emphasize the rationale of P's staying in hospital, in the presence of the patient. The patient could contradict these assertions only at the expense of departing from the role of a non-addressed participant – a move, as we see, that he opts to avoid.

Unfortunately the uses of the counsellors' statements addressed to other counsellors cannot be examined within the scope of this study.

After the co-counsellor's multi-unit turn, the main counsellor returns to the footing of questioner. Through her question, she allocates the next turn to the patient.

A formal model

Thus far it has been argued, with illustrations, that the recurrent activities in AIDS counselling – exploration of beliefs, perceptions and relations, advice-giving and information – result in a uniform and asymmetric pattern of interaction. In this pattern, the counsellors either ask questions or proffer statements, and the clients do no more than answer the counsellors' questions. To follow this pattern entails the participants organizing two central parameters of turn-taking in a distinct way. One of these parameters involves *turn types*. Counsellors produce two types of turn (questions and statements[12]), whereas the clients produce only one type (answers). The other parameter, *turn order*, is so organized that the clients' turns are produced after counsellors' questions (and therefore are answers); and these answers are followed either by a statement or a question by the counsellor. If a statement emerges, it is followed by a question, both produced by the counsellor. The pattern can be schematized in the following way.

$$[\text{Co:Q} > \text{Cl:A} > (\text{Co:St} >) \text{Co:Q}] \text{ etc.}$$

This turn-ordering applies to one-to-one sessions, as well as to the multi-client and two-counsellor sessions. In multi-client sessions, the questions are usually individually addressed, resulting in one client being selected as an answerer. In two-counsellor sessions, however, the model is expanded so that each counsellor may produce statements of his or her own, resulting in the possibility of consecutive statements.[13]

---

[12] It has to be remembered, though, that 'statement' is a relatively broad characterization of a turn type. As it has been said earlier, what here have been called statements can accommodate at least three types of activity: information, advice and commentaries. What is common to these is their position as independent first acts which do not create a strong conditional relevancy for a specific type of next act.
[13] Moreover, in the two-counsellor sessions, the delivery of the co-counsellor's questions is often managed in a particular way: the question is first addressed to the main counsellor, who then relays it to the client. This practice will be analysed in detail in chapters 4 and 5.

Varieties of the professionals' roles

The model presented above concerns the activities of the clients and the counsellors. However, apart from the counsellors, other professionals may participate in the counselling sessions as observers. Most of the time observers remain silent, but occasionally they do speak. Therefore, their role needs to be characterized. Unfortunately, this characterization has to remain brief: the observers' role will not be systematically examined in this book.

The construction of different professionals' roles involves different use of the turn-allocation techniques. As was pointed out above, the two basic techniques of turn allocation in any talk-in-interaction are self-selection and the 'current speakers selects the next' technique. Now the counsellors – both principal counsellors and co-counsellors – often self-select, and occasionally are selected as next speaker by one another. In other words, they regularly use both techniques of turn allocation.

However, as a rule with only a few exceptions, the observers speak only if the principal counsellor selects them as a next speaker. Extract (6) provides an example.

```
(6)   (E4-22)
 1    C:    ->    Jane is there anything you feel we
 2    O1:         *N:o*=
 3    C:          =haven't attended to?
 4                (1.5)
 5    O1:         No.
 6    C:    ->    Marge, (.5) any issues you wanted to raise
 7                today.
 8                (2.5)
 9    O2:         .hhh (2.0) well I think- (.3) one of the things
10                I was- (.2) thinking about was:: (2.1) had- had
11                you (.2) you and Sue ever thought if things:
12                (1.6) got worse (.) how are you going to cope
13                o:r
14                (.4)
15    P:          .hhhhhhhh[hhhhh
16    O2:                  [>I mean has< (.) has that come
17                [to your mind (.) at all?
18    P:          [hhhhhhhhhhhhh heh heh heh heh .hhhh (it must
19                have gone through) our minds but erm: (1.4) .hh
20                not particularly worried. .hh
```

In (6), the counsellor offers a turn of talk first to an observing nurse (O1) and thereafter to an observing doctor (O2). The nurse declines the offer, but the doctor asks the patient a question.

Apart from the different use of turn-allocation techniques, the observers' and the counsellors' turns are usually similar. In other words, both categories of professional participants ask questions of the patients, and proffer statements addressed to the patients and to other professionals.

The restriction in the observers' use of turn-allocation techniques (i.e. the fact that they only speak when selected by the counsellors) seems to be a *normatively based* state of affairs. Cases where the observers volunteer a turn are very difficult to find.[14] Extract (7) is one of them; and in it, the observer clearly displays the account-ability of her conduct.

```
(7)   (E4-41)
1     P:         I don't know I haven't thought about that.
2                (1.2)
3     O: –>      Can I a:sk (.) one final (0.3) I promised to
4                keep quiet but can I ask one question before
5                you move on. .hhhh If: (0.2) Mr Brown
6                ((continues))
```

In (7), a medical doctor who often works as a counsellor partici-pates in a session exceptionally as an observer. In spite of this role, she volunteers a question; but the question is marked as norma-tively accountable through the preface where O points out that she has promised to keep quiet.

The normative basis for the restrictions of the observers' activ-ities is in contrast with the *non-normative* character of the limita-tions in the clients' conduct.

Uniformity without normative basis

The [Co:Q > Cl:A > (Co:St >) Co:Q] pattern usually followed in the counsellor–client interaction in AIDS counselling sessions involves

[14] Through her turn beginning in line 5 of extract 5 the observing physician (O) seems to treat C1's preceding turn (lines 1–4) as having implied C1's selection of O as the next speaker. C1, however, resists this interpretation and does not give the floor to O.

the narrowing down of the full range of turn types and turn orders, if compared to much everyday talk. The clients adopt a responsive position, where they do not usually ask questions or produce unsolicited talk. This specification results in a likeness between AIDS counselling and the formal institutional settings where turn types and turn order are pre-specified, such as the cross-examination or news interview.

However, a closer examination of turn-taking practices in AIDS counselling reveals that the uniformity of the turn types and turn order there is achieved in a crucially different way when compared to the formal settings. In cross-examination and news interviews, there is a general rule which restricts the conduct of one party to questions and of the other to answers (Atkinson and Drew 1979; Greatbatch 1988; Heritage and Greatbatch 1991). In AIDS counselling, however, the participants do *not* orient to any such institutionally specific rule. In their turn-taking practices, the counsellors and the clients follow the rules of *ordinary conversation*. This is the paradox of turn-taking in AIDS counselling: the asymmetric uniformity is achieved without any rule prescribing it.

The asymmetric uniformity of AIDS counselling must, therefore, be a product of something else. As has been pointed out throughout this chapter, the participants' orientation to their tasks and activities seems to be the basis for uniformity in AIDS counselling.

The design and reception of the turns of talk in AIDS counselling indicates clearly that the participants do not orient to any normatively based restrictions in their turn-taking. We will first examine those cases where the course of events, by and large, follows the [Co:Q > Cl:A > (Co:St >) Co:Q] pattern; and thereafter we will turn to cases where the participants depart from this pattern.

Orientation to the possibility of other types of turn

In this section, I wish to show that during the production of interaction conforming to the above-described pattern, the participants persistently orient to the possibility that something *not* conforming to the pattern *could* very well happen. In other words, I wish to show that the participants do not orient to the type of any next turn being pre-defined, but instead they orient to an organization where the type of the turns is decided on a local basis.

Some preliminary evidence for this local allocation of turn types can be obtained from the 'non-methodical' conduct of the counsellors when receiving the clients' answers. It was mentioned above that the counsellors sometimes produce evaluations and commentaries in a third-turn position after the clients have answered their questions. These third-turn responses may then lead the clients to expand their initial answers. This is the case in extract (8) below. (For another example, see lines 20–6 in extract 5.)

```
(8)     (Section of [3])
1    C:          Do you agree with him?
2    M:          Mm::: I told the doctor to use gloves when he-
3                (.4) she was going to cut his toe:.
4    C:          Mm=
5    M:          = Or (.) look at his toe:.
6    (?):        Mm:
7                (.)
8    C:    ->    But that would be:: whether he was antibody
9                positive or not because one doesn't
10               rea[lly know:.
11   M:    ->    [(This is) why I tol[d him to.
12   C:                             [Right.
13               (1.2)
14   M:          To use glo:ves. .hhhh
15               (1.6)
```

If the counsellors were to orient to a turn type pre-allocation, allowing only questions and statements, these kinds of occasional third-turn responses would be problematic. In (8), however, and in various similar examples, they are not: the interaction moves seamlessly through them.[15]

However, more elaborate evidence for the participants' orientation to the local management of turn types comes from the analysis of the design and reception of *multi-unit turns*. Heritage and Greatbatch (1991) have shown how the management of multi-

[15] Third-turn responses may have a specific function as devices providing for a possibility of a shift of footing in the interaction. In (8) the third-turn response precedes a shift where the counsellor moves from a footing of a questioner into that of a producer of a statement (the continuation of (8) is shown in extract 3). Equally, in extract (4), lines 7–8, the third-turn response preceded the shift where C1 gave up the role of the questioner and C2 resumed it. This 'axis' function of the third-turn responses may arise from their ability to close a chain of questions and answers, as they, unlike new questions, do not project the next action of the client.

unit turns in news interviews indicates the interviewers' and interviewees' orientation to the *pre-specification* of turn types. This is most clear in the case of interviewers' questions. These often combine components other than question clauses, such as 'prefatory statements', with the question components. The interviewees' orientation to the turn type pre-allocation can be seen, Heritage and Greatbatch argue, in their withholding of any response before the question component has been spelled out. By not responding to the statement components by e.g. confirmations, the interviewees display a dual orientation to the turn type pre-allocation. On one hand they exhibit their expectation that their own activities be confined to answers, and on the other they display an expectation that the interviewer is aiming to produce a question, complying with the turn type pre-allocation.

The design and reception of the multi-unit turns in AIDS counselling are equally illuminating. Unlike news interviews, however, they bear witness to the participants' orientation to the *local* management of turn types. In AIDS counselling, multi-unit turns frequently emerge. The length of turns is most striking in the counsellors' statements, which can be seen in extracts (3), (4) and (5).

In the speech-exchange systems characterized by turn type and turn order pre-allocation, multi-unit turns are usually received without the recipients producing continuers. This is not the case in AIDS counselling. Often the clients contribute to the production of long turns by proffering continuers.[16] That is clearly the case in (4), the extract containing the longest statements: W and P don't just remain silent until the counsellors have finished, but they produce their 'Mm's and 'Yes's, usually in connection to 'transition relevance places'. Lines 27, 42, 49, 51, 58, 63, 77, 79, etc. provide examples. These small tokens appear to work as 'continuers' in ordinary conversation (Schegloff 1981): they convey the clients' consent in passing an opportunity to produce a full turn, or to initiate repair. In other words, in producing continuers, the clients orient to the possibility that they *might talk*; and by orienting to the possibility that they might talk after C has produced the statement,

---

[16] Extract (3), lines 27–37 give an example of a (shorter) statement, received without the client's continuers.

they also orient to the possibility of themselves producing other kinds of turns (at least requests for clarification) rather than only answers to C's questions.[17]

Also, counsellors' questions often stretch over several turn-construction units. Sometimes these multi-unit turns contain statement components, along with the question components. The design of these turns in many cases offers indirect evidence for the participants' orientation to the *conversational* character of the turn-taking rules in AIDS counselling.

The statement components can be located *before* or *after* the question components, or they can be inserted *within* the question components. Regarding the rules of turn-taking, the first and the last type are of particular interest. We will examine some examples of these two types.

When the statement components come *before* the question components, the participants observably orient to the possibility that the clients could respond to the counsellor's turn before she has spelled out the question. Counsellors may either *forestall* such response, or they may rely on the clients' *cooperation in withholding* their response until the question has been delivered.

To forestall clients' early responses, the counsellors often *rush through* from the statement components into the question, with the effect that there will be no space for the clients' response. Extracts (9)–(11) are examples of this.

```
(9)   (N-48)
1     P:     I feel okay, I feel ↑ fine.
2            (.8)
3     P:     ([   )
4     C1:  -> [You haven't mentioned AIDS as a concern today.
5            =How much of a conc[ern (now [it is).
6     W:                        [(   )    [I've got so many other
7            worries really t[hat that has to take a back [seat.
8     C1:                    [Uhm:                        [Uhm:
```

---

[17] An interesting topic for further study would be the way that those statements that one counsellor addresses to the other are received. In extract (5) it appears that neither the clients nor the addressed counsellor engage in 'ordinary' receipt activity. By withholding the receipt activity, the clients probably display their orientation to their 'participation status' as non-addressed recipients; and by not producing response tokens, the addressed counsellor may display her orientation to the talk being still targeted to the clients, not to herself.

(10) (N-20)
```
  1   W:        S:[:o-
  2   C1:          [I'm not quite clear about this letter to the
  3             -> building (    ) department.=.hhh[h what would=
  4   W:                                           [Well-
  5   C1:       =you- (.3) if you were writing it what would you be
  6             saying.
```

(11) (Segment of [5])
```
  1   P:        I ha[d a lot of problems,
  2   C1:           [And it's NO GOOD DIScussing what you feel
  3             like.
  4             (0.5)
  5   C1:       We have to discuss (.2) what i:s. And
  6      ->     what is is that we have a chest infection.=If you
  7             think you'll be er bored in hospital can (.) someone
  8             bring your video here for you?
  9             (.)
 10   P:        No.
```

In (9)–(11) above, the statement components in the counsellors'
turns all have some critical edge: in (9), C1 formulates the clients'
silence on a delicate matter, in (10), she indicates that she has not
quite understood what W has meant when she has requested the
counsellor to write to the building department (data not shown),
and in (11), the counsellor sanctions P's earlier talk and challenges
him with spelling out a potentially threatening diagnosis. Now the
counsellors' turn design indicates that they oriented to the relevance
of the clients' direct response to these critical statements. Due to
their rush-through from the statement components to the question
(or in (10), to the inhalation leading to the question), the counsellors in effect forestalled the clients' responses to the statements.[18]
These forestalling moves indicate that the counsellors considered
the clients' direct response as a real possibility.

All statement components preceding questions are not, of course,
of such critical quality. After producing more neutral statement
components prior to their questions, the counsellors usually trust
in the clients' cooperation to withhold any direct response. Extracts
(12) and (13) are examples of this.

---

[18] In (10), W began a response in spite of C1's turn design, through her 'Well-' in line
4. As the counsellor began her question, W aborted her response.

```
(12)  (E3-25)
1     P:              just basically the sexually transmitted [diseases.
2     C1:                                                     [O k a : y.
3     P:              Mm
4     C1:             Now other tests will be done for follow up of your
5                     health.
6     P:       ->     Mm [hm
7     C1:      ->        [What d'you know about those tests Dave?=
8     BF:             =Very little.

(13)  (SS-2-24)
1     C:              Or- or perhaps if you've had a blood transfusion in
2                     the past sometimes it's been transferred >that way
3                     because< .hhh=
4     P:              =That's rig[ht (yeah).
5     C:                         [the blood wasn't treated. We didn't
6              ->     know about it. [Have you ever had a blood=
7     P:       ->                    [Yeah.
8     C:              transfusion at all or given blood?
```

In (12) and (13), the clients produce continuers at the completion of the counsellors' statement components. Thereby they display an expectation that they in principle *could* speak at this slot. The continuers operate as devices for 'skipping' the clients' turns; and accordingly, the counsellors begin to produce their questions.[19]

Another recurrent location for the statement component is after a started but aborted question component. Typically, the counsellors begin their turn with words that project a question, but they abort this, producing thereafter the statement component. After the statement, the question is restarted and completed. Extracts (14)–(17) provide illustrations.

```
(14)  (Planning:430)
1     P:              and do the thi:ngs .hh which basically .h I am
2                     hoping to save up to do (.) later.
3     C1:             Mm:
4                     (0.2)
5     P:              uh=
```

[19] I am not arguing that there would be a 'rush-through' or clients' continuers in *every* case where a statement component precedes the counsellor's question. In a number of cases, clients simply remain silent, even when the counsellor does not make any forestalling moves. However, because the 'rush-through' and continuers recur in *many* cases, there are good reasons for arguing that the participants orient to the possibility of the clients' response to statement components.

```
 6    C1:   (1) ->   =So who do you think
 7                   (0.5)
 8    C1:   (2) ->   I think it's a very: (.) it's an interesting
 9                   dilemma.
10                   (0.2)
11    C1:   (3) ->   .hh Who do you think (.) and or what would help
12                   you most (.) to: (.) begin to clarify how you're
13                   going to resolve .hh these two rather different (.)
14                   pla:ns.
15                   (1.8)
16    P:            I think only (.) just- .hhhh only getting more
17                  information ((continues))
```

(15) (SS/2/19)
```
 1    C:    (1) ->   I mean how- how
 2                   (0.2)
 3    C:    (2) ->   well I mean there are different ways of getting HIV
 4                   if- if indeed you were to have it
 5          (3) ->   how might you possibly be at any risk.
 6    P:            uh I don't know I mean ((continues))
```

(16) (Planning:553)
```
 1    C1:   (1) ->   If Liza was here: .h[h d'you think she'd
 2    P:                                [Mm hm?
 3                   (0.5)
 4    C1:            .hhh if
 5                   (.)
 6    C1:   (2) ->   the crux of it is and it is in a bit if you're
 7                   getting a better house and you're: working longer
 8                   hour:s a:nd .hhh you're accumulating money for
 9                   the future that all means .hh it's all got to generate
10                   out of you:.
11    P:            Correct.
12                   (0.2)
13    C1:   (3) ->   If Liza was here d'you think she'd have any
14                   comment on that.
```

(17) (E4-1)
```
 1    C:    (1) ->   ↑If
 2                   (.6)
 3    C:    (2)- >   and we're just ta:lking very hypothetically
 4                   (1.2)
 5    C:    (3) ->   if you sh- (.6) yo::ur (.) em (.) T-cells did
 6                   drop an your immu:ne system (.7) began not to
 7                   work so well: an:d (1.5) you became unwell, (.)
 8                   how do you see (2.0) Tina as coping?
 9                   (1.2)
```

10	P:	Erm
11		(1.1)
12	P:	She'll r:- (.4) she'll respond to the situation

In (14)–(17), the counsellors' statement components are produced in a sequential location which discourages the clients' response to them. As the aborted turn beginnings have projected questions, the statement components are hearably ancillary to the queries that are soon to be spelled out. Thereby, the clients' response is 'directed', as it were, to the question, not to the statement. Accordingly, in (16) above, P produces only a minimal affirmation of C's statement (line 11); and in the other three cases, the clients remain silent until the questions are spelled out.

Through this practice, the counsellors seem to orient to the possibility that the clients in principle could respond to the statements. In other words, the location of the statement components after the aborted question beginnings can be seen as another technique to forestall the clients' response to the statement components. The forestalling moves would not be needed if the rules of turn-taking excluded the possibility of such response. Therefore, the turn design also here bears witness to the participants' orientation to the possibility of the clients' response to the counsellors' statement components.

In sum, both the design of the counsellors' multi-unit turns and the clients' recipient activity betray the participants' orientation to the possibility that the clients respond before the question components have been spelled out. This orientation entails two issues: (1) an orientation to the possibility that the clients produce talk in a sequential position other than after the counsellors' questions, and thereby (2) that the clients perform actions other than answering.

This kind of orientation amounts to a *local management of turn types and turn order*. In other words, the participants, in this junction, orient to the *conversational* rules of turn-taking.

To summarize: in the data analysis concerning the turn-taking practices in AIDS counselling based on Family Systems Theory, we have argued as follows. The participants usually follow a pattern of turn-taking where the counsellors ask questions and proffer statements, and the clients answer the counsellors' questions. By following this [Co:Q > Cl:A > (Co:St >) Co:Q] pattern, the participants radically narrow down the variation of turn types and turn order available in ordinary conversation. This narrowing down is, however, not normatively given but recurrently achieved 'on the spot', through the participants' orientation to *conversational rules* of turn-taking. Evidence for this was derived from the analysis of the design and reception of the counsellors' multi-unit turns.

In the rest of this chapter, further evidence for the locally achieved nature and conversational basis of the [Co:Q > Cl:A > (Co:St >) Co:Q] pattern will be presented. This evidence will come from the analysis of the *departures* from the pattern.

The absence of normative accountability

If the participants in an interaction orient to a pattern involving their conduct as a normatively sanctionable constraint, then departing from this pattern is, for the participants, a phenomenon in its own right. In other words, a departure is attended to by the participants as an observable and accountable event (cf. Garfinkel 1967). For example, in the news interviews, when the Interviewees depart from the turn type and turn order restrictions, the accountability of their conduct is regularly displayed by requests for permission and sanctions (Greatbatch 1988; Heritage and Greatbatch 1991). In the following, it will be shown that departures from the [Co:Q > Cl:A > (Co:St >) Co:Q] pattern in AIDS counselling are *not* treated as normatively sanctionable and accountable events.

The fact that the departures from the [Co:Q > Cl:A > (Co:St >) Co:Q] pattern are not treated as sanctionable and accountable indicates that the asymmetric uniformity in AIDS counselling is not a result of normative regulation. After having shown this, we will return to the argument outlined at the beginning of this chapter, where we pointed out that the asymmetric uniformity in AIDS counselling is a result of the participants' orientation to their institutionally ascribed tasks and the activities arising from those tasks.

There are five recurring types of departure from [Co:Q > Cl:A > (Co:St >) Co:Q] pattern in AIDS counselling. They all involve the clients' actions. (1) In *conversational responses to counsellors' statements*, the clients produce their commentaries after the counsellors have proffered advice or information to them. (2) In *post-answer statements* the clients use the turn of talk initially accommodating an answer for an action other than answering. (3) The clients can also ask *questions* of the counsellors. (4) In multi-client sessions, they may *answer collaboratively* to the counsellors' questions; and finally (5), they may *comment upon co-clients' answers.*

Each type of departure would deserve its own analysis. Due to the lack of space, however, we will have to limit ourselves to presenting only three types of departures: we will examine examples of conversational responses, clients' questions, and clients' comments upon co-clients' answers.

Conversational responses to counsellors' statements

The completion of a counsellor's statement is a recurring juncture where the preceding talk does not directly control the action that will follow. Unlike questions, statements do not create a conditional relevance for a specific next action. In this respect, the space after a counsellor's statement is 'free', a location where any sort of turns could be inserted.

Regularly, however, counsellors' statements are followed by counsellors' questions. The shift from a statement to a question is often achieved in a cooperative fashion: the client witholds any self-initiatory action after the statement, thus giving the counsellor an opportunity to proffer a question. Thereby, the asymmetric uniformity of the [Co:Q > Cl:A > (Co:St >) Co:Q] pattern is preserved. This is how the shift is organized in extract (18). The client responds in a minimal fashion (arrow 1) to the co-counsellor's statement, whereafter the principal counsellor produces her question (arrow 2).

```
(18)   (Segment of [4])
       ((W = P's wife))
 1     C2:        If you want to take the maximum (0.7) care: .hh
 2                then you should think about using a diaphragm or
 3                a cap, (1.0) [and a condom,
 4     P:                       [Ye:s.
 5                (.)
 6     W:         M[m hm
 7     C2:          [and crea:m.
 8                (1.2)
 9     C2:        And then (0.4) at least it (.2)preserves a little
10                bit. I don't kn[ow what the degree [is so=
```

```
11   (W):                [mhm            [
12   P:                                  [Yes.
13   C2:                 =.hhhh (.2) *but* (0.2) anything less than that (.2)
14                       condoms alo:ne (.) is not sufficient.
15   P:      (1) ->      Mm:
16                       (1.8)
17   C1:     (2) ->      Now (.3) the: (2.0) pregnancy and having the
18                       baby: (.2) uh have you (.) any idea (on) what kind
19                       of (.) tests and things we might (0.4) want to do
20                       when you've- (.) you've got your baby?
21                       (1.2)
22   W:                  *No:*
```

The clients may, however, also respond by their own commentaries on the matters raised in the counsellors' statements. Thereby, the participants depart from the [Co:Q > Cl:A > (Co:St >) Co:Q] pattern into a more conversational mode of interaction. Instead of being allocated their turn of talk by the counsellors, the clients *self-select*; and instead of answering, they produce their own statements. Regularly, departures of this kind are *not* treated as accountable or sanctionable events.

Extract (19) below is an example of this. Arrows mark the clients' response to the counsellor's information and advice concerning the prevention of sexual transmission of the HIV virus.

```
(19)  (E4-41)
  1   C2:          =A:nd (1.2) obviously (0.5) if you don't want (.2)
  2                any risk any at all (.4) you don't have penetrative
  3                intercourse at a:ll. (0.8) And you find other ways
  4                of doing it.=If you're prepared to take (.3) a
  5                slight risk .hh (.2) you would use things like a
  6                diaphragm and cream and
  7                (2.2)
  8   C2:          [c o n d o m s.=[That's not new:,
  9   P:           [Ye(hh)s .hh    [(          )
 10   P:           No[:.
 11   C2:             [that's something [that people did before the=
 12   P:                               [(It)-
 13   C2:          =pi:ll. .hhh If you want (.3) to still not take a
 14                risk you just use (1.0) a condom and crea:m.
 15                (0.6)
 16   P:           Ye:s.
 17                (0.2)
 18   C2:          And you can go right down the
```

```
19                   line [if you want    [to take some risk well=
20   W:    ->             [Yeah. I mean [it takes-
21   P:    ->                            [(I mean it's still-) Prac-=
22   C2:            =[then you do nothing. hhuh=
23   P:    ->       =[practically:
24   W:    ->       =[(there're still practicalities) [(        )
25   P:    ->       =[practically              [practically-
26   W:    ->       the effect on your [sex life general(h)y=
27   C2:                               [Mm
28   W:    ->       =of hhhh [.hhhhhhh [of having this thing=
29   C2:                     [Mm      [
30   P:    ->                         [Ye:s.
31   W:    ->       =lurk[ing in th[e
32   C2:                [Right.   [
33   P:    ->                     [That's right.=
34   W:    ->       =And it's obviously (.2) it's every period (of)
35         ->       ti:me,=
36   C2:            =Mm::=
37   W:    ->       =uhm there's- there's not just that fear there's the
38         ->       operatio:n, (.2) there's the: (.) other physical
39         ->       discomfor[t or pain that he might be i:n. .hh=
40   C2:                     [Absolutely.
41   W:    ->       =The difficulty: of (0.7) of uh- (.2) you know (0.6)
42         ->       of having sex
43                  (1.0)
44   C2:            .h[hh Look we-
45   W:    ->          [of (.) any kind.
46   C2:            We appreciate that.
```

In (19), W (the patient's wife) and P (the patient) respond to the counsellor's advice by proffering their own descriptions of the difficulties in their sex-life.

In extracts (20) and (21) below, the same pattern is replicated: the clients self-select as speakers after the counsellor's statement.

```
(20)  (SS/2/3/2)
      (Talking about how to deal with people's fears concerning trans-
      mission)
1    C1:         And I think you have to- nowada::ys you're helped
2                by the (    ) you have to be more expl[icit.=Just=
3    ( ):                                              [Mm
4    C1:         =put it right back in a very: (0.3) ca[:lm neutral=
5    P:    ->                                          [I think
6    C1:         =[way:.
7    P:    ->     [it- uh- it depends on people's motives as
8          ->     [well [doesn't it.=If people .hhhh (.5) having=
```

```
 9   C1:          [Mm: [
10   ( ):               [Mm
11   P:     ->   =see::n (.8) the facts sort of (.2) generally
12          ->   represented in a way which is reasonably calm
13          ->   (.) per[haps by you or perhaps by the- the things=
14   C1:               [Mm:
15   P:     ->   =they've read in a- a paper which is ((continues))
```

```
(21)  (N-50)
      (Talking about applying for a new apartment)
 1   C:           Your letter must go in first.=The usual routine: the
 2                copy to m[e: and then (.3) my backing would=
 3   P:                    [Mm
 4   C:           =come.=And (.4) it depends: (.2) on their reaction
 5                how hard we push them.
 6                (1.6)
 7   C:           Now just (.2) to throw it in the air. .hhh Some
 8                boroughs have a very special policy towa[rds people=
 9   P:                                                    [Mm
10   C:           =with HIV infection and will house them very
11                quickly:.
12                (1.4)
13   C:           Some may [not.
14   P:     ->             [I think- (.3) I think (there aren't) many.
15   C:           We don't even need to mention[it.
16   P:     ->                                 [No: unless we (draw
17                it back) with the housing associ[ation.
18   C:                                           [No: (.) we don't do
19                it- (.2) that is the [very last resource.
20   P:     ->                         [No (.) no (.) what I mean-
21          ->   (.2) that's right.=If we draw it back with the
22          ->   housing association they might think .hhh if I
23          ->   approach Hammersmith council (.8) which is one of
24          ->   those boroughs then I would mention it (to them).
```

It is noticeable that in (19)–(21), the clients did *not* design their turns so as to display them as accountable and sanctionable. They initiated their turns in a conversational fashion: after the previous speaker (counsellor) had reached a point where her turn could be heard as completed, the clients took the floor. No accounts, apologies or requests for permission were used. Accordingly, the counsellors aligned as recipients of the clients' turns by withholding more talk of their own before the clients had completed their turns. In (19) and (20), the clients produced multi-unit turns which were accompanied by the counsellors' continuers (in (19) lines 27, 29, 32, 36, and in (20), 9 and 14); and in (21), the patient's initial response in line 14 was designed as a single-unit utterance, whereupon the counsellor produced her response (in line 15); this led to a conversational exchange between the counsellor and the patient. In their treatment of the clients' responses, the counsellors obviously did not sanction the clients' action.

The clients' conversational responses to advice and information may be constructive and beneficial, rather than disruptive, in relation to the counsellors' activities and purposes. Especially in (20) and (21), where the counsellors are engaged in advice-giving, the clients' conversational responses seem to indicate that they have 'taken up' the counsellors' advice and treat it seriously (cf. Heritage and Sefi 1992).

These conversational responses, however, also pose a specific interactional challenge to the counsellor. If she wants to continue giving information and advice, or to explore the client's feelings, beliefs and perceptions, she has to regain a more initiatory position. This amounts to the reinstatement of the [Co:Q > Cl:A > (Co:St >) Co:Q] pattern. There are two possibilities for this: either the counsellor can resume the role of a questioner, or she can continue with a new statement.

In (22) below (the extract is an extension of extract 20), after the client's talk was first responded to by the principal counsellor in an affiliative fashion (lines 22 and 24), the co-counsellor asked a question exploring Heather's (P's wife) ways of coping. Thereby, the [Co:Q > Cl:A > (Co:St >) Co:Q] was reinstated. The co-counsellor's question is marked with an arrow.[20]

```
(22)   (Extension of [20])
 7     P:       I think it- uh- it depends on people's motives as
 8              [well    [doesn't it.=If people .hhhh (.5) having=
 9     C1:      [Mm:    [
10     ( ):              [Mm
11     P:       =see::n (.8) the facts sort of (.2) generally
```

---

[20] The co-counsellor's question here follows the 'live open supervision' format, where the co-counsellor's question is *targeted* at the client (Mr Brown) but is addressed to the main counsellor (Dr Jay). This format of questioning is analysed in detail in chapters 4 and 5.

```
12                      represented in a way which is reasonably calm (.)
13                      per[haps by you or perhaps by the- the things=
14    C1:                  [Mm:
15    P:               they've read in a- a paper which is dealing with it
16                      fairly responsibly. .hhh If they still persist in
17                      believing in the Daily Mail or the [Sunday Express=
18    C1:                                                   [Mm:
19    P:               =then there's not an awful lot of hope [for them.=
20    W:                                                      [(No)
21    P:               =.hhh [ And it- it probably causes less ]=
22    C1:                    [And maybe they're looking for]=
23    P:               =[grief on each si::de.
24    C1:              =[a n  e x c u s e anyway.=
25    P:               =Well that's right ye:s. That probably causes less
26                      grief on each side if you just lea:ve it.
27    C2:     ->       Mrs Heller if Heather (sees) back to the (1.0)
28            ->       you know (.3) how she felt when all the publicity:
29            ->       began and how- (.3) she reacted to the publi[city:
30    C1:                                                          [Mm
31    C2:     ->       Would she think) what (1.2) helped her to be more
32            ->       critical and analyse it.
```

In (23), which is an extension of (21), the participants remained on a conversational footing for a longer time, the patient and the counsellor producing their commentaries upon each other's turns. Finally, the counsellor continues with an advisory statement (marked with an arrow, below), whereby the [Co:Q > Cl:A > (Co:St >) Co:Q] pattern is re-established.

```
(23)  Extension of [21])
7     C:          Now just (.2) to throw it in the air. .hhh Some
8                 boroughs have a very special policy towa[rds people=
9     P:                                                  [Mm
10    C:          =with HIV infection and will house them very
11                quickly:.
12                (1.4)
13    C:          Some may [not.
14    P:                   [I think- (.3) I think (there aren't) many.
15    C:          We don't even need to mention [it.
16    P:                                         [No: unless we (draw
17                it back) with the housing associ[ation.
18    C:                                          [No: (.) we don't do
19                it- (.2) that is the [very last resource.
20    P:                               [No (.) no (.) what I mean-
21                (.2) that's right.=If we draw it back with the
```

```
22                  housing association they might think .hhh if I
23                  approach Hammersmith council (.8) which is one of
24                  those boroughs then I would mention it (to them).
25    C:            We[ll then we would-
26    P:               [(          ) up until-=
27    C:    ->        =And very carefully[: you would mention it.=So I=
28    P:                                [Yeah
29    C:    ->        think each step needs to be .hh co[nsidered
30    P:                                                [Mm-m
31                    (2.2)
32    C:    ->        bit by bit.=We cannot take all these pr[oblems=
33    P:                                                     [Mm
34    C:    ->        onboard at once.
35                    (1.2)
36    P:            Yeah
37    C:    ->      I mean you would find out in your area what the
38          ->      possib- there's no harm in finding out
                    ((continues with a long advisory statement))
```

To summarize, after the counsellors' informative or advisory statements, there is a juncture where the asymmetric and uniform pattern of interaction in AIDS counselling is often dissolved. The participants can briefly shift into a more conversational mode. This section has indicated that the participants do not treat the clients' conversational responses to the counsellors' statements as normatively sanctionable actions. When the clients produce such conversational responses, the counsellors align as recipients; after some conversational exchange, they regularly regain their initiatory position. Thereby, the participants return to the asymmetric and uniform pattern of interaction – without any turn-taking-related norms having obliged them to do that.[21]

Clients' questions

Clients' questions constitute a more drastic departure from the [Co:Q > Cl:A > (Co:St >) Co:Q] pattern; by asking a question,

---

[21] There is, however, a specific juncture in the session where the counsellors often actively discourage the clients' responses to their statements. This is after *the counsellors' concluding intervention* (i.e. the counsellors' summarizing statements). The active discouragement results in the turn-taking arrangements related to the closing sections having a more formal character than the turn-taking during the rest of the sessions. The concluding interventions and the closing procedures would deserve their own analysis, which, unfortunately, it is not possible to present here.

the client takes control of the selection of the next speaker. There are two ways in which clients' questions can emerge: either in a 'question time' or through volunteering. These two are very different sequential locations. In a question time, P's question is in itself a responsive next action after C's offer, whereas a volunteered question occupies the very first position in a sequence. Therefore, the volunteered question is a more radical departure from the asymmetric pattern of interaction in AIDS counselling.

Because of this more radical character, we will concentrate here on the volunteered questions.[22] Volunteered questions are often accompanied by accounts and requests for permission. These, one is tempted to argue, exhibit the clients' orientation to a normative expectation that they should not ask questions. However, a closer examination shows that the accounts and requests for permission are better explained with reference to the *local* circumstances of their production.

Extract (24) below is taken from a session with a middle-aged HIV-positive haemophilic man and his wife.

```
(24)  (E4-41i)
 1    C1:        I think uhm (2.0) we- I- I- I would like to move
 2               really (.2) more to the practic[alities. er =
 3    P:                                          [Ye:s.
 4    C1:        =uh- I- I mean (0.6) can I: (0.4) do I uh- (1.0) or
 5               can I have some kind of feedback from you[: as to=
 6    P:                                                   [Mm:
 7    C1:        =whether .hhh I mean you- you've hear:d that (0.4)
 8               that- (.2) that medically .hh er we (.) would feel
 9               that it would be appropriate to treat you with AZT:.
10               .hh [Uh:m : (0.4) gh (.2) gh (.2) gh gh wh- what=
11    P:             [Yeah.
12    C1:        =are your feelings about this,=do you want to
13               star:t? [uh:m
14    P:  (1) ->        [Can I ask some questions [first.=I mean=
15    C1:                                          [Yes.
16    P:         =it- (.2) y'know one- (.4) feels (.8) a- (.2) a need
17               for information (.) before making a deci(h)s(h)ion.
```

[22] For examples of the counsellors' offers to the clients to ask questions, see extracts (1) (lines 27–9) and (3) (line 43). In those cases – as so often in these sessions – the patients did not have anything to ask.

```
18                      That is (        ) (I could)- (.3) appreciate.
19                      (.2)
20      P:              And there's (.6) lots of that (I)- (.5) we'd like-
21                      (1.2) to know, of quite a basic nature really.
22                      (.4)
23      P:     (2) ->   (.hh) Like: (.6) what s[ort of dosage (.6) would=
24      ( ):                             [*(um)*
25      P:              =(.2) ideal >How restricted would it- (.3) .hh ar-
26                      (1.0) are th- are- are there implications, (.4)
27                      er::m (.2) and so forth.
28      C1:             .hh Well (.5) the: (1.2) dose that we start (    )
29                      normally is a thousand milligrams.
30                      (.4)
31      C1:             Which is- (.3) one (.2) tablet (.) five times a
32                      day.
```

At the beginning of the extract, C1 asks the patient whether he would like to start the treatment with AZT. In his response, the patient requests permission to ask some questions first, claiming that he needs more information before making a decision. The request for permission is marked with arrow 1, and the actual question component with arrow 2.

The first part of P's intervention is the request 'Can I ask some questions first?' The counsellor's immediate response, overlapping with 'first', is to grant the permission through 'Yes' (in line 15). This is followed by the patient's account for asking questions, beginning at the end of line 14, and continuing to line 21.

The request for permission and the account closely resemble those devices that news interviewees associate with their questions or other deviant types of turns (Heritage and Greatbatch 1991). One could argue that the request and the account, and even the perturbations in P's talk such as the various pauses and the laugh tokens in the word 'deci(h)s(h)ion' (line 17; cf. West 1983), all indicate P's orientation to his question being something potentially sanctionable and accountable. Equally, it could be argued, the counsellor's 'Yes.' as a response to the patient's initial request constitutes her as the person who usually is expected to allocate the turns and ask the questions.

However, all these features can also be explained with reference to the very local context of P's question. The key issue is that P's question entails postponement of his answer to C's question which

already has been asked. In other words, the question initiates an
insert sequence. What he orients to is not the turn type pre-allocation, but the conditional relevancy of his answer, created by the
counsellor's preceding question, and to the fact that the insert
sequence he is about to initiate is going to postpone the production
of this conditionally relevant item.

In extract (25) below, the sequential position of the patient's
question is different. We will present a rather long sequence of
interaction, leading to the client's question. Dr Moore, who participates in this session as an observer (O), is a medical doctor in
charge of P's treatment.

```
(25)  (E4-52)
  1   C:        But are there any other reasons that one might
  2              (3.1) either alter or stop the treatment that you're
  3              on at present.=That's the one reason but I don't
  4              know whether that would (.2) hold good in AZT
  5              but .hhh [anything else? Have you discussed=
  6   P:                  [Mm:
  7   C:        =anything else with Doctor Moore?
  8              (0.4)
  9   P:        Uh:m
 10   (P):      (I think that)
 11   P:        Uhm
 12              (0.8)
 13   P:        Unless of course the AZT er had m- unless there
 14              was something particularly with the er er and with
 15              the [course of treatment that was giving=
 16   C:            [Mm
 17   P:        =problems. [heh heh .hh (yeah hh)
 18   C:                   [Okay. Side    effects.=
 19   P:        =That's right [yes.
 20   C:                      [Right.
 21   P:        Ye[s (they're no-)
 22.  C:          [D'you know of any of the things that might
 23              give problem:s?
 24   P:        Uh:m
 25              (1.4)
 26   P:        Well I- I have heard of uhm of- of- of er n-nausea.
              ((5 lines omitted))
 32   P:        =And temperatures and high temperatures perhaps are:
 33   C:        D'you want to say [anything at <this stage or>=
 34   P:                          [(        )
 35   C:        no:t.
```

```
36                (0.2)
37    O:          (    ) (0.4) What about the blood counts:.
38                (.)
39    P:          [Oh I (have) to (conce[ntrate) heh heh heh=
40    O:          [huh                  [heh heh heh heh heh=
41    P:          =.hhhh heh=
42    O:          =heh
43    O:          =.hhh[h
44    P:               [This (           ) things ye:s.
45                [Of course ye[s.=(    ) (thing)-
46    (C):        [Mm:      [
47    O:                    [That's its main side effect it's on
48                the marrow.
49                (.2)
50    O:          [And that's one of the reasons why we (.2) see=
51    P:          [Mm
52    O:          =you: (0.4) so [often,=it's ju- just to check=
53    P:                         [(Quite regularly).
54    O:          =blood count's all right. And if=
55    P:          =Yes.=
56    O:          =the blood count did fall: (.) then we might want
57                to stop it or reduce (.) [the dose,
58    P:                                   [Or reduce the dosage.
59                [Yes. Okay that's what the hundred milligrams=
60    O:          [Mm
61    P:          =are for I suppose.=
62    O:          =Yes. [Yes.
63    P:    (1) ->      [Yeah. .hh [Right I actually- let me- y- y-
64    (C):                         [(    )-
65    P:          =you prompted (let me) there [actually because=
66    C:                                       [Yeah.
67    P:          =I was going to ask a[bout the er the- the bone=
68    C:                               [Yeah. Well do:.
69    P:    (2) -> =marrow. .hh Uhm uh uh What actually are the
70                effects: of the er drug >if it does affect< the- the
71                bone marrow.
72                (0.4)
73    O:          Well it has a general: (0.4) er:: depressant effect
74                on the ma[rrow:.
75    P:                   [Oh I see. [Yes,
76    O:                              [So it can drop the white cell
77                cou:nt,=
78    P:          =Right. O[kay.
79    O:                   [and it can ((continues))
```

At the beginning of (25), C is asking P questions concerning a hypothetical situation where his treatment with AZT would have to be stopped or altered. She explores P's knowledge and beliefs about the problems that could possibly lead to such a decision. After eliciting P's views about the possible problems, C gives the floor to O in lines 33 and 35. O, then, reminds P that the bloodcounts would be the most important indicator of something being wrong (line 37).

After O has explained the significance of the 'blood counts' (lines 47–57), P in lines 63–9 produces an account for a question (arrow 1), which indirectly also works as a request for permission. During the course of this account, C responds by granting the permission ('Yeah. Well do:.' in line 68). Only thereafter does P ask about the effects of the drug on the bone marrow (arrow 2).

Now it could be argued that in giving an account and in indirectly requesting permission before asking a question, P displayed an orientation to a norm restricting his right to ask questions. However, on closer examination it transpires again that more than an orientation to the activity of asking questions *per se*, the patient was here oriented to the relevancies created by the local environment of his question. A special kind of participation framework had been established during the preceding talk; and it is to this participation framework that P's request for permission primarily appears to be oriented.

C had been the conductor of the interview. Apart from asking the questions, she also allocated the next turn to O through the offer in lines 33–5: 'D'you want to say anything at <this stage or> no:t.' In allocating the turn to O, C displayed an orientation to the specific role of an Observer, who only speaks when asked to by the counsellor (see pp. 58–9 above). Before the offer, C questioned P about his knowledge of the indications of side-effects. After the last item that P supplied here (high temperatures), C did not proffer any evaluation or correction. In this context, the offer to O (a medical doctor) appears to entail that O can, if she takes the turn, add something to P's knowledge or correct it. C appears to emphasize this specific character of the offer by the slowly uttered phrase '<at this stage>', which formulates the connection between the offer and the preceding talk. And this is, indeed, the way that O uses the turn: she adds 'blood counts' to the list of items that are associated with the side-effects.

So O has spoken when invited to do so by C; and the type of her activity (indirect correction of P's preceding answer) was implicated through the sequential location and design of the offer. This amounts to C retaining a special kind of production role *vis-à-vis* O's words: she remains, at least potentially, the 'sponsor' (Levinson 1988: 172) of those words. In correcting P's answers, O does something that is motivated by co-present C.

Now, when O summarizes her statement in lines 54–7 by saying 'And if the blood count *did* fall: (.) then we might want to *stop* it or reduce (.) the *dose*,' we can hear that she has completed what she was invited to do by C. At this junction, P takes his turn, which leads to a question. My argument is that P's request displays an orientation to C's role as the 'sponsor' of O's preceding activity, rather than displaying orientation to the clients' questions in general being a sanctionable turn type.

P's postural orientation is most revealing here. It is transcribed below:

(26)   (Postural orientation in a section of [25])

```
                                          X===
P:   (o) ──────────────────,,,,.....(c) - - - - - - - - - - - - -,,,
P:   are for I suppose.        [Yeah. .hh [Right I actually- let
O:                     Yes. [Yes.
(C):                                      [(    )-

     ==============X
P:   (md/c) . . . . . . . . . . . . . . . . . . . . (c) - - - - - - - - -
P:   me- y- y- you prompted (let me) there [actually because
C:                                          [Yeah.

P:   (c) - - - ,,.(o)──────,,...(c) - - - - - - - - -,,,..(o) ─────
P:   I was going to ask a[bout the er the- the bone marrow.
C:                        [Yeah. Well do:.

P:   (o) ──────────────────────────────────
P:   .hh Uhm uh uh What actually are the effects: of the er

P:   (o) ──────────────────────────────
P:   drug >if it does affect< the- the bone marrow.
```

X=========X   indicates where P points with his right hand
              towards O

. . . .   indicates P's orientation which appears to be
                      somewhere between C and O; but may also be
                      towards C.

During his request for permission to ask a question, P's orientation alternates between C and O. In the beginning of the request, he moves away from an orientation towards O, towards C. This way he begins the new part of his turn in an orientation to C, treating her as the addressee. He remains in this orientation, or a middle-distance orientation, until the beginning of his assertion of his intention to ask a question. However, while saying 'going to *ask*', he shifts towards O for a short period, thus apparently indicating that the projected question would be addressed to O; and thereafter he returns his orientation towards C. In sum, P here appears skilfully to balance his orientation between C and O, to the effect that the indirect request can be heard to be addressed to C, while O is treated as the addressee of the question that he requests the permission for.

C indeed does treat herself as the addressee of the indirect request, when she grants the permission by saying 'Yeah. Well do:.' just after P has returned to an orientation to her. Thereafter, P shifts back to the orientation to O, and remains in that orientation throughout the delivery of his question.

By requesting permission from C to ask a question of O, P oriented to the change that his question would bring about to the participation framework. Up to this point, in spite of remaining silent, C had potentially occupied the role of a 'sponsor' of O's activity. By asking his question, P is about to solicit another kind of participation from O: something not any more sponsored by C. This would marginalize C's participation status, leaving her to the role of audience. By requesting the permission from C to ask a question of O, P seems to orient to these changes in the participation framework. And, moreover, through his request P indeed manages to alleviate the marginalization of C's participation role: through the permission that C now grants, P's question and O's subsequent answer are now spoken under the nominal sponsorship of C.

In summary, then, it appears also that in extract 25 the features that at the first sight seemed to be indications of P's orientation to normative standards disfavouring clients' questions as a turn type after a closer analysis appear to be better explained with reference to much more local issues.

A further confirmation for the primacy of the local environment in prompting the use of requests for permissions and other prefacings is provided, of course, by the cases where clients ask questions without using such prefacing. Extracts(27) and (28) are examples of this.

(27)   (N-7)
       ((W = P's wife))
1   C1:   And actually: Doctor Kaufman it's rather (strange)
2   you should .hhhh talk straight to Graham
3   the[re but .hhhh it came to my mind that Graham=
4   C2:   [( )
5   C1:   =actually: is very well trained in writing
6   W: Heh .hhh heh
7   P: Really:
8   C1:   (And really) could do it f(h)or us. ((smile voice))
9   P: Erm:
10 (C1):   .hhhhhhh
11   (.3)
12 C1:   Anyway.
13 P: -> Er:: (.6) is there any- (.2) is- (.2) is there any
14   sort of evidence about whether the: .hhhh (1.0)
15   number of people who go on to develop AIDS in the
16   haemophilics is any different or any more- .hh (.3)
17   or any less (.2) than it is in the-in the other risk
18   groups.
19   (1.6)
20 C1:   What have have you (read) so fa:r?

(28)   (E4-66)
1   C2   (...) So (1.0) I think that while I- I do
2   understand your anger I- I think (1.8) it can
3   kind of get diffused in[to- into:
4   P: [Yeah: but at the same
5   -> uh- the [(exac)- what was the exact number=
6   C2:   [(very vague things).
7   P: =of haemophiliacs who're: HIV infect-
8   who're HIV positive.
9   C1:   Well I can't tell you the exact number::

In (27) and (28), clients' questions occur in an environment where the prior talk has not created particular relevancies for the client's next action. In (27), the principal counsellor has just completed her statement, addressed to the co-counsellor. Before the client's question, there is a short gap, and then the counsellor says 'Anyway.', which seems to work as a marker for a topical shift. The client initiates his non-prefaced question in this location: after the prior business has been completed and before the next action is properly begun.

In (28), the client inserts his question in a similar kind of slot, but in a more 'imposing' manner. In lines 1–3, the co-counsellor is in the process of delivering a statement to the client. The client initiates his turn when the gist of the counsellor's statement can be comprehended, even though the counsellor has not yet properly completed her utterance. After some searching, the client initiates his question.

In (27) and (28), the counsellors' activities did not create any specific relevancies for the clients' next actions. In the absence of such local control, the clients were free to produce their questions without prefaces. This is further evidence for the primary importance of *local circumstances* in prompting the clients' requests for permission and accounts, associated with their questions.

The primacy of the local environment as a source of relevancies is further confirmed by cases where the *counsellors* use token requests before their questions. Extracts (29) and (30) are examples of this.

```
(29)  (E3-15)
 1    C2:                 (...) [I would write (.3) a- a le[tter (but I =
 2    P:                       [(    )              [(        )
 3    C2:                 =wouldn't) say I'm actually now (        ).=
 4    P:                  =Okay. Fine. .hh And then secondly: uh:m (2.0)
 5                        the: (.3) one question that my mother raised
 6                        [was .hh how (.5) is there a- (.) do you know=
 7    C1:                 [Mm
 8    P:                  =whe:n (.6) uhm: (.2) from (.3) phials of blood that
 9                        may be historic (0.8) I- (.2) that the HIV was first
10                        (.6) [like-
11    C2:                      [In you:? hh
12    P:                  [Yeah.
13    C1:   (1) ->        [Can I just (ask[ a)-
14    P:                                  [Sorry.
15    C1:   (1) ->        put a question to [Henry,=you say your mother=
16    P:                                    [(        )
17    C1:                 =wants to know:,
18    P:                  Mm hm
```

19	C1:	(2) ->	uh[:m: (.3) do you agree that (.6) [she has that=
20	( ):		[hhh [
21	P:		[( )
22	C1:	(2) ->	=informati[on.=Or do you want to know as well?
23	P:		[Yes.
24	P:		er (.2) I'd be interested,=I'm not- I'm not
25			particularly concer:ned, (.4) [er bu:t (.3) uhm=

(30)	(E4-66)	
1	P:	No they wanted to start doing- they wanted to
2		start doing tests:.=
3	C2:	=They couldn't- [they couldn't because=
4	C1:	[( )
5	C2:	=unti:l (0.5) that gene was isolate[d
6	P:	[Yeah.
7	C2:	an:d (0.5) they could sequence it no-one could
8		possibly even consider doing it.=It was a sort of
9		dream thing un[til the early eighties.=And
10	P:	[Well when:
11		(.)
12	P:	When we started usin[g-
13	C2:	[And even [now:: with]=
14	P:	[thi- this small]=
15	C2:	=[a l l : : the [c o m m e r c e available=
16	P:	=[concentrate [Yeah but when we started using=
17	C2:	=[t o-
18	P:	=[the sma[ll concentrate.=
19	C2:	[Hang on.
20	C2:	=Sorry can you just [hang on Mick. Even though=
21	P:	[Yeah.
22	C2:	=with all the- the money o- of the commercial
23		companies available (0.3) that synthetic factor
24		agent's only available in a very small amount for
25		tria:l eve[n now::. [So I mean that's something=
26	P:	[Yeah. [(But I'm not- not-)
27	C1:	[(It's on tria:l)
28	C2:	=differe[nt from using
29	P:	[(No I'm)-
30	P:	Perhaps I (.) used the wrong word when I
31		sai[d synthetic.=[I think I did. (0.2) What I'm=
32	C2:	[You have. [Mm
33	P:	=saying (.) when they- they wanted to start
34		producing their own factor eight.
35		(.)
36	P:	Rather than importing it.
37		(0.5)

```
38   P:              With- using British blood, (0.6) an::d (0.6) making
39                   ( [            )
40   C1:  (1) ->   [Can I a:sk you anoth[er
41   P:                                   [without importing
42                   [all the time.=
43   (C2):           [Mm
44   C1:  (1) ->  =Ca[n I ask-
45   P:                [And the government said no we'll keep on
46                   importing because it's cheaper.
47   C2:             No [no they were actually [making it (        )=
48   C1:  (1) ->        [Can I ask y-          [Hang on (let's get)=
49   C2:             =[(one and only)
50   C1:             =[(that)
51                   (.)
52   C1:  (1) ->  [One thing they were making it but can I (.) ask=
53   C2:             [(   )
54   C1:  (2) ->  =you what you know about our own factor eight.=Was
55        (2) ->  it completely pure.
56                   (0.5)
57   P:             Uh:m I don't know: but (.) [(          )
58   C1:                                        [Well I- I can only
59                   tell you that (0.9) there wasn't such an incident as
60                   there was in: (0.6) imported factor eight but we
61                   certainly had people infected from our own factor
62                   eight as well.
```

We will not be able to go very deeply into the details of (29) and (30). It has to suffice to say that in (29), the main counsellor, turning towards the co-counsellor, addresses to her a request to ask a question (arrows numbered 1), and thereafter she turns towards the patient and asks him a question (arrows numbered 2). The main counsellor's question is inserted between P's question[23] and an answer to it, in a situation where the co-counsellor has (through the repair initiation in line 11) shown her intention to deal with P's question. In (30), the counsellors first suppress the production of P's question (P's unsuccessful efforts to ask a question occur in lines 10, 12, 14, 16 and 18). Soon after, the main counsellor prefaces her question with a series of requests to ask a question (arrows numbered 1). Only after the preface is the question spelled out (arrows numbered 2).

[23] To put it more specifically, the question was presented as P's mother's question which P only relays.

In (29) and (30), then, the parties who in the ordinary course of events spent most of their time asking questions prefaced their questions with requests for permission. In (29), this prefacing seems to attend to the question's sequential location as an initiation of an insert sequence; and in (30), to the fact that the question interrupts P's flow of talk and sequentially deletes his earlier question.[24] These observations also emphasize the primacy of the *local* environment in the use of such prefacings. They also indirectly support the thesis put forward earlier that the *clients'* use of requests for permissions and accounts can be explained primarily with reference to the local environment.

Preliminaries, such as requests for permission and accounts, can accomplish various kinds of tasks in talk-in-interaction (Schegloff 1980). There is no reason to think that they cannot be used to display their producers' orientation to a turn-taking system precluding the type of activity that he is intending to engage himself in. However, in the single cases of AIDS counselling interaction analysed above, that seems not to be the preliminaries' main function.

Comments upon co-clients' answers

In multi-client sessions, there are many opportunities for the departure from [Co:Q > Cl:A > (Co:St >) Co:Q] pattern. One of these involves clients' commentaries upon co-clients' answers to the counsellors' questions.

The commentaries vary regarding the address: they may be addressed to the counsellor or to a co-client. There is also a difference between those commentaries which create conditional relevance of a specific type of next action from the addressee, and those which do not. Obviously those commentaries that are addressed to a co-client and which strictly control his or her next action constitute the most radical departure from the [Co:Q > Cl:A > (Co:St >) Co:Q] pattern.

---

[24] Silverman (1991) has analysed the use of requests for permission in pre-test counselling as a pre-sequence to mark an upcoming delicate question (usually related to the client's sexual contacts). That constitutes a further local environment where the party usually asking the questions marks them as potentially accountable.

In actual cases different types of commentaries are usually mixed up with one another. Extract 31 below is an occasion where a client's answer to the counsellor's question triggers off a series of commentaries from co-clients. The clients are an adolescent HIV-positive boy Richard (P), with his younger sister Penny (S) and mother (M).

```
(31)  (E3-46)
  1   C:              Who do [you go: (.3) to (.) for som[eone to be on=
  2   S:                     [.hhh hh                    [hh
  3   C:              =your si:de.
  4                   (2.0)
  5   S:              Uh:m (2.0) whuhhheh huh .hhh (1.8) (it's not)
  6                   ( ) hh
  7   C:              Mm?
  8                   (.)
  9   S:              Well I try to get mum on my side but it doesn't
 10                   (really) wor:k.
 11                   (.3)
 12   C:              It doesn't?
 13   S:              No not really,
 14                   (1.6)
 15   P:    (1) ->    [(              )
 16  (C):             [(      )-
 17                   (0.7)
 18   C:              Pardon?=
 19   M:    (2) ->    =It does work I'm- (.3) I think I'm quite (.2) er
 20                   heh [heh heh f(h)air.
 21   S:    (3) ->        [You're no::t you're always on Richard's side
 22                   and you know it's tru:e.=
 23   P:    (4) ->    =That's because I'm usually ri(h)ght a(h)ctually.=
 24   C:              =Wha[t gives you the idea mum's always on=
 25   P:                  [huh .hhhhh
 26   C:              =Richard's side when she thinks differently.=
 27   S:              =We:ll=
 28   C:              =What does she do that makes:=
 29   S:              =Well if we're arguing then I'm- (.4) I'm the one
 30                   who's told off: (.4) and (.) it's my fault. And
 31                   Richard just sort of (0.8) sits a little smug.
```

In (31), the counsellor asks Penny (P's sister) who she goes to for someone to be on her side in the quarrels with Richard, her brother (P). (Shortly before the extract S has claimed that mum takes Richard's side.) S says (lines 9–10) that she tries to get mum on

her side, but that doesn't work. After C has elicited a reconfirma-
tion to the answer (lines 12–13), P makes the first commentary
(arrow 1). Judging from P's posture, he appears to address C, as
he turns towards her at the beginning of his comment, and remains
in this orientation during his turn and most of the ensuing gap. The
comment, however, is inaudible; it appears to be so for C too,
because after a gap, she asks 'Pardon?', looking at P.

The following turn, however, is taken by mother. She turns to S
during C's 'Pardon?', and then says 'It does work I'm-'. Now it
appears that M is addressing S, challenging her preceding assertion
involving her. After a little pause, M restarts the sentence that she
had aborted, turning simultaneously with its beginning towards C.
M's postural orientation is transcribed below.

(32)   (Postural orientation in a section of [31])

M: (s) —————————   ,,.(c) - - - - - - - - - - - ,
M: It does work I'm- (- - -) I think I'm quite (- -)

M: ,.(o) - - - - - - - - ,,(s) ——— ,,,(md upwards)
M: er heh [heh heh fa(h)ir.
S: [You're no::t you're always on Richard's side and

Judging from the speaker's postural orientation, the address of M's
turn, therefore, seems to be divided between S and the practitioners
('o' stands for the observing physician, to whom M turns at the
beginning of her laughter): The turn is correspondingly divided into
two parts, separated by the 0.3 sec. pause.[25]

Mother is immediately challenged by S, who, addressing M,
renews her claim that mother indeed is always on Richard's side
(arrow 3 in extract [31]). Thereafter Richard steps in, facing Penny,
and makes his joke (arrow 4).

---

[25] Apart from the postural orientation, the change of the address in mid-turn is
observable in the different design of the two halves of the turn. The first part has
got a sharp edge on it: it is built up as a rebuttal of the accusation implicated by S. As
a sharp rebuttal, this is hearable as something spoken to S, who made the accusation.
However, the latter half is built up as a tentative description of the relations between
the family members. This appears to establish it as something spoken to a third party,
i.e. something designed for professional recipients who are observing the interaction
between the family members from a neutral position.

To summarize, in (31), S's answer to C's question, which implied a certain interpretation about the relations between S, M and P, triggered off commentaries from both P and M. The address of these comments appears to alternate between S, C, and for a little part O. Mother's initial commentary was followed by further comments from S and M, which were addressed to the co-clients.[26] It appears, then, that by the end of line 23 in extract (31), most of the structural features entailed by the [Co:Q > Cl:A > (Co:St >) Co:Q] pattern have been dismantled: clients are producing turns other than answers, self-selecting themselves as speakers and addressing one another instead of the counsellor.

However, the clients did not display an orientation to their exchange being normatively sanctionable. There were no apologies or accounts. The opportunity for the clients to produce their commentaries arose when the counsellor did not take next action immediately after the delivery of S's answer (resulting in the gap in line 14). The counsellor did not 'resist' the production of the commentaries in any way. After the inaudible first comment by P, she initiated a repair (line 18) – thus trying not to disregard P's comment. During the dispute between M and S, the counsellor remained passive. In sum, in Extract 31, the [Co:Q > Cl:A > (Co:St >) Co:Q] pattern was departed from very smoothly and without complications.

It was restored equally smoothly through C's question in lines 24 and 26. After Richard's joke C produces her question, and, therefore, she is again in control of the interaction. The clients do nothing to continue their dispute: while S aligns again as the answerer, the other clients withhold, for the time being, any competitive activity.

In (31) the clients addressed their comments to one another, triggered off by an answer to the counsellor's question. In extract (33) below, S departs one step further away from the client's role in

---

[26] Although many of the comments are addressed to co-clients and not to the counsellor, the speakers may have designed their turns so as to take into account the counsellor's presence. It appears that descriptions such as 'you're always on Richard's side and you *know* it's tru:e.' (lines 21–2) and 'That's because I'm usually ri(h)ght a(h)ctually.' (line 23) are at least partially targeted to the counsellors. M's and S's postural disengagement at the end of the exchange between them also hints at this.

the [Co:Q > Cl:A > (Co:St >) Co:Q] pattern by asking a co-client a question.

```
(33)  (E3-46)
 1    C:              D'you argue with mum?
 2                    (1.0)
 3    S:              N[o: he never does.
 4    P:               [(Maybe-)
 5    M:              He [    ↑d o e : : : s .      ]
 6    S:                   [ (He) never argue(s) with] mum.
 7                    (0.6)
 8    S:    (1) ->    [   Oh yeah:: when was the   ] last=
 9    M:              [I should kn(h)o(h)w heh heh]
10    S:              =time you had an argument with him.
11    M:    (2) ->    Well look-
12    S:              You never have a major argument. Not
13                    like you [do with me::.]
14    M:    (3) ->             [ Yes   I   do:.]=Sometimes.
15    C:              [What are the thi[ngs you two argue about then.
16    M:              [( )             [(              )
17                    (1.6)
18   (S):            *Mm*
19                    (2.0)
20    S:              Well it's because I want to go out and I'm
21                    grou:nded. hhhhh
```

Extract (33) begins with C asking a question of P. But as the beginning of P's answer is delayed, S inserts her own view of the matter (line 3).[27] S's claim triggers off an exchange of views between M and S.

S's utterance in lines 8 and 10 (the beginning of which is marked with arrow 1) is not only addressed to M, but also, being a question, projects a response from her. M's first response is minimal and apparently reluctant 'Well look-' (arrow 2). This, along with M's postural orientation where she gazes upwards at a middle distance position seems to convey her unwillingness to engage in further argument. However, as S presses on (lines 12–13), M eventually produces a response where she renews her claim that she does argue with P (arrow 3). During the renewed exchange of conflicting

---

[27] In this case the unaddressed client's answer is not sanctioned by the counsellor. However, the relative delay of the beginning of S's turn seems to indicate her orientation to P's primary right for answering.

views, M also resumes a postural orientation towards S. Consequently, S and M are in full mutual engagement during the renewal of S's accusation and M's response (lines 12–14).

Just as in extract(31), in (33) the clients did not mark their turns as accountable, nor did they produce any apologies. Equally, the counsellor allowed the exchange between the clients to take place, without imposing any sanctions on them. M appeared reluctant to escalate the quarrel at one point, but was nevertheless drawn into one more exchange of opposing views. A further similarity between (31) and (33) is in the way that the counsellor resumes her role as the questioner: after a period of exchange of turns between the clients, the counsellor intervenes and asks a question. In (33) above, the question is addressed jointly to S and M; and after some hesitation, S aligns as the answerer.

The interaction in (31) and (33) involved, as it were, a pendular movement where the counsellor's questions are first answered and then followed by a series of commentaries by the clients, after which the free flow of commentaries is interrupted by the counsellor's next question. This movement may become more observable if we follow a little further the unfolding of the interaction after extract 33. The following will be such a long extract that analysing it in detail is impossible in this context; but it will illustrate the recurrent movement to and fro of the question–answer sequence.

```
(34)   (Extension of [33])
   1   C:                .hhh Well ever since [I've known Richard (0.4)=
   2   (P):                                   [Mm
   3   C:                =he's always given me quite a good ti:me I mean I
   4                     don't get away with [anything.
   5   M:                                    [Mm:
   6                     (2.2)
   7   C:                Anything that one s:ays he has had the answers for.
   8   M:                hhem
   9   C:                And maybe Richard's:: that's one his (1.4) big
  10                     points.
  11                     (.5)
  12   C:     (1) ->     D'you argue with mum?
  13                     (1.0)
  14   S:                N[o: he never does.
  15   P:     (2) ->      [(Maybe-)
  16   M:     (3) ->     He [    ↑d o e : : : s .      ]
  17   S:     (3) ->         [ (He) never argue(s) with] mum.
```

```
18                  (0.6)
19  S:    (3) ->    [  Oh yeah:: when was the  ] last=
20  M:    (3) ->    [I should kn(h)o(h)w heh heh]
21  S:              =time you had an argument with him.
22  M:    (3) ->    Well look-
23  S:    (3) ->    You never have a major argument. Not like you
24                  [do with me::.]
25  M:    (3) ->    [ Yes I do:.    ]=Sometimes.
26  C:    (1) ->    [What are the thi[ngs you two argue=
27  M:              [( )              [(                )
28  C:              =about then.
29                  (1.6)
30  (S):            *Mm*
31                  (2.0)
32  S:    (2) ->    Well it's because I (was going ) out and I'm
33                  grou:nded. hhhhh
34  C:              You're grounded.
35  M:    (3) ->    We don't argue about that (do we).=
36  C:              =So [would
37  S:    (3) ->        [We do::.=
38  C:    (1) ->    =would [Richard have the same sort of arguments=
39  S:                     [(                            )
40  C:              =with mum about wanting to go out and mum
41                  grounding him.
42  P:    (2) ->    No:.=
43  S:    (3) ->    =( ) he never goes [ou:t.
44  M:    (3) ->                       [You: (.5) you- (.2) she
45                  wants to be grounded [there's particular friend] =
46  S:    (3) ->                         [I  don't  want  to  be] =
47  M:              =[you don't want to see him.=Say tell them I'm] =
48  S:              =[grounded anymore.=I  don't  want  to   be] =
49
50  M:              =[grounded.
51  S:              =[grounded anymore::.
52
53  M:    (3) ->    Pen(h)n(h)y heh [heh .hhhh
54  S:    (3) ->                    [I told you about [it (we)=
55  M:                                               [hhh
56  S:              =(wouldn't be [going) ( ) but you said no=
57  M:    (3) ->                  [Well you see it's not really er
58  S:              =you're still grounded.
59  C:    (1) ->    .hh So what are the other [things that Penny=
60  M:                                        [(          )
61  C:              =does that gives mum: cause to argue with her.
62                  (2.6)
63  P:    (2) ->    er:: (0.4) She- she has been known to st- (.2) st-
```

```
64                    stay out (.4) too late at night?
65                    (1.4)
66  S:    (3) ->      hh heh heh heh
67                    (.)
68  ( ):              Mm=
69  M:                =.hhhh h[hh .hhhh
70  ( ):                      [Mm
71  C:    (1) ->      So: it's: the th[ings that Penny wan[ts to do
72  M:                               [(That sort of thing). [
73  P:    (2) ->                                           [She- she
74                    malingers.
75                    (0.6)
76  C:                She malin[ger:s?
77  S:    (3) ->               [Well what does [that mea:n.
78  P:                                         [Yes.
79                    (2.4)
80  P:    (3) ->      I can't help it if you're a (malingerer) Penny.
81  S:                hhh hheh [ heh heh [.hhh
82  M:                         [ (heh)   [
83  C:    (1) ->                         [So if [you mali:ng- who's=
84  M:                                          [( )
85  C:                =missed more school in the last term you or
86                    Penny. [In your view.
87  S:    (2) ->              [(Me:).
88  P:                Penny.
89  S:                Me:.
90  P:    (1) ->      What for Penny?
91                    (1.2)
92  S:    (2) ->      (                        )
93  C:                Pardon?
94  S:    (2) ->      I had st- (.3) uhm: (0.4) I get bad stomach aches.
95                    (1.2)
96  S:                A:[nd
97  M:    (3) ->        [She's been off toda:y.
98  S:                M[m:
99  M:    (3) ->        [That's why she's come up. (Well) but you were
100                   going to come up anyway weren't you: but
101 S:                Mm:
102 M:                you didn't come out of school on ti:me.
```

In the beginning of extract (34) above, the counsellor produces a statement, where she delivers her view about Richard (lines 1–10). Thereafter the interaction unfolds as sequences consisting of the counsellor's question (arrows 1), the initial answer by one of the clients (arrows 2), and a series of commentaries by other clients

(arrows 3), triggered off by the answer and the earlier commentaries on it. The question–answer sequence in lines 83–9 appears to be the only one where the initial answer does not lead to further commentaries, even though the answer is spelled out three times, once by the addressed recipient (P) and twice by the person whom the answer primarily concerns (S).[28] The address of the commentaries varies between the counsellor and the other clients; and occasionally the commentaries involve the clients' questions to one another.

The counsellor's questions appear to be like signposts along a tortuous path. On the one hand they are designed so as to show continuity with the preceding talk,[29] and on the other they all direct the unfolding interaction towards the therapeutic direction, i.e. the exploration of relationships and perceptions. Through her questions, the counsellor recurrently puts Penny, Richard and Mum in a position where it is relevant for them to describe their relations with one another, and their perceptions and beliefs. To use the words of the counsellors themselves, in sequences like this 'questions are used in order to explore different perceptions and views of relationships' (Bor and Miller 1988: 400).

To be able to direct the interaction in this way, the counsellor has to resume, again and again, her role as the questioner. But as we have shown it in this chapter, she resumes it without recourse to a normative primacy of certain turn types or turn order. The question is the most important tool of the counsellors; the possibility of the professional use of this tool rests upon the mutually recognized turn-taking rules of ordinary conversation.

A summary of the analysis of departures from the pattern

The analysis of data in this chapter has shown that the uniform and asymmetric pattern of interaction usually followed in AIDS counselling is achieved by the participants orienting to conversational rules of turn-taking. The [Co:Q > Cl:A > (Co:St >) Co:Q] pattern does not have a sanctionable and normative character for the

---

[28] The Q–A sequence in lines 59–64 does not trigger off verbal commentaries, but non-lexical responses (laughter) from the co-clients.
[29] The first question in line 12 is connected with the talk that occurred before C's statement and is not shown in the transcript.

participants. When their conduct corresponds to this pattern, and when it departs from it, the participants' prime frame of reference appears to be the turn-taking system of ordinary conversation.

In spite of the numerous opportunities for departing from the [Co:Q > Cl:A > (Co:St >) Co:Q] format, most of the time in the sessions the participants of AIDS counselling maintain this asymmetric and uniform pattern of interaction. This entails a locally achieved specification of turn types and turn order.

During the 'ordinary' course of events, counsellors work towards the [Co:Q > Cl:A > (Co:St >) Co:Q] pattern by, first and foremost, asking a new question or producing a statement regularly after a client's answer and, after a statement, by producing a question. Correspondingly, clients comply with this by generally withholding activities other than answering questions. These choices are made, again and again, within the framework of conversational turn-taking rules.

In those cases where clients do something other than merely answer counsellors' questions, the counsellors use one of the first transition relevance places available (not necessarily the very first one) to produce a turn which brings forward the pattern once again. The techniques of reinstatement all operate within the framework of conversational rules of turn-taking.

After their departures from the [Co:Q >Cl:A (>Co:St) > Co:Q] pattern, clients by and large complied with counsellors' efforts towards the reinstatement of that pattern. In other words, after having initiated actions other than answering the counsellors' questions they were ready to return to the footing brought forward by the counsellor as soon as she made her move in that direction.

Counsellors' tasks and the opaqueness of the frame

Earlier in this chapter the distinction between 'formal' and 'informal' institutional settings (Drew and Heritage 1992) was discussed. It was suggested that AIDS counselling constitutes an informal setting; i.e. a setting in which the aggregative asymmetries in turn-taking practices are a result of the participants' *orientation to their tasks and activities*. It is time to expand that discussion now.

The counsellors' task is to conduct a session of AIDS counselling. That counselling is what they want to do, and what they are paid,

trained and organizationally accountable for. This counselling entails, among other things, advising and informing the patients about the course of their illness and its treatment, helping the patients to deal with the social and psychological strains caused by the illness, and preparing them mentally for a possible worsening of their condition at some future point in time. The counsellors in this particular clinic have also committed themselves to the Family Systems Theory approach in counselling. This means, among other things, that they believe that all the people around the carrier of the virus are somehow affected by the illness; that they each have their own cognitive, emotional and practical perspective on it; that their perspectives interact as a 'system'; and finally, that making the clients aware of this system can be helpful for them. Moreover, the counsellors' commitment to Family Systems Theory means that they want to use particular interactional techniques, such as 'circular questioning', 'hypothetical future-oriented questions', and concluding 'interventions'.

Now in order to practise AIDS counselling within the Family Systems framework, it is functional for the counsellors to operate either through questions or through statements. This entails the maintenance of the [Co:Q > Cl:A > (Co:St >) Co:Q] pattern of interaction.

To use the time available effectively, to cover all the tasks, and to encourage talk about issues that usually are difficult to address (sex, illness and death), it is useful for the counsellor to take initiatory actions and to control the agenda. This is achieved by counsellors maintaining the role of questioner and, occasionally, by giving statements. To demonstrate each client's different perspective to the shared situation, it is useful if the counsellors control the unfolding of the interaction by their questions, so that each client only speaks when questioned by the counsellor, and turns are not allocated to one another.

At a more practical level, counsellors give information and advice by first asking clients questions about their knowledge and practices, and then by offering statements tailored accordingly (cf. Peräkylä and Silverman 1991). Counsellors demonstrate clients' different perspectives to HIV-related problems by 'circular questioning' (see chapter 3); and they prepare the clients for the worsening of their situation by asking them questions about their fears concerning the future, and, if needed, by correcting misunderstand-ings (see chapters 6 and 7). These activities operate basically through questions and statements.

In sum, then, it appears that counsellors have good reason to work towards the [Co:Q >Cl:A (>Co:St) > Co:Q] pattern. It may not necessarily be the only possible pattern that is suitable for practising counselling, but obviously it is *a* suitable pattern.

The clients' cooperativeness in maintaining the asymmetric uni-formity of the [Co:Q > Cl:A > (Co:St >) Co:Q] pattern of interac-tion is perhaps more astonishing. As we have pointed out, no normative constraints seem to require the clients' collaboration. However, departures from the [Co:Q > Cl:A > (Co:St >) Co:Q] pattern are usually short, and after these departures the clients normally adopt their ordinary responsive footing.

The clients' point of view – the relevancies related to their actions – is more difficult to describe than the counsellors' point of view and their relevancies. There is no organizational accountability or body of theoretical knowledge concerned with the clients' activities. However, on a very general level it can be pointed out that the activities taking place in AIDS counselling – exploration of rela-tionships, beliefs and perceptions, and information and advice – are such that they presuppose predominantly that the clients adopt a passive and responsive footing. The clients orient to and partici-pate in these fluctuating activities, and therefore also play their part in the maintenance of the [Co:Q > Cl:A > (Co:St >) Co:Q] pattern.

The difficulty of describing in detail the clients' relevancies related to the counselling session may be symptomatic. There is no shared public understanding concerning what counselling in medical settings is about. We – as ordinary members of Western societies – do not know what happens in counselling with the same precision as we know what is going on in a doctor's surgery or in a lecture hall. For the clients, then, what the general goals of a coun-selling session are may be more or less *opaque*.[30] To put it in Goffman's (1974: 302–23) terms, there may prevail a certain ambi-guity concerning the *frame* of the encounter.[31]

[30] The clients' difficulties in orienting to the goals of their encounters with different kinds of professional have been discussed by Baldock and Prior (1981), McIntosh (1986), Dingwall and Robinson (1990), and Heritage and Sefi (1992).

[31] I make a very simple distinction between 'frame' and 'activity' here. I consider

The fact that the clients nevertheless cannot avoid knowing that something particular *is* aimed at may intensify the problem of opacity. Many things are different from everyday talk. Counselling is marked with specific location (office rooms in a hospital), time boundaries, video equipment, counsellors' unusual ways of addressing one another (see chapter 4), unusual types of questions (see chapter 3), etc. Something special is going on but, I assume, the clients do not know exactly what it is[32] (cf. Hughes 1982).

This opacity of the general frame of the activity may make certain conversational strategies attractive and others less attractive for the clients. If they are not well aware of what is going on, they may be inclined to confine themselves to *responsive* actions. If the (counsellor's) preceding turn determines the type of the (client's) current turn, then the current turn cannot be altogether off the track. Moreover, clients may want to avoid *agenda-setting* moves because they do not know what the agenda is supposed to be. Therefore, they may want to avoid initiating new topics through questions or volunteered statements. They may also want to avoid self-selecting themselves as speakers or putting co-clients in a situation where they have to speak, because they cannot know what that 'whole' is that their talk is supposed to contribute to.

Along with the opacity of the frame, the presence of delicate topics may encourage the clients to remain in a responsive position. During much of the time in counselling sessions, the participants are talking about the clients' sexual practices and about their fears

---

activities as locally varying and fluctuating. The activities taking place in AIDS counselling include exploration of the clients' beliefs, perceptions and relations, and advice-giving and information. 'Frame' is a wider concept: it refers to the overall goals of the varying activities. On the level of local varying activities, what the counsellors are doing may be more or less transparent to clients. This is indicated e.g. by clients being able to answer counsellors' questions in adequate ways. In terms of the (overall) frame, however, counselling sessions may be more opaque for the clients.

In future studies on institutional interaction, the problems related to opaqueness and transparency of action and frames deserve much more attention.

[32] In the text books of family therapy, the importance of a 'halo' around the sessions is recognized, and talked about as a therapeutic resource. In particular, the use of a 'one way mirror' (equipment that the counsellors in the hospital studied here don't have at their disposal) is supposed to raise feelings of mystery and magic, which may help to 'bring home' the therapists' messages (Hoffman 1981).

concerning the future. The etiquette of addressing topics like these is very complex in ordinary conversation (cf. Jefferson 1980). The counsellors, however, direct the talk – sometimes persistently – towards these issues (concerning the talk about the future, see chapters 6 and 7). Clients can embody their expressive caution in a strategy where they talk about delicate matters only as much as the counsellors, through their questions, create special space for such talk.

If the clients respond to the opacity of the frame and to the presence of delicate topics in the way described above, then for them to align as answerers of the counsellors' questions, or as recipients of information and advice, is a most rational strategy.

To summarize, it appears that the counsellors' orientation to their professional tasks and to their theory, along with the clients' orientation to the relative opaqueness of the frame of the encounter and to the presence of delicate topics, may be among the reasons for the participants to maintain the [Co:Q > Cl:A > (Co:St >) Co:Q] pattern of interaction in AIDS counselling.

Having said this, I have to point out the hypothetical character of these reflections. Rather than the results of a sequential analysis of data, the points raised above concerning the counsellors' and the clients' relevancies are hypotheses occasioned by the results of the data analysis proper. It would be of a great importance for the enterprise of interaction analysis if hypotheses like these could be subjected to empirical test; but I am afraid that at the current state of the art in sociology we do not have any means available for doing so.[33]

[33] Some scholars might suggest interviewing the clients and the counsellors. But unfortunately *accounts of* interactive events have a haphazard and unknown relation to the *internal organization* of those events (cf. Heritage 1984a; Silverman 1985 and 1993).

Viewing the recorded interaction with the subjects of the research constitutes a more sophisticated method. Actors can be shown recordings (e.g. video-tapes) of their own actions, and while examining these records they may disclose their own interpretations of their reasons for acting in the way they did. For the application of this method, see Erickson and Shultz (1982: 56–63).

The 'extraordinary context sensitivity' of the conversational rules of turn-taking

The pattern of turn-taking that prevails in AIDS counselling sessions is a result of an ongoing use of various conversational means available to build up interaction with a uniform shape. To apply a term associated with Claude Lévi-Strauss, we could call this ongoing organizatory activity *bricolage*.[34] Through *bricolage* the participants achieve an organization where, for the most part, counsellors ask questions or give statements, and clients answer counsellors' questions. In their *bricolage*, participants do not have a recourse to turn type or turn order pre-allocation. The uniformity, as it were, is achieved on the spot, without the help of social-normative equipment geared for generating this particular type of interaction.

Bricolage of this kind, it can be suggested, is a characteristic feature of 'quasi-conversational' (Heritage and Greatbatch 1991; Drew and Heritage 1992) turn-taking in institutional settings. The turn-taking is conversational because no extra-conversational normative equipment is used in its regulation. However, the end result (the actual interaction) achieved through *bricolage* may in its uniformity be very unlike that which constitutes ordinary conversation. In AIDS counselling, this end result is quite like – in an aggregative, distributional sense – the products of normatively sanctionable non-conversational speech-exchange systems.

The possibility for this kind of uniformity is given in the very conversational rules of turn-taking. Sacks, Schegloff and Jefferson pointed out in their seminal paper (1974: 699) that the turn-taking organization of conversation has the 'twin features of being context-free and capable of extraordinary context sensitivity'. The context-free aspects involve the universal applicability of the basic rules of turn-taking, which are oriented to across the wide variety of situations where conversations take place.

It appears that these rules are also extraordinarily context sensitive. In this chapter we have seen how they can be mobilized for organizing talk of a relatively uniform shape. The conversational

---

[34] The idea of using the term *bricolage* came from John Heritage (personal communication).

rules of turn-taking have supplied the counsellors and the clients with sufficient tools to produce talk that is relatively standardized in many aspects. This standardization makes it possible for the talk to accommodate the specific activities of AIDS counselling.

Sacks, Schegloff and Jefferson describe this context sensitivity as follows:

Hence, there must be some formal apparatus which is itself context-free, in such ways that it can, in local instances of its operation, be sensitive to and exhibit its sensitivity to various parameters of social reality in a local context . . . . We have concluded that the organization of *turn-taking* for conversation might be such a thing. (1974: 699–700)

This chapter has demonstrated the extraordinary context sensitivity of the conversational apparatus of turn-taking.

As was pointed out in the beginning of this chapter, so far the most advanced studies of institutional interaction have concerned 'formal' institutional settings. Therefore, the main general contribution of this chapter has been to cast light on the operation of a 'quasi-conversational' turn-taking system in an 'informal' setting. When it comes to understanding the specific tasks and activities in AIDS counselling, however, the results of this chapter may appear as modest. Through the analysis of turn-taking, we have outlined only a very general framework of activity in AIDS counselling.

In order to find out what makes counselling a *specific* type of institutional talk, we must, therefore, examine other aspects of it. Details of *how* questions are asked and answered, and *how* statements are delivered and received, are likely to be the site where the specific 'institutional character' can be found (see Schegloff 1987: 220). In this book I have concentrated on the questions and answers, having left the analysis of statements to future studies.

Our analysis of the turn-taking practices in AIDS counselling has indicated the ways in which the counsellors maintain their local interactional role as questioners. By studying the details of the questions and answers, new theoretical concepts will be evoked. In the following three chapters, questions and answers are studied from the point of view of *participation frameworks*: we will examine how production and reception roles are managed and negotiated in counsellors' questions and clients' answers.

3

The client as owner of experience

In this and the following two chapters, the notion of the 'participation framework', stemming from Erving Goffman's work, will provide us with the theoretical point of departure. To put it in simple terms, in these chapters we will examine how counsellors and their clients relate in various ways to the words that they utter or hear. By relating in different ways to words spoken or heard, they continuously shape, and respond to, the local contexts of their talk.

There are two questioning techniques, based on the Family Systems Theory, which make the speakers' and hearers' relation to the words spoken and heard a particularly interesting theme. Both of these techniques involve certain *indirectness*, whereby asking a question and answering a question become relatively complicated matters.

One of the techniques is called 'circular questioning'. In this type of questioning, counsellors ask questions concerning a client's feelings or beliefs, not directly from this client, but from a co-client, who usually is the first client's partner, spouse or other family member. As this co-client describes his or her relative's experience, he or she has a specific relation to the words he or she speaks; and equally, the person hearing a description of his or her own experience has a specific relation to the words he or she hears. 'Circular questioning' will be the topic of this chapter.

The topic of chapters 4 and 5 will be another questioning technique, arising from the counsellors' practice called 'live open supervision'. In this questioning practice, the co-counsellor asks questions that are meant for the client to answer – but these questions are not addressed to the client, but instead to the main counsellor. Again, the relation between speakers, hearers and the words spoken and heard becomes complicated.

Before starting to examine the data, we will need to explicate briefly Goffman's concept of 'participation framework' and its applications in earlier conversation analytical research.

Goffman's concept of 'participation framework'

A key aspect of the organization of any talk-in-interaction involves the participants' relation, as speakers or hearers, to the words that are spoken and heard. The understanding of this aspect of organization has been greatly enhanced by the work of Erving Goffman, particularly in his article Footing (1979; reprinted in Goffman 1981). More recently, Levinson (1988) has developed further Goffman's argument.

The point of departure for Goffman is that the traditional concepts of 'speaker' and 'hearer' are far too global and holistic. The interaction involved in talking cannot be satisfactorily understood unless the different variations of 'speaking' and 'hearing' are taken into account. He argues that '[w]hen a word is spoken, all those who happen to be in perceptual range of the event will have some sort of participation status relative to it' (1981: 3). People who hear an utterance may be in a very different relation to it: there is an array of possibilities ranging from a person being directly addressed in an intimate contact, to an eavesdropper, and to a receiver of a broadcast. Levinson (1988) used the term 'reception roles' to refer to these different positions. Goffman set a task to interaction analysis to codify these and to unravel 'the normative specification of appropriate conduct within each' (1981: 3).

Not only do the people who hear an utterance occupy different positions vis-à-vis the utterance: the speakers, too, can have different relations to the words that are said. Levinson used the term 'production roles' to refer to the speakers' positions. The speaker may speak, as it were, on behalf of him or herself, or on behalf of somebody else, e.g. when giving orders we often appeal to somebody in an authoritative position as the source. Moreover, people can report other people's words, or they can report their own past words, for example in the context of storytelling. Dimensions like these, related to the production of talk, set up the coordinates of what Goffman called the 'production format'.

How the production and reception of utterances is organized in terms of production and reception roles sets up the participation framework[1] related to an utterance or part of it. Goffman did not claim to have unravelled a systematic or comprehensive categorization of different participation frameworks. However, he did outline some of the basic dimensions related to production and reception roles.

Concerning the production roles, he made a distinction between the *animator*, the *author*, and the *principal*. The animator is the one who gives the voice to the words; the author is the one who has selected the sentiments which are being expressed and the words in which they are encoded; and the principal is the one whose position is established through the words that are spoken (Goffman 1981: 145). Often in conversation these production roles overlap, so that the speaker is simultaneously an incumbent of all three. But this need not be the case: the animator, the author and the principal can also be three different persons.

In terms of reception roles, Goffman (1981: 131) made a distinction between *ratified* and *unratified* participants. Ratified participants are the 'official' hearers, whereas the unratified participants are just overhearers, bystanders or eavesdroppers. Moreover, within the ratified participants a distinction can be made between *addressed recipients* and *unaddressed recipients*.

Goffman has got a mixed reception within mainstream CA research (see e.g. Schegloff 1988; Goodwin 1992 and 1993). Much of his work can be criticized because of an unsystematic use of variably recorded data and a lack of analytic rigour. That applies to a certain degree to his observations on participation frameworks, too. However, the weaknesses of Goffman's arguments do not make them useless. On the contrary, it appears that Goffman has opened up an analytic theme of crucial importance, which can fruitfully be integrated into the CA programme of more

---

[1] Goffman is not very precise in his use of concepts: it is not clear whether he relates 'participation framework' only to the arrangement of the reception of utterances, or to that of both reception and production (cf. Levinson 1988: 169). However, it appears that the term 'participation framework' has been generally used in the more comprehensive meaning.

rigorous and systematic studies. And on the other hand, writers like Manning (1989) are indeed correct when they point out that much of CA thus far has shared the traditional naive and one-dimensional conception of speaker and hearer.

How, then, could CA research make use of Goffman's ideas related to the 'participation framework'? First of all, it appears that the refinement of typologies of a general sort, concerning production and reception roles, is of limited use. (A comprehensive general typologization based on Goffman's ideas has been presented by Levinson (1988), who also notes the limits of an approach concentrating on general typologies. For a criticism of such an approach, see Hanks (1990).) Instead, the *interactive processes related to the management of different reception and production roles* could be brought into focus. Questions that could be asked, then, would be of the kind 'How does a speaker constitute himself, in an observable manner and on a momentary basis, as an animator/author/principal (or as an incumbent of any other kind of a production role which can be found in the data)?'; 'How is the recipients' collaboration achieved in this?'; 'How can the recipients challenge the production role claimed by the speaker?'; 'How do the speakers constitute the recipients, on an observable and momentary manner, as ratified and/or unratified participants, or as addressed and/or unaddressed recipients (or as incumbents of any other reception role found from the data)?', etc.

In more general terms, the point would be to treat the management of the participation framework as a generic property of talk-in-interaction (Drew 1990; Clayman 1992). In other words, it could be considered as a fundamental form of organization which is pervasively present, along with other structural features of talk such as the organization of turn-taking and the organization of repair, in all spoken interaction. How much there are uniform, cross-contextual patterns to be found in the management of the participation frameworks (comparable to those found in turn-taking and repair) remains an empirical question; but the starting hypothesis could be that wherever there is talk, it is accompanied by some sort of management of the participation framework. In other words, this means that any talk-in-interaction involves specific measures taken by the producers and recipients to constitute themselves as having a specific relation to the words that are spoken.

What, then, could be the bearing of the research of this generic form of organization on the understanding of institutional interaction? If the management of the participation framework is indeed a generic property of talk-in-interaction, then it is equally important in talk within any institutional setting as well as in ordinary conversation. Moreover, if the details of the talk exhibit the participants' orientation to any particular context, then such orientation is as likely to be found from the ways that the participation frameworks are managed as from any other aspect of conversational organization and interaction. The work of Clayman (1992) and Heritage (1985) on news interviews, Goodwin's (1992 and 1993) work on interaction in work-places, and Heath's (1986 and 1889) analyses of doctor–patient interaction have indeed indicated the centrality of the management of the participation framework in the production (and analysis) of institutional interaction.

Levinson suggests that research into assemblies like those of courtrooms, religious ceremonies and committee meetings could provide much insight into the nature of participation roles, because there 'the gross roles of producer and receiver may be surgically dissected for institutional purposes' (1988: 197). So the investigation of the management of participation frameworks in institutional settings may possibly bear a double promise: it can increase our understanding of the participation framework as a generic property of talk-in-interaction, and in so doing enhance the understanding of the specific character of the institutional talk.

A final comment is due about the relation between the system of turn-taking and the management of the participation framework. It has been suggested here that both are generic properties of talk-in-interaction. It follows that any data of spoken interaction can in principle be investigated from the point of view of turn-taking, as well as from the point of view of the participation frameworks. Moreover, the management of the participation framework and the workings of turn-taking are often tangled: for example, if a current speaker selects the next speaker by producing the first part of an adjacency pair, he will *address* the question/request/invitation or the like to a particular co-participant. Selection of the next speaker in this case involves also the allocation of a specific reception role.

Therefore, the analytic approaches that concentrate on participation or turn-taking are not mutually exclusive alternatives. The fact that news interviews have successfully been analysed with regard to turn-taking as well as to participation frameworks is an indication of this. However, particular institutional modifications of the turn-taking system appear to be more stably present in talk than those of the participation framework: long sequences of talk (such as a cross-examination or a whole news interview) may apply one institutionalized turn-taking system, whereas aspects of the participation framework (such as the Interviewer adopting the footing of an animator) can change on a momentary basis. That is why in this study explication of the systems of turn-taking was made first. But now it is time to turn to the various forms of the management of the participation framework.

'Circular questioning'

The technique of 'circular questioning', developed within the framework of Family Systems Theory, was briefly discussed in chapter 1. Following the publication of the seminal paper where the pattern of 'circular questioning' was first introduced (Selvini Palazzoli et al. 1980), much family therapeutic discussion has centred on this topic (see Penn 1982; Tomm 1985; Fleuridas et al. 1986; Feinberg 1990). Mauksch and Roesler (1990: 6) give a definition of circular questions that corresponds closely to the practice in the Royal Free Hospital:

We define a circular question as a question asked by an interviewer of a patient about a person or persons in a relationship with the patient, such as family-members, peers, or members of the family of origin. The focus of the question is the patient's perception of the experience or the belief of the third person whom the patient is discussing.

According to this definition, circular questions are questions that elicit descriptions of the client's perception of his or her 'significant others'. As it was pointed out in chapter 1, this kind of questioning is believed to help the clients to realize how the problem of one individual is embedded in his or her social relations. In other words, circular questions help the clients to realize the 'systemic' character of their problems. These questions illuminate and set in motion the family's patterns of relations, coalitions and alignments. This involves 'a deliberate effort to enable family members to be conscious of the connections between people, ideas and feelings' (Feinberg 1990: 275).

Apart from enhancing clients' understanding of their own lives, responses to these questions can also offer new knowledge to the professionals. Clients' responses to circular questions can 'illuminate the various triadic relationships' (Selvini Palazzoli *et al.* 1980: 8). As Mauksch and Roesler (1990) point out, circular questioning can help the professionals to understand and explain the clients' fears and hopes, and to identify areas where trust is either strong or lacking.

In the AIDS counselling sessions at the Royal Free Hospital, the 'significant others' of the patient are often present. These include the patients' lovers, family members, or the like. Following the practice of 'circular questioning' the patient is regularly asked by the counsellor to describe something related to the experience of the 'significant other'; and the 'significant other' is equally often asked to describe something related to the patient's experience. These descriptions may concern external states of affairs related to the other party (i.e. the counsellor may ask a mother to describe her ideas of the side-effects of a medication offered to her son), or his or her inner experiences, such as feelings or beliefs.

We will concentrate here on the descriptions of the co-clients' inner experiences, thus focusing on the issues that are central also to the above-cited definition of circular questioning. A patient may be asked to describe what his wife is worried about, or a mother may be asked to describe how the patient sees his chances of developing AIDS, and so on. These descriptions of the inner experience of other people take the participants and the analyst into the problematic of different participation frameworks.

The analysis presented below shows how the person producing a description of another's inner experience is systematically treated as having a specific relation to his/her words. It also shows how the participants systemically treat the person *spoken about* as having a particular status as a recipient. In the latter part of this chapter, it is argued that the practice of circular questioning has an important function in AIDS counselling: through circular questioning, the counsellor can create a situation where the clients, in an unacknowledged but most powerful way, elicit one another's descriptions of their inner experiences.

Let us begin with an example. This extract is taken from a session with a patient (a gay man) and his boyfriend; the patient has recently been diagnosed as HIV positive. This example sets the scene for all the forthcoming analyses in this chapter.

```
(1)     (E3.29)
        BF = Patient's boyfriend
 1  C:    What are some of things that you think E:dward might
 2        have to do.=He says he doesn't know where to go from
 3        here maybe: and awaiting results and things.
 4        (0.6)
 5  C:    What d'you think's worrying him.
 6        (0.4)
 7  BF:   Uh::m hhhhhh I think it's just fear of the unknow:n.
 8  P:    Mm[:
 9  C:       [Oka:y.
10  BF:      [At- at the present ti:me. (0.2) Uh:m (.) once:
11        he's (0.5) got a better understanding of (0.2) what
12        could happen
13  C:    Mm:
14  BF:   uh:m how .hh this will progre:ss then: I think (.)
15        things will be a little more [settled in his=
16  C:                                 [Mm
17  BF:   =own mi:nd.
18  C:    Mm:
19        (.)
20  P:    Mm[:
21  C:      [E:dward (.) from what you know:: (0.5) wha-
22        what- what do you think could happen. (0.8) I mean
23        we're talking hypothetically [now because I know=
24  P:                                 [Mm:: (well)-
25  C:    =no [more than you do about your actual state of=
26  P:        [uh::
27  C:    =health except that we do: know,=
28  P:    =uh
29  C:    .hhh you're carrying the virus::, (.6) as far as-
30        (.3) the- that first test is concerned.
31  P:    Umh
32        (1.4)
33  P:    (Well I feel) I see like two different extremes.=I
34        see [that I can just- (.8) carry on (in an)=
```

```
35   C:          [umh
36   P:          =incubation state:, [for many years [and (up)=
37   C:                          [umh            [umh
38   P:          =.hhhh you know just being very careful about (it)
39               [sexually:.
40   C:          [uhm:
41               (.4)
42   P:          [and: er (.3) can go on with a normal life.
43   C:          [umh
44   C:          umh
45   P:          And then I get my greatest fears: that- (.2) you
46               know just when I've got my life go:ing: you know a
47               good job=
48   C:          =um:h=
49   P:          things going very well,
50   C:          uhm::
51               (.3)
52   P:          that (I[::) er:: (.2) my immunity will collapse,
53   C:                 [umh
54   C:          um[h
55   P:            [you know: (and I will) become very ill:: (.2)
56               >quickly?<
57               (1.0)
58   P:          .hhh[hh an]d lose control of th- the situation,
59   C:              [um::h]
60   C:          umh:
61   P:          That's my greatest fear actually.
```

In (1) above, C makes an enquiry directed to BF, concerning the
worries of the patient. After some preparation in the beginning of
the turn,[2] C ends up asking BF simply what he thinks is worrying P.
Whereas the first part of C's turn (lines 1–3) could be heard as a
part of an invitation to produce a description of external states of
affairs related to Edward's life, the concluding line 5 unequivocally
elicits a description of his mental state. BF then produces his version
of P's worries. In line 21, C thereafter directs her enquiry to P,
asking his views about future risks. The enquiry leads P to produce
a long and detailed narrative about his fears, beginning in line 33.

---

[2] As Paul Drew has pointed out to me, these preparations would be interesting in
their own right. The statement component inserted between the two formulations of
the question may work to elicit a special kind of 'troubles-related' answer.

Owner's privileged right to the next turn

Usually in conversation, if A produces an utterance which is addressed to B, but the informational or attitudinal content concerns primarily C, C is expected to respond. That is the case in extract (2), which is an excerpt used originally by Sacks, Schegloff and Jefferson (1974), and analysed further by Levinson (1988: 166–7).

(2)   (Levinson 1988)
1   Sharon: You didn't come tuh talk tuh Karen?
2   Mark: No, Karen- Karen' I're having a fight,
3   (.4)
4   Mark: After she went out with Keith an not with (me)
5   Ruthie: Hah hah hah hah
6   Karen: Wul, Mark, you never asked me out

According to Levinson, although Karen obviously is not the *addressee* of Mark's turn above, the fact that the remark is delivered in Karen's presence and that it is a report of a 'fight' and an imputation of blame picks out her as a recipient who may be expected to respond to the complaint. In relation to Mark's utterance, Karen has a particular participation status; this is incorporated in the expectation that she will respond.

In counselling sessions, immediate responses like the one above are not regularly seen. Given that the counsellor and the client regularly are aligned as a questioner and an answerer, the counsellor usually takes (and is given) the next turn after any client turn (see chapter 2). But the person who is talked about in 'circular questioning' still has a specific participation status, comparable to Karen's in (2). This status, however, is displayed and maintained through different means than those in (2).

Most apparently, the specific configuration of participation roles entailed in 'circular questioning' is observable in the recurrent sequential patterns of consecutive questions. After having elicited a description of a client's inner experience from another client, counsellors regularly allocate the next turn to the client concerned. In other words, the standard structure of the sequence when such descriptions are made is the following:

(1) Co: Invites Client 1 to produce a description of something
            related to Client 2's inner experience
(2) Cl.1:   Produces the requested description

(3) Co: Invites Client 2 to respond to the description given by
              Client 1.
(4) Cl.2:   Produces the response.

There are two noteworthy issues in the structure of this standard
sequence. First, stages (1) and (2) regularly lead to stage (4). Indeed,
I have not come across any exceptions to this. In most cases, (4) is
preceded by the counsellor's invitation (stage 3); but it also can be
volunteered so that stage (3) is omitted. In other words, as soon as
another person's version of someone's experience is given, the person in question is due to respond.

Secondly, the other client's description of someone's inner
experience never comes *after* the description that the person him/
herself has given about his or her inner experience. In our data,
there is only one exception to this, and we will analyse it in detail
later.

The fact that the sequence in describing another's experience
regularly appears in this particular format indicates that the participants orient to a specific organization of knowledge in shaping
their interaction. The inner experience of somebody appears as a
very special kind of object: as something about which the person in
question regularly is given the opportunity to produce the final,
authoritative description (cf. Pomerantz 1980). As a speaker, somebody who describes another person's experience stands therefore in
a different kind of relation to his/her words than the one who is
describing his/her own experience; i.e. the speaker's production role
is different with regard to whether he/she describes his/her own
experience or somebody else's experience. Correspondingly, the
person who hears a description being given about his/her own
experience has a specific reception role, different from the reception
roles of those who hear somebody else's experience being described.
As a speaker or hearer, the person whose experience is described is
treated as the *owner of the experience* (cf. Sharrock 1974).

The specific configuration of production and reception roles
involved in 'circular questioning' arises, therefore, from the social
distribution of knowledge. The knowledge that the owner of the
experience has about his or her mind is systematically treated as
belonging to a different kind of category than the knowledge that
others may have about it. The difference between the owner's direct
access to his mind and the limited access that anybody else has to it

(Pomerantz 1980), is embodied in the organization of participation frameworks in counselling sessions.[3]

The analysis that follows seeks to show how the actors collaboratively, step by step, orient to these specific participation frameworks in the details of their interaction. In various details of their conduct the speakers and the hearers manage the owner's special participation status *vis-à-vis* the description of his/her experience. By so doing, the participants consistently build up the relevancy of the owner's forthcoming response. After having shown this, we will shortly evaluate the significance of these findings regarding the analysis of counselling as an institutional form of talk. It will be argued that 'circular questioning' constitutes a powerful device for eliciting the clients' talk about matters that they may initially be reluctant to talk about. The power of this device resides in its capacity to invoke simultaneously two different 'contexts': that of counselling *and* that of family/partnership.

---

[3] This particular link between the organization of knowledge and participation frameworks in conversation may apply only to the description of inner states of mind. The organization of knowledge concerning other types of objects – e.g. shared life events that both clients as spouses or partners may have their own perspectives on – is likely to be reflected in different kinds of participation framework and sequential patterns. A classic example is provided by Sacks' (1992b: 437–43) analysis of spouses telling stories, to a third party, about events they were both party to: here we find e.g. one spouse correcting the utterances of another. In our data, a client's descriptions of non-mental matters related to him/herself is sometimes followed by a description by the partner about the same issues. This is the case in the following.

```
C1:   And your [health Harry:?
( ):           [( )
      (.)
P:    Fi:ne.
      (0.2)
C1:   No [problems?
P:        [No problems.
C1:   D'you agree with hi:m?
W:    Ye:s he's been so much better since he (began to ta:ke)
      (0.4) [I- I've- well I've noticed=
C1:         [He is better now:.
W:    =the difference (anyway).
```

In this extract, the counsellor invites the patient's wife to respond to the patient's initial description of his health. The patient's health is thereby treated as a public phenomenon, on which his wife may have a valid and perhaps different perspective.

Use of agenda statements

The most obvious, and perhaps most simple, practice of displaying the specific participation framework and creating the relevancy of the co-client's response about the client's version of his experience is an *agenda statement*. Here the counsellor formulates a scheme for the forthcoming interaction in relation to the initial invitation to produce a version. Such a formulation is used in extract (3).

```
(3)    (E3.007:2-7)
       W = Patient's wife
1   C:          And how [would you see things going=
2   P:                  [heh heh heh
3   C:          =at work Mary.=D'you think- I mean
4        ->     just let's hear your view of it before we check
5               [with
6   W:          [What for him?
7   C:          Ye:s.
```

At line 4, the counsellor produces an agenda statement in connection with the initial invitation for W to produce a description related to P's experience.[4] P's authority is recognized, and his opportunity to respond later is projected, when C says 'before we check with', which refers obviously to P.

The agenda statement is here located as a self-repair. C cuts off a sentence which she has begun ('D'you think-'). Producing the agenda statement may thus be related to C's perception of some trouble in the reception of the invitation. W's repair initiation in line 6 equally hints at the existence of some troubles. For example, it may be unclear to W, whose work (her or P's) C is referring to; and C's clause serving as an agenda statement may also work to disambiguate the reference.

While projecting a space for P's response later, the agenda statement seems to have a double function. First, it picks up the invited description as something that the patient is asked to monitor in a special way in order to be able to confirm or rebut it later. This emphasizes his special recipient status regarding the forthcoming

---

[4] The semantic focus of the question can be heard in two ways. It may be related to P's inner experience at work; but it may also be related to things happening at P's work. This is not important in terms of the argument here, because in either case, 'things at work' are beyond the realm of W's own experience.

talk. Second, while locating P's response 'later', it works as a device to *delay* the production of this. By securing the delay, the agenda statement also works towards maintaining the question–answer pattern in the production of description of another's experience. The patient whom the version is about is not expected to respond spontaneously, but rather after an invitation by the counsellor ('before we check with').

As stated above, an agenda statement is the most obvious practice projecting the owner's response to the descriptions related to his/her experience. Therefore, it is also the most obvious indication of the specific participation status being ascribed to him or her, *vis-à-vis* the turn describing his/her experience. It is not, however, used in most cases; its use may indeed be related to a perception of troubles in the invitation of the version.

In the forthcoming sections we will see that *all* the participants are collaboratively occupied with displays of the specific participation statuses of the owner and the party who has been asked to describe the owner's experience. These displays also maintain the relevance of the owner's response even where no agenda statements are used.

Qualifying the descriptions

One practice displaying the speaker's specific relation to his/her words involves the design of the utterances in which descriptions of another's experience are invited or produced. Regularly, when the counsellors are requesting the clients to produce descriptions of the other's experience, and equally when clients are actually producing these descriptions, references to the other person's experience are not made in a straightforward manner. Recurrently, they are qualified in one of three alternative ways.

The first type of qualification is embedding the descriptions (or invitations to produce them) in references to the producer's own experience. That is the case in (4) below.

```
(4)    (Section of (1))
1    C:    What d'you think's worrying him.
2          (0.4)
3    BF:   Uh::m hhhhhh I think it's just fear of the unknow:n.
```

Here the counsellor does not ask BF 'what is worrying him', but rather 'what d'you think's worrying him?'. Consequently, BF prefaces his response with 'I think' rather than describing directly his partner's experience. In the first place, 'what d'you think' and 'I think' *downgrade* the knowledge claim involved in the question and the answer. This portrays BF as a speaker who is reporting something (states of P's mind) to which he has only a limited access (Pomerantz 1980). On the other hand, the use of these phrases may also betray an orientation to BF's *direct* access (Pomerantz 1980) to his *own* mind: he is requested to report, and reports, his own thoughts – and as a report of BF's thoughts, these descriptions are straightforward and not qualified.

Two further examples of this type of qualifications are provided below. In extract (5), the counsellor and the client both employ the 'I think' structure; and in extract (6), the counsellor uses this structure along with a formulation which emphasizes the client's possibly limited ability to understand his wife's experience.

```
(5)   (E3-12)
1    C:           Right. (0.6) If I ( ) hhhh if I was to a:sk you:
2         ->      (0.2) what you think uhm:: (0.6) Perry's main
3                 concern is today.=What d'you think it (.) might be.
4                 (8.5)
5    F:   ->      (        ) wedding pla(h)n(h)s I th(h)in(h)k. ( )
6                 .hhhhh heh heh heh heh .hhh

(6)   (E3-30)
1    C1:  ->      What d'you think's upsetting your wife so much
2         ->      Mister Wood?=As far as you understand it.
3                 (0.5)
4    P:           The pressure.
```

When the counsellors invite clients to describe their own current experiences, the questions and answers regularly do *not* show this embedded structure. That is the case in extracts (7) and (8):

```
(7)   (E4:16)
1    C:           ↑Can I just ask you what are your greatest conce:rns::
2                 (.) Liz
3                 ((...))
4    W:           Erm:: (.) the uncertainty?

(8)   (E4.46)
1    C1:          Can I (s[ay) what's your greatest
```

```
2    C2:          [(        )
3                 (0.6)
4    C1:          fear for th- what might happen.
5                 (0.3)
6    P:           My greatest fear:?
7    C1:          Mm
8                 (0.7)
9    P:           Uh::m (1.5) Well obviously at the moment I mean I don't
10                (.) particularly want to get AIDS or nothing like that.
11                ((...))
```

In (7) and (8) above, both counsellor and clients produce descriptions of experience in a straightforward manner.

'I think' seems indeed to be the most common way to embed descriptions of another's experience. It is very often used by clients, and almost always it appears in counsellors' invitations (as the formula 'what do you think . . . ?'). It seems to have a double function: apart from embedding the description in the describer's experience, it also downgrades the knowledge claims involved. There are, however, other ways of embedding which, on the contrary, upgrade the knowledge claim. Consider the following:

```
(9)   (E3-29)
1    C:    Carl do you th- what do you think might be Edward's
2          main concerns today. (.) I mea[n you said your=
3    P:                                  [Mm
4    C:    =health but is there anything else.
5          (0.8)
6    P:    Well of course I'm sure he's worried about his resu:lts,
```

C uses the standard 'what do you think' formula; and in addition to that, she produces another qualifier, 'might'. P, however, claims to be sure about what he is saying. But nevertheless, the description is embedded. He does not report in the first place that his partner is worried about his results, but rather that *he is sure* that his partner is worried about his results. By this choice of words, P constructs himself as a speaker who is reporting his own certainty, rather than reporting directly the other person's experience. While upgrading the knowledge claim this formulation also establishes P's specific relation to the description he is giving. By claiming certainty, P implies that this is something he can be sure or unsure about. For

Edward (the owner of the experience) such a question would not normally arise.

But in some cases speakers seem to be satisfied with a mere expression of epistemic status of their descriptions when describing another's mind. This is the second type of qualification. It is used in example (10).

(10)   (E3-45:4-10)
1   C: D'you think mum's got any concerns at the moment
2   that she would want to talk about.
3   (0.3)
4   P: ->   Oh she mi- she might be worried about the side-
5   effects.

The display of uncertainty in (10) seems to maintain the speaker's specific production role, arising from the inaccessibility of the other person's experience. Again, it would not usually make sense for P to say about himself that 'I might be worried about the side-effects', because he is expected to know what he is worried about. But concerning his mother's worries, this is a valid description.

The third type of qualification is used by the clients more than by the counsellors. After having been invited to produce a version about the co-client, the clients can transpose the focus of the discourse. Rather than describing the other's experience directly, they can describe the publicly available facts indicating the co-client's experience. Typically, this can be done by referring to the owner's earlier reports of his experience. This is the case in extract (11) below.

(11)   (E3.5)
1   C: And how do you find (.) Tom coping o:n (.) the AZT?
2   W: He seems to be all right.
3   C: Mm[:?
4   W: [He says he doesn't feel any worse than he did
5   before

In (11), W first produces a short account of Tom's experience 'He seems to be all right.' This is marked as uncertain by prefacing it with 'seems'. After W's account, C produces a continuer (line 3), which prompts an elaboration of the initial response. Now W transposes the focus of discourse by reporting Tom's own descriptions of his 'coping'. By referring to Tom's own words, W gives evidence to support her initial account. By doing this, she also displays an orientation to Tom's (the owner's) account as being more authoritative than the one she has produced.

In sum, all three types of qualification that the speakers use display their descriptions as provisional in comparison to the descriptions that the person in question – the owner of the experience – would be able to produce. The speakers display themselves as reporters of a sphere of reality to which they do not have full access. Given that the owner is co-present when the descriptions are elicited and produced, this design of turns creates the relevancy for the owner later to produce a more valid description. In other words, as soon as C has asked a question, the answer of which is based on limited access to the relevant knowledge, the expectation of a turn later by the 'owner of the experience' seems to be there, publicly displayed in the details of the design of the questions and the answers.

Speakers recognize the ownership of experience through body-movement

As a general rule, speakers in a conversation usually orient posturally to their addressees during the course of their turns. Typically, they gaze at the addressee at the beginning and/or end of the turn (see Goodwin 1981; Heath 1986). Gaze can also be used as a means of selecting the addressee if there are several people participating in the conversation (Goodwin 1979; Levinson 1988).

Apart from address, the speakers' postural orientation and gaze may be related to the content of their utterances. Goodwin (1984) provided a detailed single case analysis linking participants' postural orientation to the content of a story that was being told to them. In Goodwin's case analysis, everybody in the group who was gazing at somebody turned their gaze to the 'principal character' of the story when the punch-line was reached.

Our analysis follows the same path as Goodwin's. The speakers describing another person's inner experience display posturally their recognition of the owner's presence. Speakers regularly *divide* their orientation between the person they are describing and the counsellor who asked the questions.

Most often it seems to be the case that the client describing his co-client's experience orients to this at the beginning of the turn. There are also cases where the speaker's orientation alternates between C and the co-client during the course of the turn. An example of orienting to the co-client at the beginning of the turn is an excerpt that we examined in the previous section.

(10)   (E3.45)
1   C: D'you think mum's got any concerns at the moment
2   that she would want to talk about.
3   (0.3)
4   P: Oh she mi- she might be worried about the side-
5   effects.

On the verbal level, P's turn is obviously addressed to C who asked the question. Mum is referred to in the third person, which rules out the possibility of her being the addressee. However, the postural orientation of the participants does not fully coincide with this.

(10)   (Postural orientation)

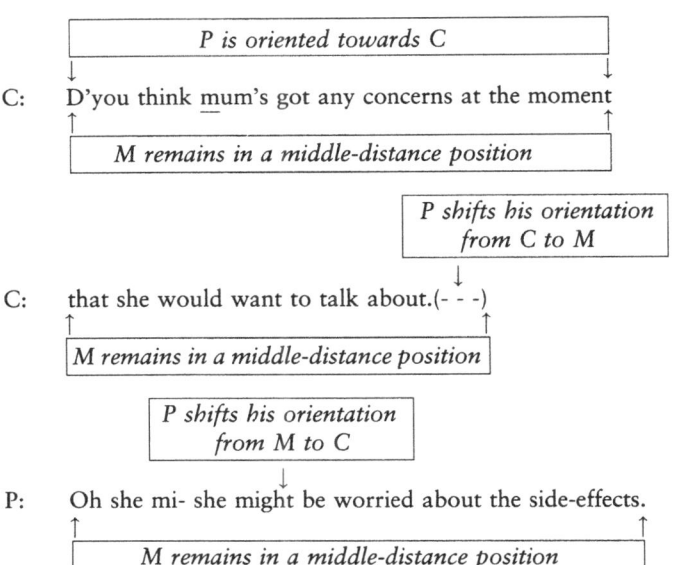

In extract (10), P turns towards his mother when C has completed her invitation for him to describe his mother's concerns. He then begins his answer to C's question in an orientation to mother rather than to the questioner. M, however, does not symmetrically orient to the speaker. She thus declines being the recipient of P's turn. P makes a renewed turn-beginning (this being a standard measure in the cases when a recipientship has not been achieved; see Goodwin 1984: 230), re-orients to C, and produces the full turn in an orientation to her.

What is of particular interest in the extract above is the *collaborative* way that the division of P's orientation between C (the addressee) and M (the party whose experience is described) is achieved. C is constantly orienting to P, thus displaying a potential recipientship throughout the excerpt. M, for her part, is displaying non-commitment all the time. P chooses to turn towards mother in the beginning of his turn, thus in body movement treating her as an addressee. P's body movement and the words he uses then with contrast each other in terms of the common-sense rule that speakers gaze at their addressees. P's orientation to M is not, however, encouraged by the other participants. Concurrently, he realigns himself towards C.

It is, however, by no means a rule that the persons described withhold their orientation from the speaker. In extract (11) below, the person described orients first to the (projected) speaker, and maintains this orientation longer than the speaker orients to him.

```
(11)  (E3.5)
1     C:    And how do you find (.) Tom coping o:n (.) the AZT?
2     W:    He seems to be all right.
3     C:    Mm[:?
4     W:       [He says he doesn't feel any worse than he did
5           before
```

The transcription of the body movement is as follows.

(11)   (Postural orientation)

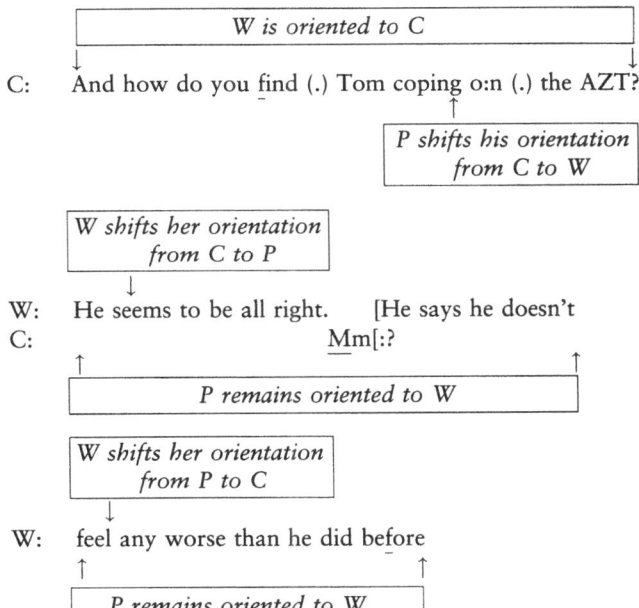

As with (10), in (11) above we have a collaborative production of the division of the speaker's orientation between C (the primary addressee of the answer) and the person the description is about. But now the collaborative component seems instead to enhance the speaker's orientation to the owner of the experience rather than to the addressee. P is the first one to reorient: he shifts his gaze to W as soon as C has made it clear that the question will be about his coping. W then orients towards P at the outset of her answering turn. After the initial gloss ('He seems to be all right') and C's continuer W continues her turn with an unpacking component ('He says he doesn't feel ...). During this component, she realigns towards the questioner (C). The questioner, however, has in the meantime aligned towards the owner.

The general pattern of the speakers' orientation in (10) and (11) is the same then: the speakers oriented at the beginning of the turn to the person whose experience they were describing, and only thereafter did they align towards the counsellors. The sequential position (following the counsellor's question) of the turns and the speakers' choice of words indicate that the counsellors are treated as the addressees. But through their postural orientation the speakers ascribe another kind of specific reception role to the 'owners'. This reception role involves other kinds of privileged relation to the words that are currently spoken. This relation arises from the organization of knowledge where the owner stands in a special relation to the objects talked about.

The owner of the experience recognizes the ownership during the course of the turn

The special reception role of the owner is not only established and maintained by the counsellor asking questions and by the co-client describing the owner's experience, but also by the owner of the experience himself. In many cases, that is, the owner produces acknowledgement tokens or other response items during the course of the delivery of the description of his/her experience. Let us return to the first extract shown in this chapter.

```
(12)  (Section of (1))
 5    C:      What d'you think's worrying him.
 6            (0.4)
 7    BF:     Uh::m hhhhhh I think it's just fear of the unknow:n.
 8    P:      Mm[:
 9    C:         [Oka:y.
10    BF:        [At- at the present ti:me. (0.2) Uh:m (.) once:
11            he's (0.5) got a better understanding of (0.2) what
12            could happen
13    C:      Mm:
14    BF:     uh:m how .hh this will progre:ss then: ((continues))
```

Here in line 8 P produces a token 'Mm:' as a response to BF's turn describing his worries. In the counsellor's query preceding BF's turn, P was not projected as the primary addressee of BF's turn (that role was allocated to C as the questioner). Usually the response items are produced by the addressees; but now P chooses to produce one as well.

The transcription of the body movement reveals how P's acknowledgement token is coordinated with the body movement of the speaker and himself.

(12)   (Postural orientation)

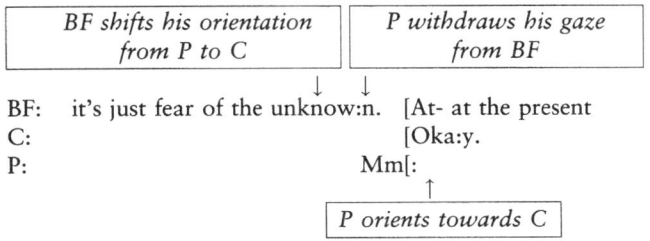

BF: it's just fear of the unknow:n.   [At- at the present
C: [Oka:y.
P: Mm[:

At the beginning of BF's turn we have the typical pattern in which the speaker (BF) divides his orientation between the primary addressee (C) and the person whose experience he is describing (P). BF begins his turn in an orientation towards P, whose experience he is describing. P, too, has shifted his orientation towards BF during the beginning of the turn (not shown in the transcript). Much of the description, then, is produced when the speaker and the person whose experience is described are mutually oriented. This is dissolved at the end of the first part of BF's turn. The speaker shifts from an orientation to P to an orientation to C simultaneously with the production of the last word of this initial gloss. At the completion of the last word, P concurrently starts to withdraw from the orientation to BF, in order to adopt a position where he gazes down.

The acknowledgement token of P (owner) is uttered in this slot: BF (speaker) has just shifted his orientation away from P, and P himself, as a response, has withdrawn from active gestural participation. At this stage it suffices to say that the acknowledgement token of P is anticipated by the speaker's orientation to him. By producing the acknowledgement token after having been gazed at by the speaker, he seems to confirm his special involvement in the issues addressed.

Another kind of acknowledgement of the ownership is done by P in extract (13). In this case, we do not examine the owner's response to a description of his mind, but something happening prior to it,

namely an owner's response to a request directed to a co-client to
produce such a description.

```
(13)  (E3.49)
 1    C2:        .hh Can you [ask Helena [whether she: .hh
 2    P:                     [not-       [not too good.
 3               (0.5)
 4    C2:        well how she thinks Mister Baker would have
 5               responded to the offer of the operation .hhhh if he
 6               was (.) had just the knowledge that we have now that
 7               we don't know whether it would (.) trigger off but
 8               it certainly was taken into consideration .hhh how
 9               would he have weighed up (0.8) would he have had the
10               opera[tion.
11    P:    ->        [.hhhh
12               (1.0)
13    C2:        [And I want Helena to [give and then=
14    C1:        [(                  ) [Helena?
15    C2:        =check (wit[h).
16    P:    ->             [*uh*
17    W:         I think he would have had the operation.
```

The participation structure of this extract is complicated indeed: C2
is asking C1 to make an enquiry to W about P's reactions in an
hypothetical situation. (See chapter 4 for the analysis of the counsellors' cooperation in this type of questioning.) C1 is then the
primary addressee of C2's turn; in addition to the third-person
form that C2 uses in reference to P and W, this is also displayed
by C2 when she directs her gaze towards C1 in the course of the
turn (data not shown).

In spite of the apparent fact of not being the recipient of C2's
turn, P chooses to produce particular activities in the course of its
production. The first indication of P treating himself as particularly
involved in C2's enquiry appears at line 5, when P nods slightly
simultaneously with the latter part of C2's word 'responded' (nod
not shown in the transcript). The core moments as regards P
acknowledging his ownership are, however, at lines 9-14. When
C2 is approaching the completion point of the first part of the
request, P lifts his head up and produces an audible inhalation.

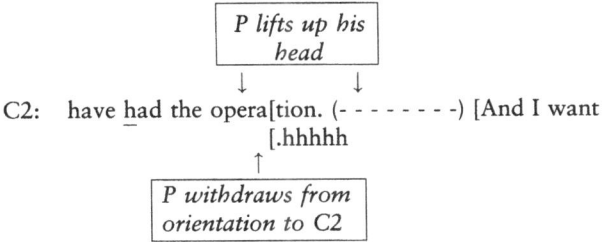

C2:   have had the opera[tion. (- - - - - - - -) [And I want
                        [.hhhhh

P here, just like P in extract (12), produces his audible response just after having abandoned the gestural orientation to the speaker, and before adopting an orientation to any other participant. A few moments later, when C2 has completed the agenda statement, P responds again, now with a subdued *uh* (line 16). My interpretation here, too, is that by his responses, P displays his involvement in the issues addressed.

As a summary of the two cases examined above, it seems that the owners, though not treating themselves as the addressees, can respond to the references to their experience in a particular way, which displays their orientation to the privileged reception role they are currently holding. The main work in the production of this kind of response is, of course, done by the owners themselves, but their activities are supported by and connected with those of the other participants. By displaying the owners' privileged reception role, these collaborative activities project the possibility of the owner producing a more elaborated response later.

Truncated sequences

The owners of the experience may, however, display an orientation to their privileged reception role and the corresponding right to respond to the descriptions of their experience also in a more dramatic way. This involves a departure from the [Co:Q > Cl:A > (Co:St >) Co:Q] pattern usually prevailing in the counselling sessions. Instead of waiting for the counsellor to elicit their response, the owners in a number of cases volunteer it. This implies that the standard four-part sequence is truncated into a three- or two-part one. The owners' self-initiatory activity reveals their expectation that their authoritative response to the description is due, regardless of the counsellor's questioning.

A three-part sequence appears when the owner of the experience makes a turn beginning immediately after the co-client has completed the description of the owner's experience. Extract (14) provides an example of that.

```
(14)   (E3-23:33-)
 1    C:           M m : .hhh Carl now that (.) (Edward) has heard that
 2                 he's positive on Friday what d'you think is
 3                 frightening?=What's his main concern. (.) About
 4                 being positive.
 5                 (1.3)

                   ((19 lines of specification of the question by C, followed
                   by the outset of BF's answer omitted.))

25    BF:          uhm basically to establish (0.5) a normal working
26                 rou[tine again.=
27    P:    ->         [Mm
28    C:             =Mm:
29                 (0.8)
30    BF:          Because that (.3) I think will help
31                 considerab[ly.
32    P:    ->               [M m : [Because these legal things=
33    C:                            [i-
34    P:    ->     =have [been tying me down (you [know b)-
35    C:                 [Is- is-                 [Is Carl ri:ght
36                 about that, that that's your main concer:n
37                 or[: would you- .hhh when you were positive what's=
38    P:             - [Mm hm
39    C:             =the first thing that came into your mi:nd.
40                 (0.2)
41    P:           Well other than sho:ck I mean uhm ((continues))
```

In extract (14), P displays his ownership of the experience under discussion in two complementary ways. First, in line 27, he produces a receipt object 'Mm' while BF (his partner) is producing the description of P's experience. The receipt object is produced in the proximity of a possible completion point of BF's utterance, and so it works as a 'continuer' (Schegloff 1981). By producing the continuer, in spite of not being the questioner, P may claim the position of a potential next speaker after BF (cf. Heritage and Greatbatch 1991). In line 32, after BF has completed the description of P's experience, P first produces another continuer, and in the absence of further talk from BF, immediately thereafter initiates his response. P's turn is designed as a continuation of BF's version of himself, as it begins by 'Because...'.

Apparently, P's self-initiatory activity here is resisted by the counsellor. After P has produced another continuer in line 27, the counsellor quickly produces another continuer in line 28. By doing this, she probably seeks to confirm her role as the intermediary of the interaction, and thereby, as the next speaker. (Note the same pattern above in extract 1, lines 8–9, where P's 'Mm:' is followed by C's 'Oka:y'.) Similarly, C resists P's uninvited turn beginning from line 32 onwards. After some overlapping talk, C manages to get the upper hand, and she then produces a question addressed to P (lines 35–7; 39).

The counsellor doesn't resist P's response as such: after having gained the floor, she herself ends up by eliciting a response from P. Instead, C seems to resist the self-initiatory production of such response. In other words, in this extract the dissonance between the activities of C and P does not concern P's right to respond to a version about himself, but rather it concerns the sequential location and thematic focusing of such a response. While P begins to tell his own experience immediately after his partner delivers a version of it, C seeks to maintain herself as the questioner and the intermediary of the interaction. As the questioner, C will be able to focus P's response to BF's initial description: she redirects P from 'these *l*egal things' towards 'the first thing that came into your mi:nd'.

In an extreme case, the owner of the experience may display his or her privileged right to produce a description of his/her experience by passing by the partner's version of it (initially elicited by the counsellor) altogether. This involves a violation of the current speaker's right to select the next speaker.

```
(15)  (E3-15:39)
      (F = Janet, P's fiancée)
1   C:          How d'you think that information would affect (.)
2               Janet's views of things?
3               (0.2)
4   P:          er[:
5   C:            [If she knew.
6   F:    ->    I think it's certainly- >sorry<
7   C:          Mm go o:n.=
8   F:    ->    hheh heh heh heh (He's fed up). .hhh=
9   C:          (A[ll right).
```

```
10    F:    ->     [I think it's so up and down that even (0.4) if
11                 (.) you were to tell me now that Gerry (was
12                 infected) over five years ago: (.) I wouldn't think
13                 oh no: it's the end of the world,
14    C:           Mm
15                 (.)
16    F:           uh:m (0.6) because (                    )
17                 (          [          ) heh heh heh=
18    C:                      [Right.
19    F:           =heh heh .hhh hhhh=
20    P:           =It's not- we're not uh:m (.) I mean you may not be
21                 able to have the answer of whe:n. So: I mean it- you
22                 know results don't matter. In a sense.
23                 ((continues))
```

Here the counsellor initially invites P to produce a version of F's inner experience, asking how it would affect his fiancée if they had been given certain information (lines 1–2). The preceding talk (data not shown) makes it clear that the question is about the consequences of knowing when P got infected; the time of the infection would have implications for P's life-expectancy. P has raised the question by reporting that his mother would be interested to know this. So he is in the process of indirectly soliciting sensitive information from the counsellors about his medical status.

After a short hesitation by P, C produces an extension of her question (line 5). After the expansion, F makes a voluntary turn-beginning, which, however, is quickly aborted and followed by an apology: 'I think it's certainly- >sorry<'. When volunteering her turn, F obviously violates the counsellor's choice of recipient of her question. This violation is recognized and repaired through the apology, and the ensuing permission given by C for F to go on speaking. Thereafter, F produces her own account of her (future) experience. As a result of this particular trajectory, the owner's version of her mind did not only end up occupying the authoritative last position among the descriptions, but it was also so located that the production of the partner's version was suppressed.

Like all other owners of experience, F in (15) oriented to her right to give the authoritative account of her experience. However, in displaying this ownership she acted differently from the other clients: she was the only one to suppress the production of the partner's description.

She may have had good interactional reasons for doing this. Her account '(He's fed up).' in line 8 probably doesn't help us very far in examining those reasons. What the account shows, however, is that F oriented to this suppression as something accountable.

F's reasons for immediately describing her own experience, instead of waiting first for the partner's description, may be related to the nature of the activity in which this exchange was embedded. P has tried to solicit sensitive information from the counsellors. C's question 'How d'you think that information would affect (.) Janet's views of things? ((...)) If she knew.' may have put P in an awkward position, regarding the display of his moral self in the conversation.

In principle, an account of 'no worries' would have been coherent with his pursuit of gaining the information. But had he answered that way, he could have been heard to be insensitive to his fiancée's possible suffering because of P's illness. In this sense, a 'no worries' report from P, given the activity under way, would have risked being heard as either insincere or insensitive. On the other hand, had he answered that F *would* be worried, then he could have been heard to have been pursuing something (information of his life-expectancy) that would cause anxiety to his partner. Also the optimism they both displayed throughout this interview would have been undermined.

In this sense, P is in a very difficult position in trying to construct an answer to C's question. A 'no worries' report would support his pursuit of information, but it would possibly be subject to negative inferences. On the other hand, F is free to report that she would not be worried. If she *herself* says that, the problems of insensitivity or insincerity don't appear. Consequently, F may have hurried to produce her response before P produces his account at all.

Regarding the issues related to the ownership of experience, this particular case shows that the participants, in orienting to the owner's privileged participation status and the corresponding right to response, can also *make use* of this right, in order to manage the interactional contingencies and sensitivities related to the issues addressed in the sessions.

A deviant case: doubt cast on owner's description

(16)   (E3-34)
         (F = Heather, P's fiancée; P = Graham, the patient;
         Cliff = F's son)

```
1    C:      Okay.And could you say that Cliff has lived .hh
2            arou:nd and with Gra[ham for 'x' number of=
3    F:                          [Mm
4    C:      =year:s. .hh And that you wouldn't allow your own
5            son [to if you weren't (.) convinced =
6    F           [Mm
7    C:      =that that was (.) all right?
8    F:      Mm
9            (0.5)
10   C:      Are you convinced that that's all right?
11   F:      I am yeah:.
12           (.)
13   C:      D'you thin[k she's convinced that =
14   F:                [(                    )
15   C:      =that's all right Graham.
16   P:      Well I think she is now:, (.) but I mean it's like
17           (you know) yes you wake up at three o'clock in the
18           morning [or you've been getting wound up for the=
19   C:              [Mm:
20   P:      =last [two weeks about it (              )=
21   C:            [Mm
22   P:      =(don't they).
23   C:      Mm:
24   P:      But I think sort of generally when things aren't (.)
25           well yeah I think Heather's convinced of it.
```

This is the deviant case referred to at the beginning of the chapter. It is the only case where the owner of the experience *first* gives her account of her experience; and *thereafter* her partner produces his version of it. In other words, here the partner's experience is given the authoritative last position.

However, there are local factors that the participants are demonstrably attending to here. In the first place, the activity under way in (16) seems to be different from that in the earlier extracts. In the cases shown earlier, the participants were involved in exploring and disclosing experience, whereas here the activity is closer to pursuit of a response, and even to what Jefferson (1985a) called an 'inquisition' and Silverman (1987) a 'charge-rebuttal sequence', as the account of one party about her mind is treated as questionable.

The conversation in (16) is about the risk possibly attached to F's son (Cliff) when being in close contact with F's boy-friend (Graham) who is HIV positive. Earlier in the session, F has expressed her worry that, given the AIDS panic in the media, Cliff's teacher might raise the question whether Cliff is at risk of getting infected (and of infecting other pupils). (The tape is from 1986, when knowledge about the transmission of HIV was not very widespread.) In lines 1–7, C suggests an argument that F could use to convince people that there is no risk attached to the boy.

F's response to this formulation is minimal. In line 8, she produces only an acknowledgement token Mm, after which a gap of half a second ensues. This vagueness and delay bears the typical characteristics of a dispreferred response (Atkinson and Drew 1979; Levinson 1983; Pomerantz 1984): a disagreement with C's formulation is hereby conveyed.

C's next turn shows that she has recognized the possible disagreement tokens present in F's initial response. She now addresses directly the possibility of F not agreeing with C's initial formulation by eliciting a focused description of F's state of mind: 'Are you convinced that that's all right.' (line 10). However, now F reports that she *is* convinced about that. But even now the affirmation in line 11 is in a minimal form, still maintaining the sense of less than full commitment by F.

It is in this local environment, characterized by ambiguity, that C chooses to elicit P's account of F's experience after F has herself reported it. P is hereby given the authorized last position in describing F's experience. P's turn between lines 16 and 22 spells out more clearly the ambiguity which was implied in F's initial response. Following the classic characteristics of delivering a dispreferred alternative (see also Sacks 1987), P first produces a hesitation ('Well'), then the agreement token ('I think she is'), and thereafter goes on spelling out the disagreement components ('but I mean . . . ')

In summary, the way that F initially responded to C's formulation cast doubt on the sincerity of her assertion. Given this doubt – which was intersubjectively oriented to by the participants – the position of being able to give the last account of F's experience was re-allocated by C to P. If the owner conceals something, she doesn't use her right to give an authoritative account of her experience – and in *that* kind of local circumstances, the partner here is given the last word.

Overcoming the clients' reluctance

We have been examining the turn-by-turn dynamics involved in 'circular questioning', where one of the clients is asked to describe the experience of another. The findings thus far can be summarized as follows: the owner of the experience is regularly allocated a privileged participation status (reception and production roles) in relation to descriptions of his/her experience. This status of him/her is embodied in the recurrent sequence structure where he/she is given the last, authoritative position in the succession of descriptions, and in various details of turn design and receipt activity related to the elicitation and delivery of those descriptions. All the participants (the counsellor eliciting the descriptions, the client giving the description and the client about whom the description is requested and given) collaboratively display the fact that the co-client's description is tentative and waiting for confirmation by the owner.

Now it is time to broaden the scope of the argument in order to examine the conditions and consequences of these displays. References to two related conversation analytical studies are due here.

Following the line of reasoning initiated by Sacks in his lectures, Anita Pomerantz (1980) was among the first to give systematic consideration to phenomena like those examined here. Pomerantz argues that descriptions of events displaying their producer's 'limited access' to the relevant facts may work as a device for inviting the other party to disclose his/her authorized version of the same issues. (Assuming, of course, that the other party is in a position of having such privileged access to the relevant facts.) Such dynamics are at work in cases like the following.

```
(17)   (Pomerantz 1980)
1    B:         Hello::.
2    A:         HI:::.
3    B:         Oh:hi:: 'ow are you Agne::s,
4    A:   ->    Fi:ne. Yer line's been busy.
5    B:         Yeuh my fu (hh)- .hh my father's wife called me .hh
6              So when she calls me::, .hh I can always talk fer a
7              long time. Cuz she c'n afford it'n I can't. hhhh
8              heh .ehhhhhh
```

In (17) above, the description, based on a limited access to relevant facts given by A (marked with an arrow), works as what Pomerantz calls 'a fishing device', successfully eliciting B's insider's report in the next turn.

Recently, Bergmann (1992) has applied a similar perspective to an analysis of psychiatric intake interviews in German hospitals. He shows how psychiatrists tell their patients something about their view of the patient's situation (the psychiatrist's view being based on direct observation, the referring doctor's notes or the like). They mark their views as uncertain. The patients respond to these accounts by disclosing their own interpretation of their situation. Bergmann concludes that presenting his knowledge as fragmentary and uncertain, psychiatrist invites or encourages the recipients to deliver an 'authentic' version. Doing this, in turn, is something that psychiatrists are expected to accomplish as a part of their professional conduct.

AIDS counsellors, just like Bergmann's psychiatrists, are practitioners whose professional task is to elicit clients' talk. Much of the time in AIDS counselling sessions is spent talking about sex, illness or dying – all topics that are difficult to address in ordinary conversation. In particular, the Family Systems Theory approach in AIDS counselling emphasizes the importance of eliciting client's own fears related to their future (Bor and Miller 1988). Much of the professional competence of a counsellor is related to an ability to break through the boundaries of not speaking (cf. Nelson-Jones 1988).

Now the simplest vehicle for eliciting someone's description of his/her fears or other inner feelings is naturally a question. Questions are, indeed, extensively used in the counselling sessions that apply the Family Systems approach. And in most cases, the questions are successful: clients answer them, and by answering questions on 'difficult' topics they produce talk on such topics.

Even though a counsellor's question creates a strong sequential implication for the client to produce an answer, it still can be circumvented so that extended talk on the topic proposed by it will not (immediately) be achieved. In extract 18, W (the patient's wife) is strongly resistant to talking further about the concerns she has just disclosed about her husband developing AIDS.

```
(18)   (E4.016)
1      C:      What's your greatest fe:ar about that?
2              (1.8)
3      C:      ( [              ) (.2) (        )
4      W:        [ T:here isn't anything (.2) specific (.) I mean it's
5              just a general abstra:ct:hh
6      C:      I mean would you: have any: mo:re worries than
7              you've got now?
8              (.4)
9      C:      when he's anti:body: positive?
10             (.6)
11     C:      (If he-) what would you know about .hh (.2) looking
12             after people with Aids,
13     W:      (Well) I don't?
14     C:      (Well) what (.3) do you
15             kno[:w (                        )=
16     W:         [I haven't even
17     W:      =I haven't even thou:ght that fa:r
```

Here W displays a reluctance to detail her fears about taking care of
her husband as a potential AIDS patient. In many cases like this,
instead of answering the counsellor's questions the clients produce
an account for not answering, thus trying to avoid disclosing their
experience or details of it. My suggestion is that asking a client to
produce a version about a co-client's experience can serve as an
applicable means of avoiding problems like this.

There seem to be two alternative formulas in achieving a client's
account of his/her experience. The apparently simpler formula is
based on question and answer:

(1)   C: Asks a question
(2)   Cl: Produces an answer

The apparently more complicated formula is based on the sequence
we have been analysing here:

(1)   Co: Invites Client 1 to produce a description of something
      related to Client 2's experience
(2)   Cl 1: Produces the requested description
(3)   Co: Invites Client 2 to respond to the description given by
      Client 1
(4)   Cl 2: Produces the response

Both formulas can be used when inviting the client to talk about his or her delicate concerns. My hypothesis is that the complicated formula can be more powerful in reaching this aim.

As we saw above, a question can be turned down by producing an account for not answering. Now, of course, the moves suggested by the counsellor in the more complicated formula can equally be turned down – but there are reasons for thinking that this will happen only at considerable moral and interactional costs.

Let us begin from the end of the more complicated formula. I have not found any cases where a client has not responded after a version of his or her mind has been given by a co-client. The only variation is that while in the majority of cases the response emerges only after the invitation has been made by the counsellor, in a minority of cases the owner responds voluntarily.

Why is there such a strong sequential implication between the description of another client's experience and the owner's response? My suggestion is that in these cases, the client is exposed to a *double expectation* to produce talk. Not only is the counsellor inviting him or her to respond (stage 3), but equally his or her *co-client is doing this*. The version of the owner's experience produced by the co-client (stage 2) works as a 'fishing device'.

As we have seen in the previous sections, *all* participants have *collaboratively* recognized the owner's privileged reception role as regards the description given by another person about the owner's experience. This recognition works now as the publicly displayed basis of an expectation for the owner to produce the authorized description of the experience in question. In other words, by having encouraged a client to give a version of another's experience, the counsellor has managed to integrate one client into the work of inviting the other to speak. The expectation to speak is then not only coming from the professional 'doing counselling', but also from the client's own partner; and this expectation has been confirmed by all participants in the verbal and non-verbal ways they used to recognize the ownership of the experience.

But there remains another question. If the occurrence of the co-client's talk on potentially delicate topics is more likely to appear after the client has given his or her version of the co-client's experience, it may be that the focus of the difficulties in inviting clients' talk is only moved in another direction. Perhaps the counsellor already encounters a problem when inviting the client to give a version of the co-client's experience?

The only empirical evidence we have here is that the clients regularly *do* give their versions of their relations when asked. Apart from adolescent clients, no 'resistance' is usually found here.[5] Our hypothesis is that the counsellor who invites the client to produce a version of another client trades off a *strong moral expectation* related to what 'proper' partners should be like.

The clients participating in each session are either members of the same family, or otherwise close partners. They come to the counselling sessions in order to find help and to support each other in their predicament. In these circumstances, being able to produce a version of another person's experience can be counted as an indication of a *close and intimate relation* between the producer of the version and the one whom it is about. To put it into the terminology of Sacks (1972), describing the experience of your partner appears, then, as a *category bound activity* based on 'standard relational pairs' like husband :: wife, or boyfriend :: boyfriend.

It may be an indication of a good partnership if you have a capacity to produce an account of the inner experience of your relation (and if you indeed use this capacity). And even more: it may be an indication of a particularly close and caring partnership if you produce an account in which her or his intimate thoughts and feelings are included in a sensitive way. Actually the fact that persuasion as in extract (18) is *not* needed when the owner is present may be additional evidence for this; when the owners are present, there is a strong and immediate expectation to display good partnership.

In these sequences, the clients giving descriptions of others' experience are engaged in an activity that resembles closely what Pomerantz (1980) called 'fishing'. The crucial difference, however, is that while persons 'fishing' pursue their own local interactional

---

[5] However, see extract (23) in chapter 7 for an example of a case where a client is reluctant to describe the (hypothetical future) experience of his co-present wife. In that particular case, the extreme delicacy of the hypothetical question (it concerns the wife's difficulties in case the client dies) appears to be the reason for his reluctance to answer.

goals, the clients describing others' experience tend to end up as part of a strategy set up by somebody else, namely the counsellor. Given the close relationship of the co-present clients, the one invited to describe the other's experience may find it very difficult not to be a part of that strategy.

As a summary, then, in the sequences examined in this chapter there are two types of extra constraints placed upon the clients to produce talk. First, there are the constraints placed upon the producer of the description of the other's experience. Not producing the elicited description would be negative evidence about the relationship between the producer and the owner. Second, there are the constraints upon the owner to respond. It is hard for the owner to say that he *cannot* answer, because the other party with the limited access to the relevant facts has already been able to talk. It is equally hard for him to resist the topics introduced in the counsellor's question and the other party's description, because now the topic already is there. Failing to respond would then be an even more accountable matter than failing to answer a straightforward question.

The success of C in extract (1) in eliciting P's fears may be gained through the exploitation of this kind of constraint. P's revelation of his 'greatest fear' is preceded by the elicitation and production of P's boyfriend's version of P's worries. Given this background C, when finally eliciting P's response, does not need to ask sensitive questions which might possibly carry a sense of intrusiveness. C does not even focus on P's inner experience in her question; she simply enquires about P's knowledge of the future possibilities. This question triggers off the extended account by P about his fears.

Sometimes the use of 'circular questioning' in overcoming the clients' initial reluctance to talk can be very transparent. This is the case in extract 19 below. This segment is from the very beginning of the session with Heather and Graham.

```
(19)   (E3-31)
1      C1:        Well,=in coming today::hh (.6) Heather what-
2                 (.5) m:os:t- (.5) would you now like- (.5) to
3                 discuss.
4                 (.2)
5      C1:        Because it's six months (till)- si[nce we saw=
6      F:                                           [umh
```

```
 7   C1:              =you last,
 8                    (1.0)
 9   C1:              What are the main issues
10                    (1.2)
11   F:      (1) ->   .hhhh I don't (know really)? I mean- (.6)
12                    things haven't changed that much (.) (have
13                    they)?
14                    (.8)
15   F:               (I think I am)- (.3) *(     )*
16                    (1.4)
17   C1:     (2) ->   .hhh Well let's put it this way: erm: WE
18                    ARRANGED (.2) for this meeting (.3) an:d (.)
19                    erm (1.4) .hh in agreeing to come today.=what
20                    would you most want to talk about.
21           (3) ->   (11.0)
22   C1:     (4) ->   Can I make it easier [can I ask it in=
23   F:                                    [(          ) heh=
24   C1:              =[another way:.]
25   F:              =[heh heh heh h]eh
26   ( ):             .hhh
27   C1:              What d'you thin[k Graham would most want to=
28   F:                             [hhh hh
29   C1:              =about toda:y.
30                    (0.2)
31   P:               I thought you said you were going to make it
32                    ea[sier.
33   F:                 [heh heh .hh heh heh (did you) .hh[hhh
34   P:                                                   [.hhhh
35                    (2.0)
36   (F):             hhhh
37                    (.)
38   F:               .hh I don't know I- I don't (.3) know whether
39                    we spoke to you about it last time (is it)- I
40                    suppose (.2) the things that we've been
41                    talking about to each other (at [home).
42   ( ):                                            [(   )
43   C1:              What are one of those thi:ngs.
44                    (2.5)
45   F:               Publicity.
46   C1:              Publicity.
47   F:      (5) ->   The tremendous stra:in
```

In (19) above, F's initial response (arrow 1) to the counsellor's topic elicitation is reluctant and delayed. Before F responded, the counsellor had to re-complete her question twice (lines 5–7 and 9); and in her response, F fails to name any topic. After the initial reluctant response, the counsellor reformulates her topic elicitation (arrow 2). The reformulated topic elicitation, however, is no more successful, as an extraordinarily long gap ensues (arrow 3). In this environment, the counsellor resorts to 'circular questioning', and asks for F's version of P's concerns (arrow 4). After some laughing, this enquiry proves productive, as F names 'publicity' as a strain (arrow 5). Thus, in (19) the counsellor uses 'circular questioning' quite manifestly as a means for overcoming the client's reluctance to speak.

Theory and practice of 'circular questioning'

The upshot of the empirical analysis presented in this chapter is that in AIDS counselling 'circular questioning' constitutes a most powerful device to elicit clients' discussion of matters that they may initially be reluctant to talk about. Through circular questioning, the counsellors can create situations where the clients, in an unacknowledged but most compelling way, elicit one another's descriptions of their inner experiences.

After having completed the empirical analysis, it is possible to return to the ideas presented in Family Systems Theory. The theoretical justification for the use of 'circular questioning' was briefly introduced at the beginning of this chapter. According to the theory, the main function of 'circular questioning' is to help the clients to realize how the problem of one individual is embedded in his or her social relations. Circular questions are asked in order to help the clients to realize the 'systemic' character of their problems.

There is an apparent incongruence between the results of our empirical analysis and the statements of Family Systems Theory. The empirical analysis, however, does *not* call into question the ideas of Family Systems Theory. The functions of 'circular questioning' suggested in Family Systems Theory, and in our analysis, belong to different levels of analysis, as it were.

It is quite likely that the circular questions asked by the AIDS counsellors in all the extracts shown above contributed to the clients' understanding of the systemic network of social relations that their AIDS-related problems are embedded in. Apart from this, however, asking these questions serves a more primary purpose, related to the momentary management of the unfolding interaction.

In order to be able to do anything at all with the clients, the counsellors must, in the first place, engage them in talk, into answering the questions. This is the fundamental task, the accomplishment of which we have analysed in this chapter. It appears, then, that 'circular questions' have a *double function*. They are a device for demonstrating the systemic nature of problems; but on a more basic level, they are also a device for eliciting talk.

This view is not completely alien to Family Systems Theory. In their seminal paper 'Hypothesizing – Circularity – Neutrality', the founders of the Milan School point out that

One will readily agree that it is far more fruitful, in that it is effective in overcoming resistance, to ask a son, 'Tell us how you see the relationship between your sister and your mother', than to ask the mother directly about *her* relationship with her daughter.   (Selvini Palazzoli *et al.* 1980: 8)

For the Milan associates, however, the effectiveness of 'circular questioning' in overcoming resistance is an obvious fact of less analytical interest. The primary focus of the Milan associates' interest lies elsewhere, for example, in the 'efficiency of this technique in initiating a vortex of responses in the family that greatly illuminate the various triadic relationships' (Palazzoli *et al.* 1980: 8).

In this chapter, we have shown *how* circular questioning operates in 'overcoming resistance'. Conversation Analysis is primarily interested in analysing the 'obvious facts'. What is 'obvious' in the practice of everyday living – or in the practice of counselling – may indeed be a methodic achievement, brought about by complicated cooperative effort. In this chapter, we have analysed the cooperative efforts that lie beneath the effectiveness of 'circular questioning' as a means for overcoming clients' reluctance to talk.

'Counselling' and 'family' as parallel contexts

Asking clients to describe the experience of their relations can be a powerful way of inviting their talk on sensitive matters. In the ordinary question–answer sequence, responding to an invitation to talk is a moral matter within the framework of a conversation in general, and probably a client–professional relation in particular. In the sequences analysed here, it is also a moral matter within the framework of relations between lovers, family members and the like. Exploiting *this* moral sphere within the counselling session seems to be very effective, and is perhaps a characteristic feature of the approach of Family Systems Theory.

A final comment, concerning the invocation of contexts, is due here. It was emphasized in chapter 1 that the context of interaction should be treated as something achieved locally rather than externally imposed. Social analysts should try to find out how the participants of an interaction 'display in their conduct which of the indefinitely many aspects of context they are making relevant' (Schegloff 1987: 219).

In the sequences analysed here, the participants skilfully interlock invocations of two different contexts and related identities: a professional–client encounter and a family/partner interaction. By asking questions about delicate topics, the counsellor displays professionality and invites others to constitute themselves as 'clients'. The clients collaborate by providing opportunities for the counsellor to ask questions and by answering them. Simultaneously, the counsellor treats the co-participants as 'family' or 'partners' by asking one to tell the experience of the other. In a similar fashion, the clients treat themselves as 'family' or 'partners' by disclosing the other's experience or allowing it to be disclosed.

Managing and making use of the simultaneous invocation of these two contexts is one of the admirable aspects of the professional activity of counselling.

4

The management of co-counsellors' questions

In the preceding chapter, we examined how the participants of the multi-client counselling sessions manage the participation frameworks in a particular questioning practice arising from Family Systems Theory. The following two chapters will apply a similar perspective. However, we will now examine another questioning technique, and thereby move the focus to the *counsellors'* production and reception roles in *two-counsellor* sessions.

In two-counsellor sessions, the activities of the counsellors are basically the same as in one-counsellor sessions. Regardless of their number, counsellors mainly ask questions of the clients, or produce statements conveying information or advice. When there are two counsellors present in a session, the co-counsellors' contribution to these activities is organized in a particular way.

In what follows, we will focus on co-counsellors' questions which employ a specific questioning format based on Family Systems Theory. This arises from a practice called *live open supervision*, and it involves the co-counsellors' questions being targeted to the client(s) but addressed to the main counsellor.

Live open supervision

'Live supervision', the principles of which were briefly described in the Introduction, is an important part of Family Systems practice. To apply live supervision in the ordinary way, the professionals need to use two adjacent rooms, connected by a one-way screen. The counsellors of the Haemophilia Centre, however, do not have such facilities at their disposal. Therefore, they use their own application of live supervision, which could be called 'live open supervision' (Olson and Pegg 1979; Smith and Kingston 1980). In the absence of the one-way screen, the counsellors and other professionals at the Haemophilia Centre sit in the same room with the family.

When more than one professional is present at the session, the counsellors decide which of them is to work as the principal counsellor (C1). She is in charge of the session, having thus approximately the same role as the therapist conversing with the family in family therapy. The other counsellor present, called here the co-counsellor (C2), is in principle doing the same job as the supervisory team behind the mirror in family therapy. This means that she may proffer statements to the client, give her view of the client's problems to the principal counsellor,[1] or she may suggest some questions that the principal counsellor should ask the client. In practice, the bulk of co-counsellors' activity consists of proposing questions to be asked.

The separation of the counsellors' roles achieved through this mediated pattern of interaction is expected to have the same advantages as the division of roles between the therapist and the rest of the team in 'ordinary' family therapy. Most importantly, therefore, these arrangements are supposed to give the co-counsellor a genuinely different perspective on what the clients are saying as well as on the interaction between the clients and the principal therapist.

Because of the uniqueness and unfamiliarity of this kind of arrangement, counsellors regularly have to explain the conventions of this system to their clients. This is done with all new clients. In the following, a co-counsellor describes their way of working to a patient at the beginning of a session.

```
(1)    (Planning 1:8-24)
1    C2:      [And if I can just remind you of the=
2    C1:      [(    )
3    C2:      =way we work uhm (0.6) I'm sitting ba:ck,
4             (.)
5    P:       Yeah.
6             (0.2)
7    C2:      and only (0.3) will interrupt if (1.2) and I won't
```

---

[1] Unfortunately, due to lack of time and space, we will not be able to analyse the participation framework related to these commentaries. For an example, however, see extract 5 in chapter 2.

```
8                    (0.7) ask you any quest[ions because (.) ( )=
9    P:                              [Ri:ght.
10   C2:    =(                    ) and we do it this way
11          which ever one is doing the interview does the
12          questions and if [I think of anything I'd like=
13   C1:                       [That's right.
14   C2:    =her to ask I'll ask her and she'll decide whether she
15          wants to ask you or not.
16          (0.5)
17   P:     Can I smoke?
```

Following the technique they have developed, then, C1 ought to be the only one among the professionals who asks questions in the session. If and when C2 feels that something else should be asked, she turns to C1 and proposes that she asks the question. C1 may ask it, or turn it down.

In this chapter and in chapter 5, we will analyse in detail how these arrangements work in practice. The focus in this chapter is on the technical details whereby the counsellors *achieve* and *sustain* the 'live open supervision' questioning format. The aim of chapter 5 will be to examine the *interactional functions* that this type of questioning may have.

The data used in these two chapters consists of all cases of co-counsellors' questions that appeared in our data base. From the 15 interviews conducted by more than one counsellor, a total of 110 questions were collected and analysed. Out of these 110 questions, in 42 the co-counsellor addressed the client directly – thus abandoning the 'live open supervision' questioning format.[2] We will see some non-mediated questions below, in extract 33. In the remaining 68 cases, the co-counsellors initially addressed the main counsellor. The central focus of our interest lies on the sequences triggered off by these turns.

In these cases C2 gets the floor usually through self-selection in the course of a question–answer sequence between C1 and the

---

[2] The numbers, however, may not give a fully accurate picture of the counsellors' ability/willingness to follow their own policy. Namely, out of 42 occurrences where the co-counsellor addressed the patient directly, 20 were from one very unusual interview. In that interview, the main counsellor was a rather inexperienced medical doctor. Her inexperience made it difficult for the co-counsellors (who were more experienced) to apply the ordinary pattern of questioning. Extracts from that particular interview are shown in cases (24) and (25).

client.[3] C2 then addresses C1, producing a turn which contains a question which concerns primarily the client(s). Extracts 2–8 provide examples of these turns.

(2) (E4-8:37-94)
     W = Patient's wife
1   C1:   But then let's take [ourselves- let's-]
2   W: [(   ) be ru]de
3   but (.) I (.) just how [I feel   ] at the moment.
4   C2:   [DO THEY-]
5   C2:   ->   ( ) do they want to know the results, have
6   they not been told the result.

(3) (E4.72:151-172)
1   P: Just [that-
2   C2:   ->   [Who do you think Doctor Kaufman will suffer
3   most over the next few day:s if (0.2) Doug goes
4   home without the treatment that we know might
5   have a chance of helping him,=will it be hi:m? .h
6   Will it be Philip having to bring him again?=Will it
7   be his mother?=His father?
8   P: .hhhh=
9   C2:   =( )

(4) (E4.46: 1-25)
1   P: No well I'll keep walking (.3) anyway (.2) (which
2   will make me a) (   ).
3   C2:   ->   Doctor Kaufman I'd (.3) like (.3) to a::sk (3.0)
4   what (.4) at the moment hh (.2) is Michael's main
5   concern.

(5) (E4-50/1)
1   C1:   So who is there in [your fam-
2   C2:   ->   [Mrs Walker does Mr Joseph
3   think there's any less dissent in the views now than
4   there was. [(On HIV)?
5   C1:   [Mm

(6) (E4.46/7)
1   C2:   ->   Doctor Kaufman one of the things that (.) I think we

---

[3] Sometimes, however, C2 obtains the floor as a result of C1's request for her to produce any questions or comments she feels she would like to say. Typically, this happens as a part of the closure of the session. The dynamics related to these invited questions are not unlike those of the volunteered questions. In what follows, however, we will use only the more frequent volunteered questions as our material. For an example of an invited question, see extract (10) in chapter 7.

```
2                    need to get clear (.) if Michael and Harry don't
3                    talk that's (.) oka:y. .hhh I'm not sure whether
4                    we've talked (0.6) to Michael or Harry about this
5                    I've got (.2) muddled up.
6                    (0.4)
7    C2:   ->        But who does Michael (.2) consider as his next of
8                    *kin:.*
```

```
(7)  (E4-46/2B)
1    P:              ((...)) but I don't know how far (.5) into
2                    AIDS I a:m. (.6) Yet.=So:
3                    [I don't know. (I don't [like to be).
4    C2:             [Does-                  [s-
5    C2:   ->        How much does (0.2) Michael want to know about
6                    (0.8) how far he's (into AIDS)
```

```
(8)  (E4-72:3-8)
1    P:              ((...)) my sister's down from (Lancaster). (.6) And
2                    the childre:n.
3    C2:   ->        How does (.3) Phili:p Doctor Kaufman (1.1) see:
4                    (0.2) if one is HIV positive as Doug is very clear
5                    and understands (0.6) if people get (.3) small
6                    symptoms how does he see them as (0.4) being
7                    treated. Do you wait or do you come quickly,
```

Two features are common to all the extracts above. First, they are co-counsellors' turns addressed to the main counsellor; and secondly, they all contain questions which concern issues about which the clients have the primary competence to speak.[4] Therefore, we see here a type of questioning that seems rather alien to ordinary conversation. The production and reception roles of the utterances are subjected to systematic manipulation in a way which is unusual in casual conversation.

[4] In most extracts, the questions in one way or another concern the clients' inner experience: their beliefs, feelings and preferences. In (2), however, the question is also partially about the clients' biographical events. Extract (3) is different from all the others, because in it the focus of the question is on hypothetical future events concerning the whole family, most members of which are not present in the session. The question in (3) is also, unlike the other extracts, embedded in C1's experience ('Who do you think Doctor Kaufman . . . '). Apart from (3), all questions concern issues to which a particular co-present client (in (2) a married couple) has got 'privileged access' (Pomerantz 1980) and therefore is primarily competent to speak. Even in (3), one or the other of the co-present family members could be expected to be more competent to speak than the counsellor to whom the question is addressed.

The co-counsellors' questions in extracts 2–8 set up a particular triangle consisting of the two counsellors and the client. C2 is talking to C1; i.e. C2 treats C1 as the addressee of her turn. But in C2's turn there is a question that is observably meant for the client to answer. To put it in terms suggested by Levinson (1988), there are two distinctively different *reception roles* related to this turn. C1 is treated as the addressee. However, she is not the destination of the whole content of the turn, because the turn contains a question which the co-present client is primarily competent to answer. These two aspects of organization – the choice of address on one hand and the epistemic structure related to the partipants' relative competence to answer on the other – therefore maintain different aspects of recipientship. In Levinson's (1988) terms, C1s could be called the *Intermediaries*, while the clients are the *Indirect Targets* of C2s' questions.

This unusual participation framework is related to the sequential structure of the interaction in a particular way. The co-counsellors' initial turns project some activities in response: as questions they are first parts of 'adjacency pairs' in which second parts are due. Because the questions concern issues that the clients are primarily competent to talk about, a conditional relevancy is created for the clients' answers. However, as C1 has been treated as the addressee, there is an overlapping expectation for C1 to respond. This ambiguity is indeed reflected in the actual course of the interactions following these turns.

To put it crudely, the initial turns by the co-counsellors can trigger off two kinds of trajectories of interaction between the counsellors and the clients. In one trajectory, the initial question is rephrased by the main counsellor, and thereafter the client produces an answer. In another trajectory, the client's answer follows the initial turn by the co-counsellor without the interception of the main counsellors' talk.

In what follows we will explore how the participants set up and maintain specific participation frameworks at different stages in these sequences. It will become clear that the standardized, institutionally specific participation frameworks are achieved by the counsellors and their clients consistently using the tools and practices of *ordinary conversation*. These include *address terms*, *body posture* and *third person reference*. Through these ordinary conversational resources, the counsellors repeatedly set up the production and reception roles, and the sequential patterns of talk, constituting the 'live open supervision' questioning format.

We will follow below, step by step, how the interaction unfolds, diverting into different trajectories, all beginning from similar kinds of initial turns by the co-counsellors. However, before examining the subsequent turns, we will first analyse briefly the initial turns by the co-counsellors.

Design and delivery of the initial turns

The unusual type of participation framework related to the co-counsellors' questions is set up and maintained in the fine details of participants' action. In ordinary conversation, our questions are usually produced from a different footing: if the target is present, we usually address the questions directly to him or her. (This is not to say that other practices would not be possible: in interaction with children and elderly people, for example, there are often different practices, too.) Deviation from the 'ordinary' pattern in AIDS counselling is accomplished through the systematic use of a number of linguistic devices.

In all cases shown above, the co-counsellors referred to the clients (to whom the questions were targeted) in the third person, either with the use of their proper names, or the third person pronoun, or both.[5] By doing so, they excluded them from the address. This use of third person forms in referring to clients is in contrast with the content of the co-counsellors' turns, as these turns include questions the content of which concerns exclusively the co-present clients.

Correspondingly, the address of the main counsellor was actively maintained with the use of names and titles. In most of the cases, the co-counsellor mentioned the main counsellors' name at the beginning of her turn.[6] This use of a vocative singled out the main counsellor as the addressee right from the beginning of the turn.

Gaze and body posture were also used in all the cases above: the co-counsellors oriented posturally towards the main counsellors during the delivery of their initial turns. In this way they also

---

[5]   In the last sentence in C2's turn in extract (8) the second person pronoun 'you' is used in a context which makes it possible to hear it as referring to the client (lines 6–7). However, the usage of 'you' here is ambiguous: it is equally possible to hear it as a passive form.

created a contrast between the content of their turns (questions targeted to the client) and the management of the address.

Extract (2) may serve as an example of the body posture of the participants during the delivery of the initial turn of the co-counsellor. The transcription below shows that C2 turns towards C1 well ahead of her initial turn. A continuing line (———) indicates a participant's postural orientation to C1; a broken line (- - - -) indicates an orientation to C2; a line of 'plus' signs (++++) indicates an orientation to W and a line of asterisks (****) indicates an orientation to P.

```
(2)    (postural orientation)
       C1:   (p)************************  (c2) - -
       C1:   But then let's take  [ourselves- let's-]
       C2:   (p)************ (c1) ———————————
       W:                    [(        ) be ru]de

       C1:   (c2) - - - - - - - -  (w)+++++++++++++   (c2) - - - - - -
       C2:   (c1) ——————————————————————————————————
       C2:                   [ DO THEY-]
       W:    but (.) I (.) just how [    I feel     ] at the moment.

       C1:   (c2) - - - - - - - - - - - - - - - - - - - - - - - - - - - -
       C2:   (c1) ————————————————————————————————————
       C2:   (    ) do they want to know the results, have they

       C1:   (c2) - - - - - - -      (w) +++++++++++++++++
       C1:                    [Have you not been told.
       C2:   (c1) ———————————————————  (w)++++++++
       C2:   not been told the [result,
```

C2's initial turn is uttered from a postural position where she is oriented towards C1. This was the case in all the extracts shown above. Here C1 is reciprocally oriented to C2 most of the time; this was equally the case in most of the extracts – we will analyse the deviant case in detail later. Through this postural orientation, the

---

[6] Note also how these vocatives were designed to convey the 'official' or 'professional' role of the counsellors. They did not use their first names but used surnames and titles instead.

co-counsellors selected the principal counsellors as addressees of the turns that contained questions targeted to the clients.[7]

Reception of the initial turn

In the previous section we examined what co-counsellors do in order to set up a particular participation framework, where C1 is the intermediary, and P the indirect target of their initial question. Before moving to focus on the events following the initial turn, we will shortly examine how the main counsellor and the client collaborate in the maintenance of this participation framework during the initial turn.

The main counsellors collaborated in the maintenance of the participation framework in two ways. First – apart from the deviant case that we will examine later – they gazed at the speakers. An example is provided in the transcription of the body movement of extract (2) presented above. The main counsellor's postural orientation constitutes the classic 'display of recipiency' (Heath 1986) whereby the addressee can acknowledge his/her conversational role.

However, in many cases, even if not as persistently as the main counsellors, the clients also displayed postural orientation to the co-counsellors during the initial turns. Again, if we look at extract (2), we can see that during the latter part of C2's turn, W reaches an orientation to her. But W's postural orientation does not challenge, or fail to comply with, her role as an indirect target; rather it shows that she monitors the fact that C2's turn is designed to be targeted at her. It is important to notice that W adopts a postural orientation towards C2 relatively late.

---

[7] Still another technique the counsellors can use in establishing this unusual participation framework is related to the *preliminaries* that often accompany the co-counsellors' questions (see extracts 4 and 6 above). The preliminaries, unlike the questions that they foreshadow, are unambiguously targeted to the principal counsellors, not to the clients. The work that the preliminaries do would deserve an extended analysis which cannot be presented here.

(2)   (postural orientation)
      W: (c1) ————————————————————
      W: [(   ) be ru]de
      C1: But then let's take [ourselves- let's-]

      W: (c1) ——————————————————————————
      W: but (.) I (.) just how [I   feel   ] at the moment.
      C2:   [DO THEY-]

      W: (c1) ——————————— ,,,,
      C2:   (   ) do they want to <u>know</u> the results, have they

      W: ...(c2) - - - - - - - - - - - - - - - -,..(c1) ————
      C2: not been told the [result,
      C1:   [Have you not been told.

When we examine the vocal response items, where they appear, the picture is more unequivocal. Throughout our data, the main counsellors are the only subjects producing receipt tokens or continuers during the co-counsellors' initial turns. Above, in extract 5 (line 5), the main counsellor produced 'Mm' in response to the co-counsellors' question. Also in extract (9) the main counsellor produces vocal response items when C2· is delivering her turn.

(9)   (E4-8:177-218)
1   C1:   (...) but I want to be <u>reas</u>[sured that=
2   P: [umh
3   C1:   =she (.8) understands the <u>facts</u> as we
4   have them now.
5   P: Umh
6   C1:   .hh And-
7   C2:   Mrs Heller you asked Mr Wood if he'd do
8   anything differently if he was po[sitive an̅d̅=
9   C1:   ->   [umh
10   C2:   =he said <u>no</u>. Would Mrs Wood want to do
11   anything [differently *if he was positive.*
12   C1:   ->   [umh

Through the response tokens in (9), the principal counsellor collaborates in being the addressee of the co-counsellors' turn; and conversely, through withholding vocal recipient activity, the patient displays an acknowledgement of not holding the role of addressee. However, the fact that most of the questions, even if consisting of more than one turn constructional units, are delivered *without* any response activity from C1 *or* the clients (see extracts (2)–(8) shown earlier), perhaps betrays the participants' orientation to the 'formality' of this participation framework: neither the clients nor the main-counsellors are actively claiming ordinary, 'full' addressee status.

C1 rephrases the question

After the delivery of C2's initial turn, the trajectories that the interaction follows divert into the two paths mentioned above. Following one of the paths, C1 takes the next turn. Usually C1 uses her turn to rephrase the initial question, addressing it now directly to the client; but she can also use her turn for some other purposes to be specified below. In the following, we will examine C1's turns that follow the co-counsellors' question. The usual 'standard' procedure (where C1 rephrases the initial question in her turn) will be analysed first, and thereafter we will turn to the alternative ways that C1s may use their turns.

The cases shown below are examples of the 'standard' procedure.

```
(10)   (Extension of [2])
       W = Patient's wife
  1    C1:            But then let's take [ourselves- let's-]
  2    W:                                 [(        ) be ru]de
  3                   but (.) I (.) just how [ I     feel    ] at the moment.
  4    C2:                                   [ DO THEY-]
  5    C2:   (1) ->   (       ) do they want to know the results, have
  6                   they not been told the [result.
  7    C1:   (2) ->                          [Have you not been told.
  8    W:    (3) ->   Yes we've been told we've been negative as far
  9                   as I'm awa:re

(11)   (Extension of [3])
  1    P:             Just [that-
  2    C2:   (1) ->        [Who do you think Doctor Kaufman will suffer
  3                   most over the next few day:s if (0.2) Doug goes
  4                   home without the treatment that we know might
  5                   have a chance of helping him,=will it be hi:m?
  6                   .h Will it be Philip having to bring him
  7                   again?=Will it be his mother?=His father?
  8    P:             .hhhh=
  9    C2:            =[(                    )
 10    C1:   (2) ->   =[Who will have the worst Christmas if you (0.2)
```

```
11                      go ho:me Dou:g?
12      P:    (3) ->    Well if I go ho:me (0.2) .hh and I do what I do:
13                      (0.8) normally (0.5) it won't affect anybody. (.)
14                      Because-
```

```
(12)    (Extension of [4])
1       P:              No well I'll keep walking (.3) anyway (.2) (which
2                       will make me a) (        ).
3       C2:   (1) ->    Doctor Kaufman I'd (.3) like (.3) to a::sk (3.0)
4                       what (.4) at the moment hh (.2) is Michael's main
5                       concern.
6                       (.2)
7       C1:   (2) ->    Yes.=Michael what's your main concern today.
8                       (3.5)
9       P:    (3) ->    It depends (o:n) I suppose what you (.3) mean by
10                      concer:n,=I'm not really uh:m
```

```
(13)    (Extension of (8))
        ((B = Philip, the brother of the patient))
1       P:              ((...)) my sister's down from (Lancaster). (.6) And
2                       the childre:n.
3       C2:   (1) ->    How does (.3) Phili:p Doctor Kaufman (1.1) see:
4                       (0.2) if one is HIV positive as Doug is very clear
5                       and understands (0.6) if people get (.3) small
6                       symptoms how does he see them as (0.4) being
7                       treated. Do you wait or do you come quickly,
8                       (.)
9       C1:   (2) ->    What would you:
10-                     (.3)
11      B:              N[o I:'ve-
12      C1:              [think was the right thing to do.
13      B:    (3) ->    No I've got to: (0.6) I've got to the stage when:
14                      (2.2) this isn't something that you: (0.2) play
15                      patterball with. (0.4) You know:. Uh:m
16                      (2.8)
17      B:              I know it's difficult (.) Christmas and all that,
18                      (0.4) (              ), but er: (1.2) he:ll (.2) you
19                      know I want to be around to see next Christmas
20                      and all you know. hhh hh .hhh
```

```
(14)    (E4.46:156-84)
1       P:              Yeah. (0.2) If it was (0.5) trust- er tried an:d
2                       trusted yeah.
3       C2:   (1) ->    Doctor Kaufman I('m) still (0.3) would like you to
4                       pursue (this a bit). (1.7) I don't know: and I'm
5                       talking to you now as well as to Michael but .hhh
6                       (0.2) will he- does he think that everything we
```

```
7                       gi:ve is (0.8) that we know exactly what the
8                       outcome is.
9                       (.)
10    C1:   (2) ->      Do you think that all the tablets we offer to people
11                      with AI:DS are te- are tried and trusted and that
12                      we know the outcome.
13                      (1.5)
14    P:                Well obviously not all of them I suppose uh:m
15                      (0.4) but er a few of them yeah. (              )
```

The participation framework of the interaction is once more transformed when C1 rephrases the question initially suggested by C2.
Now C1 is saying something that has its origin in the preceding talk
of another participant; she passes C2's question over to the client.

C1's production role in relation to her words comes close to
what Levinson (1988) has called a *Relayer*. She is transmitting
something the form and motive of which were initially shaped by
someone else. Again, given that the initial deviser of the question is
present, this is a rather unusual footing in talk-in-interaction.
Therefore, it is interesting to see how the role of the relayer is
accomplished in the details of the interaction.

In the first place, this role is accomplished by the main counsellors through a careful design of their turns. They construct their
turns so that they are hearably produced, not only as 'next' actions
after the co-counsellors' questions, but more importantly so that
instead of providing an answer, they *maintain* the conditional relevancy of an answer in the *following* turn by *renewing* the initial
question and by *redirecting* it explicitly to the client. This is
achieved by the main counsellor through producing her turn in
close reference to the co-counsellors' turn.

Extract (12) is most straightforward in this respect. The question
component in C2's turn 'what (.) at the *mom*ent is Michael's main
concern.' is almost echoed by C1, who addresses the patient with
the question 'Michael what's your main concern to*day*'. In this way,
C1 reanimates what has already been said by C2, the difference
being that now the patient is treated as the addressee.

However, C1 is not acting like a tape recorder mechanically
repeating C2's question. In a potentially significant detail, she transforms the temporal reference from 'at the moment' into 'today'.
Through this transformation it appears that C1 avoids mechanically

repeating C2's question. Apart from that, she also adds a potential new ingredient to the meaning of the question: 'at the moment' can be heard as more existential than 'today', which is more instrumental. (We will return to this difference in chapter 5.)

Extract (10) is relatively straightforward as well. C1's initial turn was

DO THEY- ( ) do they want to *know* the results, have they not been told the result,

The question consists of two different clauses:

(1) do they want to know the results,

and

(2) have they not been told the result.

Of these clauses, (2) 'logically' precedes (1), because if the answer to (2) is that they *have* been told, then (1) is irrelevant. Moreover, the central objects of these two clauses also invoke different spheres of reality: 'wanting to know' is linked with the clients' subjective worlds, e.g. their fears and choices, whereas 'being told' can be heard as a reference to the external reality of biographical events. The subsequent turn by C1 very much echoes the part (2) in C2's initial turn. C1 simply substitutes 'you' for 'they', and drops 'the result' from the end of her question:

'Have you not been told.'

In this way, C1 reanimates what has already been said by C2; the difference being that now the clients are treated as the addressees. But in choosing to reanimate the component of C2's initial turn which primarily relates to the world external to the clients' minds, C1 also ends up *not* renewing the relevancy of the subjective world of fears and personal choices. Accordingly, W focuses her response on the 'external' world (being told), thus leaving aside the subjective world that appeared in C2's initial enquiry.

In extract (14), the distance between C2's initial turn and C1's subsequent question addressed to the patient was much greater. But there also the main counsellors' turn is constructed according to the same procedure. The co-counsellors' initial turn was:

Doctor Kaufman I('m) still (0.3) would like you to pursue (this a bit). (1.7) I don't know: and I'm talking to you now as well as to Michael but .hhh

(0.2) will he- *does* he *th*ink that everything we *gi:*ve is (0.8) that we know exactly what the outcome is.

Crudely, this turn consists of four parts. A request, a description of C2's state of knowledge and a formulation of the address together make up the preliminary; and the final part of the turn contains the question. C1 picks up the question and echoes that in her turn.

C1's subsequent turn ignores the hesitation that appeared in the beginning of C2's question component, but otherwise it reproduces

Table 1: Continuity between the co-counsellor's question and the main counsellor's reformulation of it in extract (14)

Co-counsellor's turn	Main counsellor's turn
(0) .hh will he-	
(1) does he think that	(1) Do you think that
(2) everything we gi:ve	(2) all the tablets we offer to people with AI:DS
(3) is (.8)	(3) are te-
(4) that we know	(5) are tried and trusted
(5) exactly	(4) and that we know
(6) what the outcome is.	(6) the outcome.

all the elements of C2's initial question. The correlation between the two questions can be displayed in a table:

In table 1, the question component of C2's initial turn is divided into parts. Apart from the hesitation in the beginning, there is a counterpart in C1's turn to each of these parts; the counterparts are marked with corresponding numbers. Interestingly enough, there is a symmetry even between the occurrence of self-repairs in these two turns: in C2's question a pause leads to self-correction; and in C1's turn, a cut-off word leads equally to self-correction (numbers 3 in the table).

Apart from the hesitation in the beginning, the only part in C2's initial turn that has not an apparent counterpart in C1's turn is the qualifier 'exactly' (number 5). But a similar sort of work that C2 does with the qualification 'exactly', C1 does with the idiom-like expression 'are tried and trusted': both emphasize, or upgrade, the degree of knowledge that the medical team, according to the argument, has about the medicines they are giving to patients.

Potential transformations of meaning can be seen here, too. C1 substitutes 'all the tablets we offer to people with AI:DS' for C2's initial object 'everything we gi:ve'. C2's initial formulation is hearable as a reference to *all medication* given by the clinic, whereas C1 can be heard as talking about one sort of medication given only to a limited set of patients. 'Offering' something can also be different from 'giving': 'offering' presupposes negotiation and consent of the patients (e.g. in drug trials) whereas 'giving' can take place without the patient being asked anything at all. Therefore, C1's version of the question clarifies some aspects of C2's initial turn; and it seems to treat the patient more like a partner in mutual cooperation.

In sum, it seems that C1 in (14) is also careful to design her turn so that it is hearably a renewal of C2's question, rather than a fresh question of her own. In doing that the main counsellor, here as well as in the other cases, avoids mechnically repeating C2's words, which also provides for the possibility of slight transformation of the meaning of the question.[8]

Extract (11) is another case where the initial turn by C2 is long and complicated and not wholly rephrased by C1. The initial turn consists of two kinds of question – an overarching WH-question and four clarifying yes/no questions – and two statement components, one tagged to the WH-question and another to one of the yes/no questions:

Who do you think Doctor Kaufman will suffer most over the next *few* day:s if (0.2) Doug goes home without the *t*reatment that we know *m*ight have a chance of helping him,=will it be *hi*:m? .h Will it be *Phi*lip having to bring him again?=Will it be his mother?=His father? ((...))

Now the main counsellor picks up the WH-question in C2's turn, whilst leaving aside the statement component initially tagged onto it. This is echoed in the subsequent turn, as table 2 below shows.

Apart from the statement component, the only part of C2's turn that is not echoed in C1's turn is the second part. This is a component that embeds the initial question in the main counsellors' thoughts; and this, naturally, cannot be transmitted further to the

---

[8] Notably, P's response (lines 14–15) is targeted at the transformed version of the question: by choosing the plural in 'not all of them' (line 14), P appears to refer 'all the tablets' (C1's version in line 10) rather that 'everything we gi:ve' (C2's version in lines 6–7).

Table 2: Continuity between the co-counsellor's question and the main counsellor's reformulation of it in extract (11)

Co-counsellor's turn	Main counsellor's turn
(1) Who	(1) Who
(2) do you think Doctor Kaufman	—
(3) will suffer most over the next few day:s	(3) will have the worst Christmas
(4) īf (0.2) Doug goes home	(4) if you (0.2) go ho:me Dou:g?

clients. However, in the main counsellors' question, 'having the worst Christmas' substitutes the original 'suffering most in the next few days'. Given that the session took place a few days before Christmas, and that the participants were discussing whether or not Doug should go home for Christmas, this change preserves much of the situated meaning of C2's words: C1 substitutes a non-deictic expression to C2's initial deictic one (cf. Levinson 1983). But again a potential transformation of meaning takes place, too: the explicit reference to Christmas can possibly be heard as emphasizing, more than did the initial formulation, the special importance and character of the few days that could be spoiled.

In (13), unlike the other cases examined this far, C1 does not reiterate any individual parts of C2's turn. However, she achieves the renewal and redirection of the original question through alternative, situationally composed means. The co-counsellors' turn culminates in a question component setting up two alternatives: 'Do you *wa*it or do you come quickly,'. The main counsellor produces her turn with a close reference to this. By asking 'What would you: (...) *th*ink was the right thing to do.', C1 refers to the alternatives proposed by C2, inviting P to choose the right one.

To summarize, the main counsellors accomplish the role of a relayer by producing their turns in a close reference to the co-counsellors' initial questions – the whole question (as in extract (12)), or a core part of the question (as in the other extracts). The main counsellors' turns renew and redirect these. In renewing the questions, the main counsellors can alter some of the words of the initial questions, or they may use their own formulations altogether; preserving, though, the close and hearable link between their turn and (the core component of) the preceding turn. The main counsellors' choice of the core component to be relayed and their alternative lexical choices may result in slight transformations of the meaning of the questions along with the relay.

In a number of cases, the principal counsellors observably orient to the fact that the clients have heard and understood the co-counsellors' initial versions of the questions. This orientation is visible when the principal counsellors' version of the question is so designed that it presupposes something that has been said in the co-counsellors' question. Thus, in (10), C1 merely asks 'Have you not been told', whereby she presupposes that the client has understood from C2's preceding turn that the question is about the test result. Similarly, in (13), when referring to the 'right thing to do', C1 presupposes that B has understood from C2's question that the issue is whether you '*wa*it or do you come quickly'.

The techniques that the main counsellors adopt in relaying the questions also betray an orientation to a problem of *redundancy*. It is one of our basic maxims in conversation that talk should be recipient designed. This entails, among other things, that speakers avoid saying anew things that have already been said and that have been understood by the recipients (Sacks 1992b: 438; cf. Grice 1975). The technique of questioning developed in the clinic we are studying puts the main counsellor regularly in a position where she has to break this rule. The manner in which the principal counsellors relay the co-counsellors' questions can be seen to attend to this problem of redundancy. Confining herself to relaying only one component of the co-counsellors' turn, and by transforming some of its words, the counsellor manages to avoid mechanical repetition, but nevertheless conveys the (original or slightly transformed) meaning of the co-counsellors' initial words.[9]

---

[9] I am not saying, however, that certain types of repetition could not be used as a resource in conversation. For example, Tannen (1990) argues that repetition can be a poetic device creating mutual attachment between the conversationalists. Also in AIDS counselling, the consecutive production of two slightly different versions of the same question actually enables the counsellors to do things that they otherwise might not be able to do (see chapter 5 below); but this does not eliminate the fact that the counsellors *also* have to deal with the problem of redundancy here.

Alterations and rejections of C2's questions

In the section above, we saw how the main counsellors often slightly transform some aspects of the meaning of the co-counsellors' initial questions through alternative lexical choices and through choosing the component to be rephrased. It has to be pointed out, however, that this transformation of meaning is implicit, as it were: the difference between the two versions of the question is not brought to the attention of the participants. The main counsellors' *overt* action involves just the renewal and redirection of the initial question; the change of meaning of the question is a 'side product' that is not emphasized or overtly attended to by the participants.

However, there is a very limited number of cases in our data base where the main counsellors overtly do something other than merely renew and direct the initial question. They may change some aspects of the question, or they may turn the question down altogether. In extracts (15) and (16) below, the main counsellors overtly change aspects of the questions. The co-counsellors' questions are marked with arrows numbered 1, and the alterations with arrows numbered 2.

```
(15)  (N-2)
      ((W = P's wife))
      ((Talking about the AIDS hysteria in the media))
 1    W:           .hh I tried I- (.8) I tried very hard to
 2                 ignore: (.2) the Daily Mirror and the
 3                 [Daily Mai(h)l heh .h[hh erm:
 4    C1:          [Mm:              [:Mm
 5                 (.4)
 6    W:           (              ) Report Guardian.
 7    C1:          (Mm And [what would happen-)
 8    C2:  (1) ->          [(    ) how is it (that) Heather
 9                 became (.8) able to differenti[ate between=
10    C1:                                        [Mm
11    C2:          =what was fact and what was hyste:ria.=What-
12                 (2.2)
13    C2:          The reason I'm asking is
14                 [that (   ) (.2) (   )
15    C1:  (2) ->  [Well I'd like (.) eh- (.2) (to come) one back
16                 and ask whether you a:re able to
17                 (.3)
18    C2:          Mm[:
```

```
19   C1:   (2) ->   [d[istinguish betw[een fact and hysteri[a.
20   C2:            [distinguish    [              [
21   W:                             [Mm            [.hhh
```

(16) (N-44)
((Talking about P's fear that people would 'panic' if they knew that
he is HIV positive.))

```
1    P:            of perhaps (.2) having (.2) s:omebody: .hhh who
2                  would be over reacting and [panicking. [.hhh
3    C1:                                       [Mm         [M[m
4    C2:                                                     [Mm
5    C2:   (1) ->  Mrs Heller [if that happened (.6) could=
6    C1:                      [Mm
7    C2:           =John (1.0) having experienced [panicking=
8    C1:                                          [Mm
9    C2:           =himself .hhh could he think of ways to allay
10                 th[e other persons panic.=by information?
11   C1:             [Mm
12   C1:   (2) ->  Can I just add to that that it might be that
13                 you had to allay the- (1.5) f:ears and panics
14                 even with professionals.
```

In (15), the co-counsellors' initial question presupposes that
Heather has become able to differentiate between fact and hysteria,
whereas the main counsellor asks whether that actually is the case.
Thus the main counsellors' turn renews the conditional relevancy of
the client's answer, and it preserves the focal object of this expected
answer, approaching it, however, from another direction. In (16),
the main counsellors' activity is of a different kind: instead of
rephrasing the question, she produces a statement. This statement
can be heard as a re-specification of some aspects of the co-counsellors' question. Thereby, in an indirect way it preserves the conditional relevancy of the client's answer, simultaneously re-directing
the focus of this answer.

In exceptional cases like (15) and (16), the participation framework related to the questions becomes very complicated indeed. In
these extracts we have questions initially shaped by the co-counsellors, but thereafter partially *reshaped* by the main counsellors.
Therefore, the main counsellors are not just relaying questions
initiated by another participant; they have overtly given their own
contribution to these questions. However, in reshaping the questions, the main counsellors still observably treat them as questions

that initially belonged to someone else; i.e. they do not present the renewed questions as being in the first place their 'own' questions.

This peculiarity of the participation framework is displayed in the prefaces that the main counsellors attach to the questions. The prefaces *mark* the changes by pointing out that the main counsellors are the sources of new aspects of the questions. In (15), C1 begins by saying 'Well I'd like (.) eh- (...) (to *come*) one *back* and ask...', and in (16), C1 begins by requesting 'Can I just *add* to that...'. In an interesting way, these prefaces seem to orient to an expectation that the main counsellors relay the questions 'intact'; changing the question is presented as an *observable* and *accountable* event.

If it is observable and accountable to change the co-counsellors' questions, *turning down* these questions could be expected to be even more problematic. This seems to be confirmed by the two single cases in our work where the main counsellors reject the questions suggested by the co-counsellors. These cases are presented below; the initial questions are marked with arrows numbered 1, and the rejections with arrows numbered 2.

```
(17)   (E4.74-1)
  1    C1:              You say the .hhh the rest of your health is
  2                     fi:ne uh:m
  3                     (1.0)
  4    C1:              [(that)-
  5    C2:   (1) ->     [Sorry could we just hear what his new job is.
  6 -  C1:   (2) ->     I'm going to (come to that). You say the rest
  7                     of your health is fi:ne uh:m .hh have you had
  8                     any worries about HIV at all?

(18)   (N-41)
       ((Talking about the GP's role))
  1    P:               Haemophilia: I (.8) don't want him to ge[t=
  2    C1:                                                       [No
  3    P:               =involved wit[h haemophilia:.=I want to=
  4    C1:                           [O:kay.
  5    P:               =come up here,
  6                     (.)
  7    P:               Er:::m
  8                     (.5)
  9    C1:              But w[hat would it be-
 10    C2:   (1) ->          [Mrs Heller how much information does a
 11                     GP need to f[unction adequately.
 12    C1:   (2) ->                 [*I'll a:sk later that.*
```

13   C1:   I was just wondering: (.) (yeah) ( ) (.3)
14   how: (.2) I mean what would be: (.2) the worst
15   effects do you think of the GP knowing.
16   ((continues))

In turning down the co-counsellors' questions, the main counsellors observably orient to the expectation that they should relay these questions to the clients. This orientation is displayed in the main counsellors' turns marked with arrows numbered 2. In both cases, the main counsellors assert that they will return later to the issues raised by the co-counsellors. By these assertions, they indirectly give a reason for not relaying the questions now. And more importantly, perhaps, the main counsellors design their turns so as to indicate that they do not *reject altogether* the co-counsellors' questions, but rather *postpone* relaying them.[10]

The analysis of the four 'deviant' cases presented above suggest that the main counsellors *oriented to an expectation* that they should relay the co-counsellors' questions without changing them. Deviations from this expected course of events were attended to as observable and accountable events.

Use of non-verbal means in relaying the question

It has been argued above that when relaying the co-counsellors' questions, the main counsellors attend to the problem of redundancy: they avoid mechanical repetition of the co-counsellors' words and sentences. On the other hand, it has also been argued

---

[10] The design of the initial questions in (17) and (18) may have made these queries 'easier' to be turned down than many other co-counsellors' questions. This is most clearly the case in (18). The question 'how much information does a GP need to function adequately' does not (unlike the other co-counsellors' questions) concern issues that the client is primarily competent to talk about. C2 is probably willing to elicit *P's view* about the matter, but that is not explicated in the question. P's role as the target of the question is weakly established, and thereby it may be easier for C1 not to relay this question. In (17), the question is more indirectly expressed than in most of the other cases. C2 does not spell out a question but rather expresses her willingness to know something related to the patient. Because the question has not been spelled out 'on the record', it may be easier for C1 to resist relaying it.

that the main counsellors orient to an expectation that they should relay the co-counsellors' questions in an overtly intact form, without changing them. These two expectations – to avoid redundancy and not to change the questions – are of course potentially difficult to reconcile: the measures that are used for avoiding redundancy (alternative lexical choice and confinement to one component that is passed over to the clients) seem almost inevitably to entail some degree of transformation of the meaning of the initial question. The *ad hoc* solution, which in many cases seems to be good enough for all practical purposes, is for the main counsellor not to focus on the transformation of meaning, i.e. to leave the transformation implicit, as it were.

However, there is also a more radical solution available. In a number of cases, the client's answer follows the co-counsellors' initial turn without the interception of the principal counsellors' talk. In these cases, the principal counsellors observably relay the co-counsellors' questions using non-verbal means. In so doing, they can manage to reconcile the dual expectation of not changing the questions and of avoiding redundancy.

Extracts below represent this trajectory. In these data segments, the co-counsellors' questions are marked with arrows numbered 1, and the clients' ensuing responses with arrows numbered 2.

```
(19)  (Extension of (5))
 1    C1:           So who is there in [your fam-
 2    C2:   (1) ->                     [Mrs Walker does Mr Joseph
 3                  think there's any less dissent in the views now
 4                  than there was. [(On HIV)?
 5    C1:                           [Mm
 6                  (3.0)
 7    P:    (2) ->  I'm not sure really.=From the stuff I've read it
 8                  seems to be: you know one- one thing if I've read
 9                  sort of (0.2) an American science magazine Nature
10                  ((continues))
(20)  (Extension of (6))
 1    C2:   (1) ->  Doctor Kaufman one of the things that (.) I think we
 2                  need to get clear (.) if Michael and Harry don't
 3                  talk that's (.) oka:y. .hhh I'm not sure whether
 4                  we've talked (0.6) to Michael or Harry about this
 5                  I've got (.2) muddled up.
 6                  (0.4)
```

```
 7   C2:              But who does Michael (.2) consider as his next of
 8                    *kin:*.
 9                    (1.7)
10   P:      (2) ->   Obviously it has to be Harry I suppose.

(21) (Extension of (7))
 1   P:               ((...)) but I don't know how far (.5) into
 2                    AIDS I a:m. (.6) Yet.=So:
 3                    [I don't know. (I don't [like to be)
 4   C2:              [Does-                   [s-
 5   C2:     (1) ->   How much does (0.2) Michael want to know about (0.8)
 6                    how far he's (in[to AIDS)
 7   P:      (2) ->                  [Well I think I should know
 8                    everything.=I think it's only- only right. (Isn't it
 9                    really).


(22) (E4.66-67/1)
 1   C2:     (1) ->   Mrs Heller I've I've got [another =
 2   C1:                                       [Mm
 3   C2:              =question.=(That) Don say:s (0.5) that they
 4                    wouldn't have hesitated if (.) Ted annoyed them to
 5                    tell him.
 6   C1:              Mm:
 7                    (0.2)
 8   C2:              Did they feel (0.2) better for having brought that
 9                    annoyance out into the open.
10   C1:              Mm
11   C2:              And if they did (.) how do they think it would be
12                    bringing grief out into the ope[n.
13   C1:                                             [Mm
14                    (0.5)
15   P:      (2) ->   er We:ll as far a:s (0.6) I think a lot of it i:s
16                    (0.5) before: (.) you could tell when Teddy was
17                    dow:n,=you could tell when he was all right.
18                    ((continues))


(23) (E4-8:122-62)
 1   W:               (...) I can't eh (1.0) take onboard (.) any
 2                    more (.) complica[ted though
 3   C1:                               [uhm
 4   C1:              Well can I [just
 5   C2:     (1) ->              [(    ) Mrs Heller could I [just=
 6   C1:                                                    [uhm
 7   C2:              =ask, (.2) (is it-) (1.0) (a little bit) confused-
 8                    .hh (.4) is it the case that Mr Wood doesn't
 9                    know the results:, or is it that they don't want
```

```
10                      to know the results (      ) up (to them)
11                      know the results even (   ) up to
12                      [them to look them up [(                )
13    C1:               [umh              [
14    W:    (2) ->                        [I: (.) I thought
15                      we knew (.5) I thought that we knew that we were
16                      both ne:gative.
```

To refrain from rephrasing the co-counsellors' question, although the co-counsellor has treated the main counsellor as an intermediary, can be seen as an ultimate solution to the dilemma of the conflicting expectations of avoiding redundancy and leaving the co-counsellors' question 'intact'.

The first impression from the data may be that the main counsellors treated the dilemma so seriously that they chose to be totally passive, and not to relay the co-counsellors' initial turns at all. In some cases a gap ensued, after which the client took the next turn and produced the answer; and in other cases, the client produced the answer immediately. However, as the transcriptions of the body movement of the participants show, the main counsellors are *not* refraining from all activity: they systematically turn to the clients after having received the co-counsellors' turn. By doing this, it will

(19)   (Postural orientation)

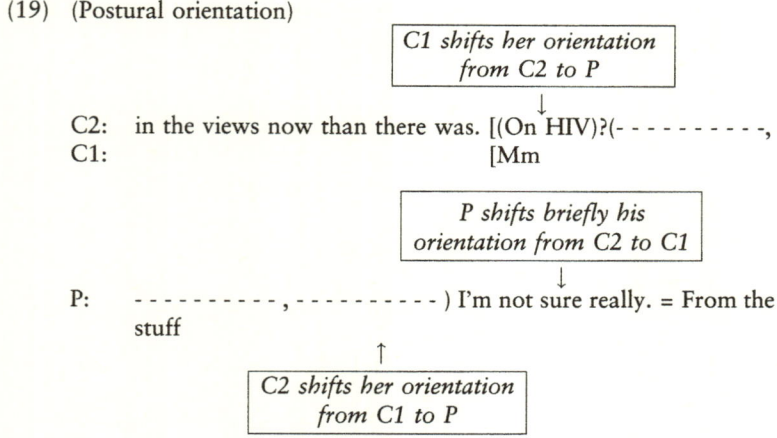

```
C2:    in the views now than there was. [(On HIV)?(- - - - - - - - - -,
C1:                                      [Mm
```

*P shifts briefly his
orientation from C2 to C1*
↓

```
P:     - - - - - - - - - -, - - - - - - - - - -) I'm not sure really. = From the
       stuff
                           ↑
```

*C2 shifts her orientation
from C1 to P*

(20)   (Postural orientation)

> P adopts a
> middle-distance position

↓

C2:   But who: does Michael (- -) consider as his next of *kin:*.

> C2 shifts her orientation
> from C1 to P

↓

P: (- - - - - - - - - - , - - - - - - -)Obviously it has to be Harry I suppose.

                  ↑   ↑

> C2 shifts her orientation   P orients towards
> from C1 to her notes   C1

(21)   (Postural orientation)

> C1 shifts her orientation
> from C2 to P

↓

C2:   know about (- - - - - - - -) how far he's (in[to AIDS)
P: [Well I think I

                                               ↑

> C2 gazes down

(22) (Postural orientation)

> C1 shifts her orientation
> from C2 to P

↓

C2:   bringing grief out into the ope[n.
C1:   [Mm (- - - - -)
P: er We:ll as far

                                            ↑

> C2 shifts her orientation
> from C1 to P

(23)   (Postural orientation)

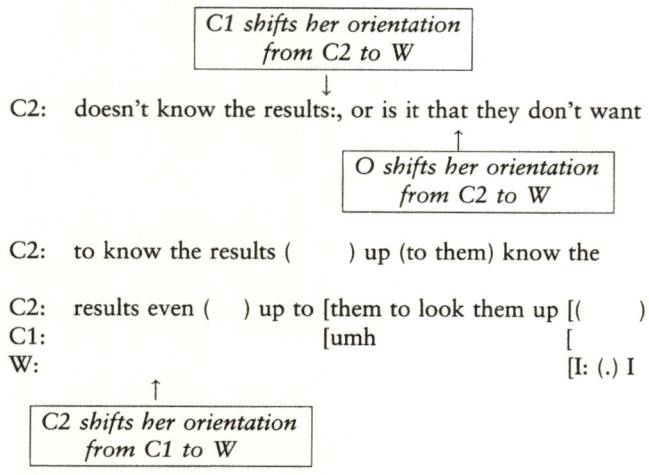

C2:   doesn't know the results:, or is it that they don't want

C2:   to know the results (   ) up (to them) know the

C2:   results even (   ) up to [them to look them up [(   )
C1:   [umh   [
W: [I: (.) I

be argued, they try to accomplish the role of a relayer in a manner that both avoids redundancy, and leaves the content of the initial question intact. We see this pattern in all the cases presented above.

As noted before, turning towards somebody often counts as a *display of recipiency*, i.e. it conveys that the non-speaking person turning to the other is expecting this other to speak next (Goodwin 1981; Heath 1986). In this context, the display of recipiency takes place in a very sensitive environment. The person who turns to the client has been allocated the role of intermediary for a question in the co-counsellors' previous turn. Now the intermediary orients to the client, without beginning a turn of her own. This little gesture is then subject to the interpretation that by making it, the main counsellor *actually seeks to relay* the question initially expressed in the co-counsellors' turn. By relaying the questions using non-verbal means only, the principal counsellor also leaves the content, or the meaning, of the question intact.[11] But, as we will see, the main counsellors' success in

---

[11] There is, of course, the possibility that the main counsellor might 'punctuate' the question, or express her own position *vis-à-vis* it, by e.g. raising her eyebrows. The data we have, however, do not give any hints about this being done.

relaying the questions through non-verbal means is only partial. Among the cases above, in (20), (21) and (23) this interactional technique seems to work well. In (20), at the end of the co-counsellors' initial turn, C2 is oriented to C1 and C1 is oriented to C2. In other words, C2 is treating C1 as the addressee of her turn (intermediary), and C1 responds accordingly. P is just shifting from an orientation to C2 into a middle-distance position, perhaps in response of not being allocated the role of the addressee of a turn which nevertheless contains a question targeted to him.

After the completion of C2's turn, a gap of 1.7 secs. ensues. During the gap, two significant moves take place. First, C1 departs from an orientation to C2, and adopts instead an orientation to P. Thereafter C2 reorients towards her notes. After these moves, P begins his answer to the question initially embedded in C2's turn. At the end of his answer, he orients posturally to C1.

The patient seems to treat the main counsellors' postural moves as having relayed C2's initial question. There are two reasons for thinking so. First, P did not begin his turn before C1 had oriented towards him. A display of recipiency by C1 thus preceded P's turn-beginning. And, second, P oriented to C1 at the completion of his answer, thus treating C1 as the addressee of his turn. This means that P 'gave his answer to' C1 and not to C2.

However, C2's collaboration seemed to be crucial in this management of the participation framework. She did her part by *withdrawing from postural participation* after having produced her initial turn. By turning towards her notes she obviously discouraged P from addressing her. It may also be significant that P began his answer only after C2 had withdrawn from postural participation. P may have been waiting for displays of recipiency from C2; in which case C2's withdrawal would indicate to P that such displays were not to be expected, and thereafter P began his turn, addressed now to the main counsellor.

Extract (21) is another case where the transmission of C2's question through C1's body movement seems to work equally well. There C1 orients to P when the completion of C2's initial turn is approaching. As a response to this shift in C2's posture, P begins his answer.

In (23), C1 orients to W at the completion of the first question component of C2's turn. A few seconds later, the nurse who is observing the session also orients towards W. Even C2 orients to

W before she has completed her turn. Perhaps as a response to all the professionals present displaying recipiency to her in this way, W initiates her turn already before C2 has completed hers.[12]

In the remaining two cases, however, the main counsellors can be seen to run into trouble in eliciting the clients' answers through their body movement. In (19), C1 orients to P during the last two words of C2's question, immediately after the continuer that she produces. P, however, does not begin his turn until 3 seconds have elapsed after the completion of C2's turn. P's turn seems to be triggered only when C2 also orients to him, thus also displaying recipiency. P's own postural orientation seems to confirm that he expected a display of recipiency from C2: until the beginning of his turn, he remains oriented to C2.

In (22), the pattern is essentially the same as in (19). Now, however, C2 orients more quickly towards the patient, and accordingly, only a half-second pause ensues. Moreover, the patient remains persistently oriented to C2.

Concerning the main counsellors' role as the relayer of the co-counsellors' questions, we have argued thus far five points. First, the participants orient to an expectation that the principal counsellors relay the questions without changing them. Second, relaying the question is potentially problematic because it may lead to massive redundancy in the interaction. Third, when the main counsellors relay the question verbally they design their turns so as to minimize redundancy. Fourth, the main counsellors can also try to relay these questions by using non-verbal means only, which eliminates the problem of redundancy, and also leaves the content of the question intact. Fifth, client collaboration in the non-verbal transmission of the questions is potentially difficult to obtain.

The claim that the main counsellors seek to accomplish the role of the relayer of co-counsellors' questions through non-verbal means may appear to be a speculative one. It could be argued that it is an analyst's construction rather than something that the participants themselves are oriented to. However, there is additional evidence about the participants interpreting the main counsellors' body movement in exactly that way. That evidence is provided by two deviant cases.

---

[12] An interesting detail of this extract is how W ends up being chosen as the answerer, even though the beginning of the question was targeted to P. We cannot examine this further here.

Deviant case analysis: the passive main counsellor

In one session in our work the main counsellor is a medical doctor who (at the time of the interview) lacked experience and training in this type of counselling. Consequently, when the co-counsellor (who was one of the experienced professionals) tried to ask her questions using the live open supervision format, the main counsellor neither displayed reci-piency to C2's initial turn, nor did she orient towards the patient after the completion of it. This resulted in obvious difficulties.

```
(24)  (E3-49/P3B)
1     C2:    I have one question more Doctor (Jay) and (then) (.)
2            perhaps then more questions need to be asked.=I'd
3            like to know: (1.0) wh-what Mister Brown thinks: (.)
4            Helena's greatest concern is having heard this
5            conversation toda:y?
6            (2.0)
7     C2:    And then vice versa.
8            (3.0)
9     C2:    If you could just (.) (put it to [him).
10    C1:                                      [What- what-
11    P:     hhhh
12    C1:    .hh What is your (0.2) greatest conce[rn
13    C2:                                         [No:.=
14    P:     =What- [ what do I- do I think   ]=
15    C2:           [does- what does he think his]=
16    P:     =[Helena's greatest concern.
17    C2:    =[wife's is.
```

In what follows, I will concentrate on lines 1–12. The body move-ment of the participants during this episode is as follows.

(24) (Postural orientation)

```
          ┌─────────────────────┐
          │ C2 shifts her orientation │
          │ from C1 to her notes │
          └─────────────────────┘
                     ↓
C2:  I have one question more Doctor (Jay) and then (.)
     ↑                                                    ↑
     ┌──────────────────────────────────────────────────┐
     │            C1 remains oriented                     │
     │               to her notes                         │
     └──────────────────────────────────────────────────┘
```

C2: perhaps (then) more questions need to be asked.=I'd

> C1 *and* C2 *remain oriented*
> *to their notes*

C2: like to know: (- - - - - - - - - -) wh-what Mister Brown thinks:
     x- - - - >

> C1 *and* C2 *remain oriented*
> *to their notes*

C2: (.) Helena's greatest concern is having heard this

> C1 *and* C2 *remain oriented*
> *to their notes*

C2: conversation toda:y? (- - - - - - - - - - , - - - - - - - - - -) And

> C1 *and* C2 *remain oriented*
> *to their notes*

> C2 *shifts her orientation*
> *from her notes to* C1
> ↓

C2: then vice versa. (- - - - - - - - - -, - - - - - - - - - -, - - - - - - - - - -)
     ↑   ↑

> P *glances at* W   P *shifts his orientation*
>   *from* W *to* C2

> C1 *shifts her orientation*
> *from her notes to* P
> ↓

C2: If you could just (.) (put it to [him).
          <- - - -x
C1:   [What- what-
                                          x===
P: ↑   hhhh

> P *shifts his orientation*
> *from* C2 *to* C1

> C2 *shifts her orientation*
> *from* C1 *to* P
> ↓

C1: .hh What is your (- -) greatest concern
    =============x

Notes:
(1) For some time, C1 arranges her note sheets in a ringbinder on her desk. The beginning of this activity is indicated with x- - -> and its completion a few lines later is marked with <- - -x.
(2) x====x indicates the time when P smiles.

Outside the transcription, we must first note that there were two other persons present in the room as well. The wife of the patient and an observer both remained in a non-participatory middle-distance position during this exchange.

In terms of body movement, relatively little happens in the long transcript of (24). The principal counsellor remains oriented to her notes most of the time. She had adopted this orientation a few moments earlier in the session, while the patient was producing an answer to the co-counsellors' preceding question (data not shown). In the beginning of the transcript, C2 gazes at C1 while beginning her initial turn. However, C1 does not reciprocally orient to her, and perhaps as a result of this C2 also drops her gaze to her notes. Consequently, the bulk of C2's initial turn is delivered in an awkward position where both the speaker and the addressee are looking down at their notes. The sense of awkwardness is sharpened when C1 begins to arrange her note sheets in a ringbinder while C2 is speaking. The only participant who *is* gazing at somebody at this time is P, who is persistently oriented to the co-counsellor.

After the co-counsellor has finished the question part of her initial turn, a gap ensues. According to the pattern seen in other extracts, an action by the main counsellor would have been due here, either in the form of rephrasing a core component of C2's question, or in the form of a postural shift towards the patient. C1, however, keeps on arranging her notes, and does not say anything. After 2 seconds, C2 re-completes her preceding turn, after which a new gap emerges. During this gap, postural activity intensifies. First the patient turns briefly towards his wife, and then back to C2. During the latter half of the 3-second gap, the co-counsellor orients to the main counsellor, and the silence is broken with her request: 'If you could just (.) (put it to him).' During the delivery of the co-counsellors' words, the patient first orients to C1, and then C1 orients to P, whereafter C1 puts the question to the patient. As it

turns out later (see the transcript of the talk only), C1's understanding of C2's question failed. P and C2 engage in overlapping talk,
both in an effort to correct C1's understanding of C2's question.[13]

At least two things are notable in this extraordinary episode.
First, P obviously orients to the unusual participation framework
that C2 seeks to build up. This orientation is clearly displayed by
him when he withholds an answer until C1 has rephrased the question. By refraining from answering at the completion of C2's initial
turn or its continuation, P shows that he expects somebody else to
act first. Plainly, his having with held an answer does not arise from
him having not understood the question: the proof that he did
understand being that he is able to correct C1 at the end of the
extract. Second, both P and C2 orient to the lack of activity from
C1. P displays this by withholding an answer. C2 shows this by
producing the request 'If you could just (.) (put it to him).' when no
activity appeared after the second gap.

During the same session, there was a similar type of episode
triggered by C2's question. Also in this case, C1 remained looking
at her notes throughout the sequence; and the other participants
oriented to this as her having not relayed C2's question. In the
absence of C1's activity, C2 recompletes her turn twice (arrows
numbered 1 and 2); and P orients to the lack of activity by C1
first by withholding an answer, and thereafter by asking whether
the question is meant for him (arrow 3).

```
(25)  (N-52)
 1    P:           Well hh .hh you see- (.4) this is a- (.3) this is a
 2                 problem.=You get (1.0) you get told (.) things
 3                 which are actually .hh
 4    C1:          Mm[:
 5    P:              [not (.2) completely compatible.
 6                 (1.2)
 7    P:           Er[m
 8    (C1):          [Well-
 9    C2:          Can you [ask Mr B[rown how he
10    P:                   [(Now)hh [What is the case.
```

<hr />

[13] C2's question was not about P's greatest concern, but instead, following the
pattern of 'circular questioning' it was about P's assumptions about W's greatest
concerns. C1's reluctance in transmission of the question may be related to her
difficulties in understanding it.

```
11   C1:              Mm:
12   C2:              Can you ask Mr Brown how (1.2) how he
13                    accounts for the fact that (.8) in this situation
14                    things are told that are incompatible.
15                    (2.8)
16   C2:   (1) ->     (He has) asked an interesting question *I mean
17                    it's:*
18                    (2.0)
19   C2:   (2) ->     I mean how come things are told that are
20                    incompatible.
21                    (.5)
22   P:    (3) ->     Is that a question to me. =
23   (C1):            =[Mm-m
24   C2:              =[Mm-m
25   P:               .hhh Well (.2) differen- (.2) different people's
26                    different (.2) pers- (.) er: interpretations
27                    ((continues))
```

The only way that C1's behaviour in these two deviant cases
departs from the behaviour of the main counsellors in extracts
(19)–(23) is that in the deviant cases the main counsellor did not
orient posturally to C2 during her initial turn, and to P after it. This
indicates that this postural orientation really serves as the accomplishment of C1's participation roles, first as the intermediary and
then as the relayer.

Clients' orientation to the dual problem of relaying C2's question

We argued above that the participation framework involved in C2
addressing to C1 her question targeted at the client leads to a
dilemma between the need to avoid redundancy and the expectation
not to change the initial question. C1s have been shown to orient to
these problems either by the special design of their turns or by an
effort to relay the questions through non-verbal means. In the following, we will examine two single cases where the *clients* seem to
orient to the same problems.

In three cases in our work, the interaction after the initial question by the co-counsellor followed a 'mixed' trajectory. In each of
these cases, the main counsellors started their turns after the co-
counsellors' initial questions. However, the main counsellors' turns
remained uncompleted, because the clients began their answers at

the earliest opportunity. In what follows, we will examine two of these cases.

```
(26)   (Extension of (9))
 1    C1:              (...) but I want to be reas[sured that=
 2    P:                                         [umh
 3    C1:              =she (.8) understands the facts as we
 4                     have them now.
 4    P:               Umh
 5    C1:              .hh And-
 6    C2:              Mrs Heller you asked Mr Wood if he'd do
 7                     anything differently if he was po[sitive and=
 8    C1:                                               [umh
 9    C2:              =he said no. Would Mrs Wood want to do
10                     anything [differently *if he was positive.*
11    C1:                       [umh
12    C1:    (1) ->    Would [ you ( )-]
13    W:     (2) ->          [ Well   ] (.2) I don't think
14                     so.=Because I think we've been careful
15                     wi[th everything now:.
16    C1:                [Yes.
17    C1:              Oka[y.
18    W:                 [So I don't think that ((continues))
```

In (26) above, C1 begins her turn (arrow 1) following the 'standard' pattern we identified earlier in this chapter. It appears that she has picked up the question component (lines 10–11) from C2's initial turn, and is going to rephrase it. We can hear the first two words 'Would you', which correspond to the words 'Would *Mrs* Wood' in the initial question. If C1 had produced the whole turn, designing it following the same principles as C1s in extracts (10)–(14), she would have ended up saying something like 'Would you want to do anything in a different way?'

After the first word of C1's turn, however, W (Mrs Wood) begins her turn by saying 'Well' (arrow 2). W's 'Well' bears the typical characteristics of a 'pre-start' accomplished using an 'appositional beginning' (Sacks, Schegloff and Jefferson 1974: 719): by saying 'Well', W claims the floor, without yet revealing what she is going to say.[14]

---

[14] This is not to say that 'Well' does not convey anything at all. 'Well' often starts a dispreferred turn (Levinson 1983). It appears that 'Well' here is related to a normatively based acceptability of an affirmative answer to C2's question. By

After having heard W's pre-start, C1 abandons the turn she had begun, thus giving way to W's talk. After a pause of 0.2 sec., W then delivers her answer to C2's initial question. The way in which the interaction between W and C1 unfolds, however, betrays that both of them orient to the rephrasing of C2's question as something redundant. W shows this orientation through initiating overlapping talk while C1 is in the course of producing her turn. W does not wait for C1 to relay the whole question of C2's, but produces her answer after having heard C1's first word. By doing this, she treats C1's turn as something that can be glossed over. C1, in her part, shows the orientation to the redundancy of rephrasing C2's question by giving up the floor to W. Usually in the counselling sessions the counsellors win the competition for the floor, but here it goes the opposite way. By giving up so readily, C1 shows that she considers what she was going to say as something which was not necessary.

Another perspective on the problems related to C1's role as a relayer is provided by the other single case where the client begins his answer before the completion of the main counsellors' turn. In extract (27) below, the main counsellors' turn is marked with arrow 1, and the client's response with arrow 2.

```
(27)  (Planning 663)
 1    C2:           Would it be [possible for=
 2    (C1):                      [(      )
 3    C2:           =John to make (0.2) sets of alternative plans if
 4                  this .hh (.) (yeah u)- (0.2) what sort of symptoms
 5                  would have to happen to make him change to
 6                  plan 'b' or plan 'c'.=I mean is that something he
 7                  can envisage doing with Liza?
 8    C1:    (1) -> I'd like to (.4) [a-
 9    P:     (2) ->                  [I think I can a- answer that (0.2)
10                  very simply.
11                  (1.5)
12    P:           If I: (0.2) had fe:lt (0.6) .hh .hh (0.9) eighteen
13                  months ago (1.1) maybe not as long as that (.) just
14                  after May was born because this is relative
```

wanting to do something differently, W would display how responsible she is and how much she cares about P. By saying, however, that they have already been careful, W proffers an account for an answer that initially appears less acceptable.

```
15   (C1):         Mm
16                 (0.6)
17   P:            If I had felt then how I feel now (1.0) bottom line
18                 we would never have moved.=[I would never=
19   (C1):                                     [No.
20   P:            =have gone ahead with it. (0.2) .hhhh (.) If I'd
21                 ((continues))
```

At the beginning of her response in (27) (arrow 1), the main counsellor describes her *own intention*: 'I'd like to'. This 'self-attentive'
turn-beginning resembles closely the main counsellors' prefaces to
their turns in extracts (15) and (16) analysed earlier; as we saw,
these prefaces were attached to turns where some aspects of the
initial questions were overtly changed. Indeed, by focusing on her
own intention in this way, the main counsellor departs from the role
of relayer: she is hearably beginning an action of her own, not
merely relaying the other participant's turn. Even though the
turn-beginning does not yet define the action to come, it seems to
exclude the possibility that C1 would merely aim at relaying C2'
question intact.

Following the 0.4 sec. gap after C1's turn beginning, P start
talking (arrow 2), overlapping the continuation of C1's turn
Now P produces a preface to his action: 'I think I can a- answer
that (.2) very simply.' Through this preface, P creates a connectic
between his turn and the earlier question of C2: he is going
answer the co-counsellors' question. This connection is support
by P's hand movement: during the five first words of his turn,
points towards C2 with his hand (not described in the transcrip
The location of P's turn-beginning and his way of prefacing
talk seem to disclose P's orientation to the possiblity that C1
indeed aiming at some action other than merely that of relay
C2's initial question. By taking the floor and producing the expl
action projection, P indirectly claims that C2's initial questio
something to which he can legitimately respond. As soon as
has started a turn that seems to be leading her either to by
C2's initial question or to change it, P intervenes, with the dem
strated intention to answer.

Again, we see the main counsellor accepting the client's clai
the floor. Thereby, C1 displays an understanding that the client's

answer at this slot is indeed legitimate, and that her own projected alternative action is to be postponed.

In sum, our analysis of extracts (26) and (27) suggests that the clients also orient to the dual expectation that the main counsellor should avoid redundancy and leave the initial question intact. Extract (9) demonstrates that from the client's point of view C1's rephrasing of C2's question is a redundant activity, which can simply be glossed over. On the other hand, extract (19) shows a client observably orienting to the expectation that the co-counsellors' question be relayed to the client intact, without any active intervention by the main counsellor.

Restoration of the ordinary footing

After the main counsellor has relayed the question to the client, who has subsequently answered it, a further interactional task faces the participants. If the main counsellor is going to conduct the rest of the interview, her role as the questioner – not only as the relayer of questions, but as deviser of them as well – has to be restored. The triangular footing and the mediated format of action have to be dismantled for the main counsellor to regain her full control of the interview.

In what follows, I examine three interactional trajectories through which the main counsellors' control is restored. In one of them, the main counsellor re-establishes her initiatory role immediately after the client's answer; in another, the restoration is delayed. In the third trajectory, the live open supervision format of questioning *collapses* when the *co-counsellor* acquires the initiatory role, and the main counsellors' control is restored only after that. The examination of the restoration of the principal counsellors' initiatory role will indicate some further intrinsic difficulties in the operation of the live open supervision format of questioning.

1. The main counsellor re-establishes her initiatory role immediately after the client's answer. The restoration of the ordinary footing often takes place in the next two turns following the client's answer to the co-counsellors' question. After the client's answer, the main counsellor asks the following question, and the client provides an answer to that. The main counsellor is now fully in control of the

interaction; and the co-counsellor has returned to the role of audience. In the following three cases, this pattern is followed. The main
counsellors' first 'own' questions after P has answered C2's question are marked with an arrow.

```
(28)   (Extension of (2))
       ((W = Patient's wife))
  1    C1:          But then let's take [ourselves- let's-]
  2    W:                              [(      ) be ru]de
  3                 but (.) I (.) just how [ I feel ] at the moment.
  4    C2:                                 [ DO THEY-]
  5    C2:          (      ) do they want to know the results, have
  6                 they not been told the [result.
  7    C1:                                 [Have you not been told.
  8    W:           Yes we've been told we've been negative as far as
  9                 I'm awa:re
 10                 (.9)
 11    C1:    ->    Who's been negative y[ou::-
 12    W:                                [I (.) I have (.) because I
 13                 had (.2) ( [ ) another test done.


(29)   (Extension of (3))
  1    P:           Just [that-
  2    C2:               [Who do you think Doctor Kaufman will suffer
  3                 most over the next few day:s if (0.2) Doug goes
  4                 home without the treatment that we know might
  5                 have a chance of helping him,=will it be hi:m? .h
  5                 Will it be Philip having to bring him again?=Will it
  6                 be his mother?=His father?
  7    P:           .hhhh=
  8    C2:          =[(              )
  9    C1:          =[Who will have the worst Christmas if you (0.2) go
 10                 ho:me Dou:g?
 11    P:           Well if I go ho:me (0.2) .hh and I do what I do:
 12                 (0.8) normally (0.5) it won't affect anybody. (.)
 13                 Be[cause-
 14    C1:    ->       [But if you go home and you can't do what you do
 15                 normally: and you get more breathless and you need
 16                 everybody doing everything for you: (1.0) how will
 17                 that be that Christmas for- for you: and for
 18                 everybody else.
 20    P:           ((Coughs)) .h Well I'll spend mo(h)st of the
 21                 ti(h)m(h)e .hhhh ((Coughs)) in my room anyway
 22                 ((continues))
```

(30) (Extension of (6))
```
1   C2:          Doctor Kaufman one of the things that (.) I think we
2                need to get clear (.) if Michael and Harry don't
3                talk that's (.) oka:y. .hhh I'm not sure whether
4                we've talked (0.6) to Michael or Harry about this
5                I've got (.2) muddled up.
6                (0.4)
7                But who does Michael (.2) consider as his next of
8                *kin:..*
9                (1.7)
10  P:           Obviously it has to be Harry I suppose.
11               (0.4)
12  C1:   ->     Well is that your view. (.) [er That he is,=[and=
13  P:                                       [Yeah.        [Mm
14  C1:          =does he think that about you?
15  P:           Yeah.
```

In all the cases above, C1's role as the conductor of the interview is restored in a seamless way. C2s collaborate in the restoration by withholding further action of their own; and Ps collaborate in it by aligning as answerers to C1's questions.

Restoring the main counsellors' control of interaction may require extra effort even in those cases where she asks the next question following the co-counsellors' intervention. The management of the reception roles of the client's answer is one potentially problematic issue. The more unambiguously the main counsellor acquires the role of the addressee of the client's answer to the co-counsellors' question, the better she is able to preserve her central position in the interaction, and the more smoothly she can thereafter claim back her initiatory role. However, this can prove problematic. Problems may become manifest especially if the main counsellor has not rephrased the co-counsellors' question, and if P's answer is long. In extract (31), it seems that the main counsellor is involved in specific 'alignment work' during the delivery of the client's answer – and these efforts are not very successful.

(31) (Extension of (5))
```
1   C1:          So who is there in [your fam-
2   C2:                             [Mrs Heller does Mister Joseph
3                think there's any less dissent in the views now than
4                there was. [(On HIV)?
5   C1:                     [Mm
6                (3.0)
```

```
7   P:              I'm not sure really.=From the stuff I've read it
8                   seems to be: you know one- one thing if I've read
9                   sort of (0.2) an American science magazine Nature
10                  or whatever it says [one thing. .hh [you can read=
11  C1:  ->                            [Mm              [Mm
12  P:              =another review
13  C1:  ->        Ye:s.
14  P:              a:nd you know (0.7) er [sort of clippings or=
15  C1:  ->                                [Mm
16  P:              =whatever (I [read) that sometimes are=
17  C1:  ->                     [Mm
18  P:              going (0.8) and there's (0.8) there don't seem to be
19                  any sort of any great correlation in the views in my
20                  [er
21  C1:  ->        [Mm
22  P:              you know but I'm not- [I'm not (a doctor or)=
23  C1:  ->                              [Mm
24  P:              =( ) (0.5) er specialist so [I wouldn't know=
25  C1:  ->                                     [Mm
26  P:              =really. (1.0) But as a layman [I'd say (yeah:).
27  C1:  ->                                        [Mm:
28                  (1.0)
29  C1:  ->        M[m
30  P:               [I mean I wouldn't say it was: you know
31                  one [or- or either really.
32  C1:  ->             [Mm
33  C1:              If there was for instance more certainty that we
34                  (0.2) could say from tests and things you're
35                  definitely going to .hh get AIDS would that help you
36                  more: or would it be more difficult.
37                  (1.0)
38  P:              Well d'you mean in respects with AZT or:
39                  ((continues))
```

If we examine the transcription of the vocal activities only, this case seems to flow as smoothly as any of the other cases where the main counsellor acquired back her role as the conductor of the interview immediately after the client's answer. The patient's turn is rather long; but during it, the main counsellor displays her alignment as the addressee through active production of continuers and other response tokens (marked with arrows).

However, the transcript of the body movement reveals that there is a mismatch between the main counsellors' recipient activity, and the postural orientation of the speaker (the patient). During most of his turn, the patient is posturally oriented to the *co-counsellor*, the initial deviser of the question. Through his body movement, the patient treats the co-counsellor, rather than the main counsellor, as the principal addressee of his turn.

The origin of the mismatch may lie in the very beginning of P's turn. As noted above, he didn't initiate his answer before C2 (in addition to C1) had oriented posturally towards him. He waited for the co-counsellor to display recipiency before starting. In the beginning of his answer P turns for a little while towards C1; but thereafter, he soon realigns himself towards C2. He remains in this posture throughout most of his turn.

A transcription of P's postural orientation during the delivery of the answer is shown below. Orientation towards C1 is shown by a dotted line (- - - -) and orientation to C2 by a continuous line (——). When there is no line above the transcript of the talk, P is in a middle-distance position, not being oriented to anyone.

(31) (Postural orientation)

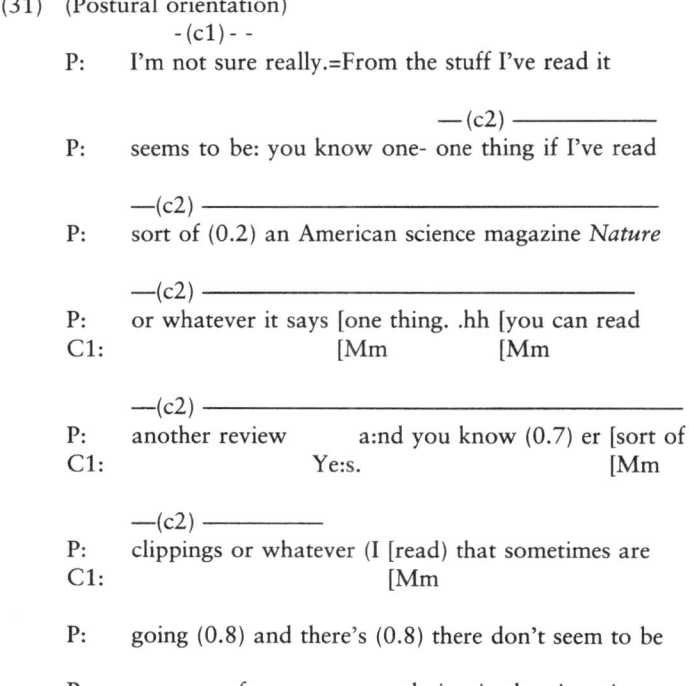

```
        -(c1)- -
  P:    I'm not sure really.=From the stuff I've read it


                       — (c2) ———————
  P:    seems to be: you know one- one thing if I've read


       —(c2) ———————————————————
  P:    sort of (0.2) an American science magazine Nature


       —(c2) ————————————————————
  P:    or whatever it says [one thing. .hh [you can read
  C1:                       [Mm            [Mm


       —(c2) ——————————————————————
  P:    another review        a:nd you know (0.7) er [sort of
  C1:                  Ye:s.                          [Mm


       —(c2) ————————
  P:    clippings or whatever (I [read) that sometimes are
  C1:                            [Mm


  P:    going (0.8) and there's (0.8) there don't seem to be


  P:    any sort of any great correlation in the views in
```

```
            —(c2) ————————————————————
P:    my [er you know but I'm not-   [I'm not (a doctor or)
C1:       [Mm                        [Mm


        —(c2) ————           - - (c1) - -
P:    (    ) (0.5) er specialist so [I wouldn't  know
C1:                                 [Mm


    - (c1) - -                        - (c1) - -
P:    really. (1.0) But as a layman [I'd say (you know).
C1:                                  [Mm:


    (c1) - - - - - - - - - - - - - - -      — (c2) —
P:    (1.0) [I mean I wouldn't say it was: you know
C1:         M[m


    — (c2) ————————————————  - - (c1) - - - - - -
P:    one [or- or either really.
C1:        [Mm                    If there was for instance
C2:                              x====x
```

Note: x====x indicates when C2 nods towards P.

The transcript shows that P vacillates between an orientation to C1 and to C2; choosing, however, to be oriented mostly to C2. He seems to try to include both counsellors as addressees of his turn, the emphasis being on C2 rather than C1. But all vocal response items are produced by C1. She appears to be engaged in active 'alignment work' to regain her central role *vis-à-vis* the patient. The sense of active alignment work stems from the contrast between P's postural orientation and C1's acknowledgement tokens: most of C1's acknowledgement tokens are produced while the speaker is oriented to another recipient (C2).

C2 collaborates in C1's alignment work by refraining from the production of any response items of her own. Her only activity to acknowledge P's turn is a slight nod towards him, appearing right after the completion of P's turn and simultaneously with the beginning of C1's question to P. This nod seems to serve as an acknowledgement of P's turn, but being just a silent gesture, it also reaffirms the secondary reception role of C2.

In spite of all the alignment work by C1 and C2, P completes his turn whilst orienting towards C2. Only the next question by C1 (lines 33ff in the original extract) successfully restores her central role. The persistence of the mismatch betrays some inherent problems of this type of questioning.

2. *The restoration of main counsellors' initiatory role is delayed.*
The main counsellors' central role is not always restored through the turn immediately following the client's answer. There are cases where the triangular footing persists over the next turns.

   In extract (32) below, the triangular footing lasts over an additional question–answer pair, after which it is dismantled in an orderly fashion. The beginning of the co-counsellors' second question is marked with arrow 1, the patient's answer to it with arrow 2, and the beginning of the subsequent question by the main counsellor by arrow 3.

```
(32)  (Extension of [7])
 1    P:           ((...)) but I don't know how far (.5) into
 2                 AIDS I a:m. (.6) Yet.=So:
 3                 [I don't know. [I don't [like to be)
 4    C2:          [Does-          [s-
 5    C2:          How much does (0.2) Michael want to know about
 6                 (0.8) how far he's (in[to AIDS)
 7    P:                               [Well I think I should know
 8                 everything.=I think it's only- only right. (Isn't it
 9                 really).
10    C2:  (1) ->  [One other question first before we =
11    C1:          [Mm
12    C2:          =go into (what he might be doing) is that .hhh
13                 (0.7) what if he did get AIDS,=what does he think
14                 (0.7) will be: (0.2) the hardest thing for
15                 him.=What does he fear most.
16                 (0.8)
17    P:   (2) ->  I think (.) accepting it I suppose. (.) That's going
18                 to be quite- and I know I've accepted it this far.
19                 (0.7)
20    C1:  (3) ->  Is thi[s accepting AI:Ds or the- the=
21    P:               [Mm
22    C1:          =outcome of AIDS.=Is it (0.9) the [things that=
23    P:                                            [Mm
24    C1:          =might happen to you like happened to Harry or is
25                 it [dying in the en:d.
26    P:           [Mm
27    P:           I think probably a bit of both really.=I mean I've
28                 s- (.) I've seen what Harry's gone through and
29                 ((continues))
```

C2 seems to orient to the extension of her questioning in the triangular footing as something which is interactionally problematic.
This orientation is displayed in the design of the preliminary she
attaches to her question: by saying 'One other question first before
we go into (what he might be doing)', she seems to convey her
commitment not to continue in this footing any more than over
the forthcoming question. By projecting the end of her questioning,
she anticipatorily contributes to the restoration of the main counsellors' initiatory role at the end of the extract.[15]

3. *The co-counsellor acquires the initiatory role before the main
counsellors' control is restored.* Sometimes, however, the restoration of the main counsellors' initiatory role is delayed even longer.
The co-counsellor may continue asking questions, but from a different footing, addressing the client directly. This entails the collapse of the 'live open supervision' questioning format. That
happens in extract (33). C2 responds to the client's initial answer
with a follow-up question. Its delivery leads to a shift of footing.

```
(33)   (Extension of (23))
 1    W:              (...) I can't eh (1.0) take onboard (.) any more (.)
 2                    complica[ted though
 3    C1:                     [uhm
 4    C1:              Well can I [just
 5    C2:                        [(     ) Mrs Heller could I [just=
 6    C1:                                                    [uhm
 7    C2:              =ask, (.2) (is it-) (1.0) (a little bit) confused-
 8                    .hh (.4) is it the case that Mr Wood doesn't
 9                    know the results:, or is it that they don't want
10                    to know the results (      ) up (to them)
11                    know the result even (    ) up to
12                    [them =to look them up [( )
13    C1:              [umh                  [
14    W:                                     [I: (.) I thought we knew
15                    (.5) I thought that we knew that we were both
16                    ne:gative.
17    C2:  (1) ->     Were you told you were both nega[tive?
18    W:                                              [As far as I
```

---

[15] The preliminary also does another kind of work: it separates C2's forthcoming
turn from the preceding question and answer. By characterizing her turn as 'one
other question', C2 emphasizes that she is introducing *new issues* rather than
following up what has been said earlier.

```
19                          re[member.
20    C2:                   [in the last test
21    W:                    And (.) it was
22                          [so long ago I wouldn't have [thought.
23    C2:                   [(            )             [( ).Now if (1.5) if
24                          there are new results (.) >I mean<
25                          [(             )]
26    W:                    [We would want] to know.
27    C2:                   You haven't heard the last results of last time
28                          (you) we had have you?
29    P:                    As far as I know not no.
30    (?):                  No no:
31    C2:                   I mean I [don't kno:w them I have to tell you=
32    W:                             [I'm
33    C2:                   =[(                )=
34    W:                    [I'm so totally-
35    C2:                   =( [                            )]=
36    W:                       [I'm so totally lost with ('em]=
37    C2:                   =[(      )] I just want to know=
38    W:                    =[(entirely).]
39    C2:                   =whether you want to know or not
40                          because [(      )later.
41    W:                            [Oh I would want to
42                          know.=[Rather than [not.
43    P:                          [yes          [
44    C2:    (2) ->                            [(All right that's-) that's
45                          good.
46    C1:    (3) ->         Well I think ↑one of the reasons Mrs Wood really
47                          (.5) for exploring a little bit today: is that (1.4)
48                          I (1.0) am impressed with how (.4) you are dealing
49                          with things: we are ((continues))
```

In line 17 (arrow 1), C2 asks a follow-up question after W has answered her initial enquiry. This follow-up question leads to others; in all of them, the interactants are aligned into an 'ordinary' questioning footing, where C2 poses her questions directly to W. (In lines 29 and 43, P also makes his contribution.) The 'live open supervision' format has collapsed, and the co-counsellor has taken control of the interaction.

The participants, however, find a subtle way to restore the main counsellors' control. After having completed a series of enquiries, C2 produces an assessment (arrow 2). This turn of hers is different from the preceding ones, because it does not project a responsive action from any of the others present. This assessment is a backward-looking item, which closes the line of enquiry that C2 has just been involved in (cf. Jefferson 1981). By using such a closure, C2 relinquishes the floor as a questioner, which allows room for the other participants to step in. Consequently, C1 starts a turn of talk, leading to a formulation of the preceding conversation and description of the counsellors' perception of the clients (arrow 3). Through this turn, C1 regains her initiatory role and control of the interaction.

Two practising family therapists who use live open supervision in their work have pointed out that '[a]voiding direct interaction cannot be carried to absurdity' (Smith and Kingston 1980: 384). They suggest that abandoning the triangular footing is occasionally needed for the supervisor (or co-counsellor) to show his or her alignment with the clients or to produce lightness or intensity. After his or her direct contribution, 'the supervisor can then withdraw from the central arena of interaction through the therapist' (ibid.).

Our data analysis presented above suggest a conclusion that is not far from Smith and Kingston's position. The analysis of extract (33) has demonstrated that the live open supervision format may be difficult to preserve over a number of questions and answers. A direct response by C2 to the client's initial answer to her enquiry may create a tendency for the participants to abandon this format of action. Should that happen, the participants may need to engage in specific interactional manoeuvring to restore the the principal counsellors' control of the interaction.

Management of the participation framework as 'bricolage'

The sequences examined in this chapter have been related to an effort by the counsellors to standardize some conversational features in the counselling sessions. In ordinary conversation, participants move freely between the different production and reception roles regarding their utterances (cf. Goffman 1974: 496–544). In the counselling practice examined in this study, an effort has been made to standardize the participation framework related to co-counsellors' questions.

In their seminal paper on turn-taking, Sacks, Schegloff and Jefferson (1974: 730) argued that other speech-exchange systems differ from conversation in the respect that they pre-specify some of the features of the turn-taking system that conversation allows to vary. This same point of view can be applied to the allocation of production and reception roles in institutional talk (Garcia 1991). Certain forms of institutional talk can be distinguished from conversation by having pre-specified some aspects of a participation framework, which are more freely transformed in ordinary conversation. For example, the reader in a church service, the defence counsel talking on behalf his or her client to the jury, or the priest declaring absolution after confession all display different, pre-specified production roles in relation to their words.

In the first place, the arrangements regarding co-counsellors' questions to their clients represent another variation of the standardization of the participation frameworks in institutional talk. However, what makes these arrangements particularly interesting is the fact that this standardization relates in the first place to one particular local culture only. 'Live open supervision' is a theory-based practice that is followed only in a few clinics. Many aspects of the arrangements discussed in this chapter were developed by the very counsellors whose work we have been analysing.

Hence, we cannot properly speak about *pre-specification* of participation frameworks here, if pre-specification presupposes shared, public norms about proper conduct (such as the norms regulating a reader's, defence counsel's or priest's conduct). Even if the counsellors have 'pre-specified' these practices amongst themselves, the clients are most likely to encounter them for the first time when they have their first counselling session.[16]

The management of participation frameworks related to live open supervision represents, therefore, another aspect of *bricolage* in the production of institutional talk in the context of AIDS counselling. This standardization is achieved primarily on a local basis by the counsellors using consistently the tools and the practices of ordinary conversation, such as address terms, gaze and third-person

---

[16] This does not mean to say, however, that arrangements comparable to the 'live open supervision' format of questioning could not be found elsewhere. Possible settings include consecutive interpretation and service encounters with children, the elderly or people with disabilities. In these environments, questions may be phrased twice, first addressed to an intermediary, and then to the target of the question.

reference. Through these tools of ordinary conversation, they repeatedly set up the unique configuration of production and reception roles, and the corresponding sequential patterns of talk.

Because of the uniqueness of this standardization of the participation framework, the counsellors have actively and persistently to work towards its maintenance. In this chapter, we have seen how hitches can occur despite constant vigilance: the clients may interrupt the counsellors before the questions have been rephrased, or they may not answer even though an effort has been made to relay the questions. Occasionally the live open supervision format breaks down altogether.

Despite these hitches, the sequences analysed above bear witness to the possibility of *creativity* in conversational practice in general, and to the *professional creativity* of the subjects acting in these sessions in particular. Participation frameworks *can* be systematically manipulated on a local basis, leading to unique patterns of interaction to emerging. In their professional practice the counsellors in this clinic, together with their clients, have locally produced something not previously seen.

Functionality of live open supervision

In this chapter, we have seen how complicated interactional arrangements are needed to establish and maintain the questioning pattern employing the live open supervision format. It has also been shown how the counsellors often face difficulties in the management of this questioning technique. We have seen how the participants orient to two conflicting expectations, one of which requires the main counsellor to avoid redundancy while the other requires her to relay the co-counsellors' question intact. A major solution to this problem appears to be that the main counsellor seeks to relay the co-counsellors' question using her postural orientation only; but this leads to a risk that the clients will fail to treat the shifts in the main counsellors' body posture as acts of relaying the question. Another difficulty is related to the follow-up questions and other immediate responses to the client's initial answers, which lead easily to the collapse of the live open supervision format.

In spite of its interactional complexity, and the difficulties in its employment, counsellors continue to apply the questioning technique based on the live open supervision format. This suggests that it may have significant interactional functions, or 'pay-offs', related to the professional role and tasks of the counsellors.

The theory that informs the counsellors' work – the Family Systems Theory – suggests some 'pay-offs'. As noted at the beginning of this chapter, the major intended function of the separation of the roles of the main counsellor and the co-counsellor is to give the co-counsellor a specific perspective, from which she can observe the clients-plus-main-counsellor system.

On the other hand – given the counsellors' persistent application of this format – it is also possible that this questioning format may have some additional functions which are not necessarily discussed in the Family Systems Theory textbooks. One of the classical teachings of sociology is that a given social arrangement also can have unacknowledged pay-offs, or latent functions, other than the functions that the operators of this arrangement say and believe that it has (Merton 1957).

Therefore, it will be the task of the next chapter to explore the 'pay-offs' and functions, manifest and latent, which may make it useful for counsellors to apply this pattern of questioning in spite of its complexity.

5

Some interactional uses of co-counsellors' questions

In the preceding chapter we examined in detail the management of participation frameworks related to co-counsellors' questions applying the family therapeutic technique called 'live open supervision'. At the end of that analysis, the question was raised whether the complicated way of delivering the co-counsellors' questions could have functions other than those referred to in the Family Systems Theory textbooks. The purpose of this chapter is to explore empirically the interactional uses of co-counsellors' questions, both those that are referred to in textbooks and those that are not.

Like any CA work, my analysis of the uses of co-counsellors' questions employing the live open supervision format progressed in an inductive fashion. In other words, I examined all my data where this type of question was asked, identifying the recurrent patterns of interaction in different types of cases. In organizing the presentation of my results in this chapter, however, I use a somewhat more deductive approach. In presenting some of the recurrent patterns, I use the counsellors' theory as the point of departure. This is possible because it happened in the data analysis that some of the interactive uses of co-counsellors' questions were nicely in line with this theory. However, there are other interactional uses of the co-counsellors' questions which seem to transcend the theory. In presenting those, the theory of course cannot be used as the point of departure.[1]

---

[1] There are also such Family Systems theoretical discussions related to the advantages of live supervision which seem not to be relevant to my data. I have not referred to those discussions in this book, but a brief note may be needed. For

In what follows, I present first those interactional uses of the co-counsellors' questions which seem to conform to the ideas presented in the Family Systems Theory texts. There are three different uses of this kind: *first*, the intervention can topicalize an item from the client's talk; an item to which the principal counsellor has not attended. *Secondly*, the intervention can constitute an interpretative operation *vis-à-vis* the client's talk elicited by the principal counsellor. And *thirdly*, the intervention can involve an effort to open up an alternative route towards the direction that the principal counsellor's questions have aimed at. We will now examine some cases of each type.

Topicalizing passed-by items

Discussions based on Family Systems Theory on 'live supervision' emphasize that the primary rationale for the use of teams and supervision – either with a one-way mirror or without – is it allows the primary therapist (principal counsellor) and the supervisor (co-counsellor) to have *different perspectives* to the issues at hand. To put it simply, the assumption is that 'two heads are better than one' (Selvini and Selvini Palazzoli 1991: 34). In other words, if only one member of the team is actively conducting the interview, and the rest follow it either from behind the one-way mirror, or have an observatory role while being in the same room, then the observer(s) can achieve a distinctly different perspective on the clients and the interaction between the therapist and the clients. The supervisor/co-counsellor will be able to 'obtain a clearer view of the processes which are occurring, both within the family and between the family and the therapist' (Smith and Kingston 1980).

The term 'meta-position' has been commonly used (see e.g. Burnham and Harris 1985: 61; Cade and Cornwell 1985: 56) to describe the supervisor's wider perspective. Even though it is arguable whether or not the supervisor(s) should be emotionally

---

example, Hoffman (1981: 333–4) suggests that the team can act as 'a dissenting voice', forcing the clients to take sides. In my work, consisting of the co-counsellors' questions, I did not find cases where that kind of a process would have taken place. Among the co-counsellors' utterances *not* packaged as questions, however, there might also be cases of 'dissenting voices'; but I have not examined these cases systematically.

'detached' from the clients (see Selvini and Selvini Palazzoli 1991), there seems to be an agreement in the Family Systems literature that the *difference in perspective* constitutes the core rationale for live supervision. The supervisor (or the co-counsellor) is able to observe not only the clients, but the family-plus-clients system which is operating during the session. Live supervision is, then, a practice that can enhance the observatory or perceptual capacity of the team: the supervisor (or to use our term, the co-counsellor) can *see differently.*

My data analysis coincides with this assumption. There are two types of co-counsellors' questions in which this kind of different perspective is clearly manifested. In the first (and most simple) type, the co-counsellor topicalizes from the client's prior turn an item which has not been noticed by the main counsellor. Extracts (1) and (2) provide examples. In these extracts, the 'topicalizable' items are marked by arrows numbered 1, the principal counsellors' turns showing no intention to topicalize these items are marked with arrows numbered 2, and the co-counsellors' subsequent interventions are marked with arrows numbered 3.

```
(1)   (E4-74-1))
 1    P:              (...) if I just think it might be a blee:d.[Now=
 2    C1:                                                         [Mm
 3    P:              =I'll wait (.) and make sure it is, then treat
 4                    it [properly.
 5    C1:                [Mm
 6    C1:             Have you ever missed- have you missed any time off
 7                    work because of blee:ds.
 8    P:              No. None.
 9    C1:             None at all.=
10    P:      (1) ->  =No. I've just started a new jo(h)b actual[ly
11    C1:                                                        [Mm:
12    P:              a few weeks ago but (.) I haven't missed any.
13                    (0.8)
14    C1:     (2) ->  You say the .hhh the rest of your health is fi:ne
15                    uh:m
16                    (1.0)
17    C1:             [(that)-
18    C2:     (3) ->  [Sorry could we just know what his new job is.

(2)   (E4-50)
 1    C1:             So er do you think there's been anything since
 2                    you've been HIV that has actually helped you to do
```

```
 3                        things differently and perhaps better than you did
 4                        before:.=Being less concerned about some things.
 5                        (0.3)
 6    P:                  Uh:m (0.4) not really I think initially it was it
 7                        slowed me down a bit be[cause (        )=
 8    C1:                                        [Mm:
 9    P:                  =mental stop-check I think really
10    C1:                 Mm:=
11    P:                  =slowed me down because it's: (0.5) y'know in
12                        [fact with haemophilia I'm capable because=
13    C1:                 [Do-
14    P:                  =[I've grown up with i[t (              )=
15    C1:                 =[Mm                  [Ri:ght.
16    P:                  =(all going [all together:)
17    C1:                            [Mm
18    C1:                 mhm:=
19    P:                  =which no-one seemed to know a lot.=
20    C1:                 =No:.
21    P:     (1) ->       You know there's a lot of dissonance in all the
22                        view:s,
23    C1:    (2) ->       So who is there in your [fam-
24    C2:    (3) ->                               [Mrs Walker does Mister
25                        Joseph think there's any less dissent in the views
26                        now than there was. [(On HIV)?
27    C1:                                     [Mm
```

Extracts (1) and (2) have similar structures. In both, the patients expand their answers to the principal counsellors' questions, by adding (after the reception of the first parts of the answers) some materials that move the answers away from the questions. In (1), P mentions that he has a new job, and in (2), P points out the dissonance in the (public) views, probably concerning AIDS. After this, the principal counsellors initiate their turns,[2] in which items introduced by the patients in their expansions observably are not intended to become topicalized. Before the principal counsellors have completed their actions, however, the co-counsellors intervene with queries which topicalize just these items.

Extract (3) has the same key features, but it is more complicated. The arrows are numbered in the same way as in (1) and (2).

---

[2] In (1), the principal counsellor's turn begins with a statement format. The statement seems to work, however, as a preface for a question: a few lines later, when C1 resumes her question, it is prefaced by a statement which seems to be 'redoing' the statement initially spelled out in line 14 (data not shown).

```
(3)     (N-40)
 1      C1:             Is there anything you feel that Liza (1.0) can do
 2                      (1.4) to make life easier for you now.
 3      P:      (1) ->  No.
 4      C1:     (2) ->  Is there anything- (.2) you f(h)ee(h)l y[o(h)u=
 5      ( ):                                              [hhh hhh
 6      C1:             =c(h)ould d(h)o .hhhh h for Liza to make
 7                      her life easi[er now.
 8      P:                           [Yeah.
 9      C1:     (2) ->  What do you think [(might) that be.
10      P:                                [Pull myself together,=and if it
11                      me:ans: (.) using a s:tructure.=having .hhhh
12                      err::::hh .hhhh erm:: (.3) these tablets which (.3)
13                      Doc[tor (Kleinman's) given me.=And it means that=
14      C1:                [Mm-h,
15      P:              =I can (.2) therefore (.5) cope, .hhh and keep on
16                      top of the problem, .h[hhh and it doesn't (.3) make=
17      C1:                                   [Mm:
18      P:              me a misery which in turn upsets Liza and the kids?
19                      .hhhh
20                      (1.0)
21      P:              Then that's what I got to do:.
22      C1:             Mm::
23                      (.8)
24      C2:     (3) ->  Mrs Heller you('ve) asked (1.2) John if there was
25                      anything Liza can do to help him.=he said
26                      no:.=Does L:iza agree with that.
27                      (.)
28      C1:             Yes (sorry) (.2) Do you agree with
29                      ((continues))
```

In (3), the potentially topicalizable object brought in by the client is
his answer to the principal counsellor's question: an abrupt negation, 'No.', when asked whether his wife could do anything to make
his life easier. The principal counsellor does not invite any elaboration of this 'No.',[3] moving instead to a closely related but different
question: she turns around the positions of Liza and John, and asks
now whether *he* could do something to make *her* life easier (lines 4
and 6–7). This question leads to a longer exchange between P and

---

[3] The abruptness of P's 'No.', however, seems to elicit an indirect response from C1,
whose next question is accompanied by laugh-tokens (lines 4 and 6). This kind of
unilateral laughter is very seldom produced by the counsellors; in this case, it
seems to convey that C1 orients to P's abruptness as a 'quasi-joke'.

C1, in which P describes in more detail what he could do to help his wife (up to line 21). C2 does not intervene before this sequence is observably completed through P's summarizing statement in line 21, and C1's declination to produce a follow-up question (lines 22 and 23).[4] In her intervention, C2 first rephrases C1's initial question and P's response (thus retrieving a context that had been passed by), afterwards producing her question, which preserves P's 'No.' in the topical focus.

In all three extracts, the co-counsellors' questions indicate that they have observed the interaction between the clients and the principal counsellors. The topical foci of the interventions arise from the clients' turns. The interventions are produced, however, only after the principal counsellors' actions have made it clear that they are not going to topicalize these materials. Therefore, the co-counsellors in these interventions reveal and trade off a position where they are able to observe the workings of the 'clients-plus-counsellor-system', just as it is suggested in the Family Systems Theory textbooks.

Interpretative operations

Another type of intervention that transparently indicates the co-counsellor's specific perspective involves interpretative operations. In this type of intervention, the co-counsellor links the client's prior talk to a suggested underlying mental pattern or disposition.[5] In her question, the co-counsellor describes this mental disposition, thus eliciting the client's confirmation or rejection.

Extract (4) below is an example of interpretative operations in the co-counsellor's intervention.

---

[4] The delay in C2's intervention may be related to the fact that C1's questions in lines 4 and 9 are topically connected to P's utterance in line 3. In extracts (1) and (2), the principal counsellors' next actions (lines 14–15 and 23 respectively) proposed *a definite move away* from the issues brought in by the clients. In (3), however, the topical movement is less 'disjunctive'; and perhaps because of that, C2 waits until C1 and P have completed their action before intervening. I wish to thank Marja-Leena Sorjonen for pointing this out to me.

[5] Garfinkel (1967) suggests that an interpretative method of constructing underlying patterns, where the single observable facts are elaborated (the 'documentary method of interpretation'), is used both by 'ordinary' members of society and social scientists.

(4)   (E4-66-67:366-)
      ((P has expressed his fear that he couldn't maintain his composure if
      his brother died. This has led to a series of questions and answers,
      revolving around P's wish to be brave and not to show emotion.))

1	P:	If I thought my being upset would upset mum and da:d
2	C1:	Right.
3	P:	and Ted
4	C1:	Mm:
5	P:	I'd bottle it u:p.
6		(0.2)
7	C1:	So if Ted wasn't there: and- (.2) would you st- do
8		the sa[me for your parents?
9	P:	[I'd-
10		(0.2)
11	P:	Yeah. (.) I: I've always: (.) as I say I always
12		won't sh- I won't show my feelings [if I think=
13	C1:	[Mm:
14	P:	=that it'll upset other [people. (0.2) But I=
15	C1:	[Mm
16	P:	=think (.4) in the event of Ted's death (.4) I
17		think (.4) my parents (2.6) will take it hard
18	C1:	M[m:
19	P:	[And I know my father (1.4) won't be able to
20		handle it. I know that- I know [that he [will=
21	C1:	[What are [you =
22	C2:	[Mrs =
23	P:	=[have a really hard of time of i[t.=And I think=
24	C1:	=[most- [Mm?
25	C2:	=[Heller
26	P:	=that that's what'll get me.
27	C2:	->	I would [like to ask a question.=Does Don think=
28	(?):		[( )
29	C2:	->	=that (0.4) showing emotion when som[eone dies=
30	C1:		[Mm
31	C2:	->	=means you (just) can't handle it.=
32	C1:		=Ye:s that's (what-)/(it-)[6]
33	P:	No:. I don't think that at all:. Bu:t at the same
34		ti:me (0.6) I think (0.5) once it- once again if I
35		show: that I'm upse:t (0.3) I know it'll upset (0.9)
36		my parents and Jill and everybody else.

---

[6] It is impossible to hear whether C1 says here 'Ye:s that's it-' or 'Ye:s that's what-'.
Therefore the notation '(what-)/(it-)'.

The co-counsellor's intervention in (4) involves a shift from detailed description of feelings and plans into a more abstract discourse. In lines 1–26, P and C1 discuss P's ways and preferences of responding to distressing events. In this context, P expresses his fear that his father and himself will have serious trouble if Ted (P's brother) would die. The co-counsellor's intervention (marked with arrows) *discontinues* this talk about concrete objects. Her question treats the client's descriptions of his feelings and the (anticipated) events as possible indications of his underlying thoughts and beliefs. The preferences and fears that P has just expressed are thus connected with his suggested belief that '*show*ing emotion when someone dies means you (just) can't handle it'. Through creating this connection, the co-counsellor's intervention in (4) hearably accomplishes interpretative operation: the client's prior talk is now treated as an indication of an underlying mental disposition. Interpretative operations exhibiting a similar pattern are shown in extracts (5) and (6) below.

(5)   (N-37-9 and 50)
       ((W and P have expressed P's fear that if he came to the haemophilia
       centre complaining of flu symptoms, the staff there would 'panic' and
       they would want to take him in and put him into an isolation room))

1	C1:	You know what (.2) would (.) what else would make
2		us panic.
3		(1.8)
4	C1:	If you're coming in.
5		(.6)
6	C1:	If you think we'd do that.
7		(1.0)
8	C1:	Do you think there's ([ )?
9	P:	[No: of course I mean
10		if you'd be sensible abo:ut it and I- I-I have (.2)
11		I have ( ) I mean just (.) just ( ) anybody
12		on the (whim:) .hhh of having flu: and because
13		they're in an (.2) so called .hhhh high risk area-
14		>>we'd better take them in.
15	C1:	([ )
16	P:	[I mean being s:::ensible about it. Being
17		realistic about it >>I've got a- .hh
18		(1.0)
19	P:	If (.2) if I had these concerns (.2) (of coming up)
20		.hhhhh and you kn- (.2) an-an-and actually saying to

```
21              you, .hhhh Just check my weight (.) just check my
22              back (.) just-just (.2) tell me I'm being s:tupid.
23              .hhhh
24              (1.0)
25    C1:       Wel[l- (.2) (   )
26    C2:  ->       [Mrs Heller is th- John's fear of coming up
27              ((Infant making noises))
28    C2:  ->   really- (.6) because he doesn't want the answers
29         ->   rather than
30              (.3)
31    ( ):      (   )
32    C2:  ->   >>because (.2) unless he can be sure that he
33         ->   [gets a reassurance he doesn't want to=
34    C1:       [I actually-
35         ->   know.[(=No matter-)
36    C1:            [(liked)
37    W:        He want's to hear the answers he wan[ts. ( )
38    C1:                                          [(Can) let's ask
39              John.((continues))
```

```
(6)   (N-35 and 48)
 1    W:        Everybody we kno:w (.) had the same cough.[=And=
 2    P:                                                  [Yes.
 3    W:        =it's been- and it's- and eve[rybody has had it
 4    P:                                     [It's (ramped) and
 5              (ramped)
 6              (.3)
 7    C1:       Mm[:
 8    W:          [for weeks and weeks.
 9    P:        Right.
10    C1        I'd like to get-
11    W:        And the doctors aren't (.) the GPs aren't giving
12              anybody [anything because they say its a virus.
13    (C1):             [(Mm)
14    P:        And th- a[nd  t[he truth i:s:
15    (C1):              [(Mm)[
16    W:                      [So they don't give (you)
17              antibio[tics.
18    P:               [The truth is (.4) that I've had one
19              (1.2) ↑Okay (.3) do the obvious (.2) go to the
20              G[P
21    W          [(But he puts a block of) [(     )
22    P:                                   [Perhaps get a vi- er: er
23              er (.2) Penicillin (.) or whatever. .hhh And then
24              (   ) is it gonna work. No .hhhh it's not working,
25              .hhh (.2) er this is because I've got this problem.
```

```
26              (.3)
27    P:        Right? er- (.2) Everyone else's cough's getting
28              better,
29              (.5)
30    P:        Min[e isn't.
31    W:            [But-
32    W:        But you'd probably been told that- (.3) there's
33              nothing to give anyway.
34    P:        Fine.
35              (1.0)
36    C1:       John (.) can I get ba[ck to my (original)
37    P:                             [((It's that- it's that)
38    C1:       que[ s t i o n.= I' v e heard what Doctor Kaufman=
39    P:           [(It's the fear.)
40    C1:       =said,=.h[hhh
41    C2:  ->            [Can I ask you to ask you some- to ask
42       ->   something (rather) first. .hhhh Does John (.2) think
43       ->   (.3) that you go from being antibody positive to
44       ->   having AIDS: or are there other stages on the way:
45       ->   before you get something ( [          )-
46    P:                                 [The answer to that is
47              I'm under the impression that from (.) being
48              antibody positive ((continues))
```

In the talk preceding C2's question in extract (5), P unpacks his thoughts about the staff's panic, thereafter describing how he would want the staff to respond if he came to the Centre with flu-like symptoms. In (6), P and W describe the cough P has had, and the fears that it aroused.

Again, the co-counsellors' questions indirectly suggest a connection between the clients' concrete descriptions and their underlying thoughts and beliefs. In (5), P's ideas about the staff's panic and his wishes for how he should be treated are linked with him not actually wanting the answers and not wanting to know; and in (6), P's fears concerning his cough are connected with his thoughts about the progression from being antibody positive to having AIDS. The interpretation operates through establishing the linkage between clients' descriptions of their feelings and activities, and these underlying mental dispositions.[7]

---

[7] It is a further challenge for the conversation analyst to show exactly *how* this interpretative character of C2's questions is achieved. Why are these questions

When C2's interventions have an interpretative character, they incorporate their producers' specific position and perspective upon the interaction during the session. The co-counsellors view the clients' talk from a distance, as it were, suggesting links between issues that neither the clients nor the main counsellors had on these occasions connected.

It is also notable that in all three cases shown above, the co-counsellors' questions constituted an *alternative action*. In each case, the principal counsellors had already begun a turn when the co-counsellors intervened. Because the principal counsellors' activities were not completed, we do not know exactly what they were aiming at; but it seems likely that their turn-beginnings did not project any interpretative operations.[8] By intervening at this point the co-counsellors exhibited that they follow the counsellor-client

hearably 'interpretative questions', and not just innocent, straightforward questions concerning the clients' emotional dispositions? The following considerations are relevant here.

(1) For the co-counsellors' interventions to be heard as interpretative operations, the hearer must orient to a *link* between the clients' concrete talk prior to the intervention, and the interventions' abstract content. In the first place, this link is established by the sequential location of the interventions. Because the interventions follow the clients' talk; because this talk has not suggested a topic termination; and because the co-counsellors' interventions do not include any 'misplacement markers' (Schegloff and Sacks 1973), they are heard to be connected with the clients' prior talk.

This connectedness is enhanced by variable means in each case. In (4) and (5), the co-counsellors repeat or rephrase key objects of the clients' preceding talk: in (4), P's 'show my feelings' (line 12) and 'handle it' (line 20) are echoed by C2, and in (5), P's 'concerns (.2) (of coming up)' (line 19) are reproduced by the counsellor in the form of 'fear of coming up'. In (6), C2 produces her intervention only after C1 has expressed her intention to shift the topical focus away from P's prior talk (by prefacing her turn 'can I get back to my (original) question.' in lines 36–8). By producing her intervention in a location *before* moving away from the issues that the clients have talked about (this 'before' character is expressed by C2's request 'Can I ask you to ask (...) something (rather) first' in lines 41–2), C2 can be heard to suggest that her intervention is connected with the clients' prior talk.

(2) There is a shift of focus – from concrete to abstract – between the clients' prior talk and the co-counsellors' interventions. However, when a sequential link has been established between these two, an interpretative relation can be established between the two levels of description, and thereby the co-counsellors' questions are heard to suggest an interpretation of the talk that the clients produced prior to these interventions.

8   The following observations can be made. In (4), C1 seems to be heading towards a follow-up question (lines 21 and 24); in (5) the principal counsellor seems to be beginning a turn responding to P's prior talk in a dispreferred or unexpected way

interaction from a specific position: they do their interpretations only when the principal counsellors' turn-beginnings have already suggested that they are not going to give such interpretations.

Finding an alternative way

In Family Systems Theory literature, the most often discussed advantage of live open supervision is that it gives a specific perspective to the supervisor/co-counsellor. The two types of co-counsellors' questions described above were manifestations of such a 'meta-position'. However, the supervisor's/co-counsellor's different perspective is not the only advantage mentioned in these texts. One of the other advantages that the Family Systems Theory texts suggest is related to the possibility that interaction between the therapist/principal counsellor and the clients 'gets stuck' (Speed *et al.* 1982: 279). In such a situation, the supervisor/co-therapist can intervene. This intervention can give new direction to the interaction, and thus it 'often elicits more cooperation and can resolve an apparent impasse' (Cade and Cornell 1985: 50; see also Smith and Kingston 1980: 380).

In the data analysis, I have identified some cases where the interactional environment for the co-counsellor's intervention has involved observable difficulties in a series of questions and answers between the principal counsellor and the client(s). As the counselling theories suggest, the co-counsellors' questions can establish a way out from such deadlocks. However, these interventions seem not to give an entirely new direction to the interaction; rather, they constitute an alternative route towards the same goal that the principal counsellor was (unsuccesfully) aiming at.

Extracts (7) and (8) below are examples of this type of an environment. Extract (7) includes material that we have seen in extracts (2), (10) and (28) in chapter 4; and (8) includes material from extracts (3), (11) and (29) in that chapter. C2's interventions are marked with arrows; the long sequences of talk preceding them are

---

(with 'well', line 25; cf. Pomerantz 1984) and in (6), the principal counsellor appears to be heading towards a topical shift by retrieving a question that has been discussed earlier (lines 10 and 36).

presented to demonstrate how the interaction between clients and
main counsellors drifts into difficulties.

```
(7)   (E4-8)
  1   C1:    Did you know that (.) Mrs Wood, (.3) .hh that S:ay:
  2          I mean we're talking hypotheticall[y now.=because=
  3   W:                                        [uh-hum
  4   C1:    =I don't know- (.4) ex[act=
  5   P:                           [Mm
  6   C1:    =details say: .hhh Mr Wood was (.) negative.
  7   W:     Um:
  8   C1:    Have yo- (.2) did you understand what he said (.)
  9          that he could be negative at the m[oment and-]
 10   W:                                       [ Oh yes.   ]
 11   C1:    Rig[ht.
 12   W:        [Yes.
 13   C1:    S[o if:: (1.2) the test came out positive.=I mean=
 14   W:     [(        )
 15   C1:    what are the thing:s- (1.5) how would you conduct
 16          your life.=What are the thing:s
 17   W:     hhhhhhhh [I don't know hh         ].hhh ((teary voice))
 18   C1:             [IF I WAS TO (SAY IT-)]
 19   C1:    We[ll-
 20   W:       [I just don't know. ((teary voice))
 21          (.4)
 22   C1:    Well (.2) just have a guess?=I mean what- (1.0)
 23          Mr Wood i[s sa- (                    )
 24   W:              [I think (I'm at a stage) (     ) AIDS
 25          just another thing.hh
 26          (2.0)
 27   W:     .hhhhh I'm at a stage where: I feel's if- (1.0)
 28          (there) would just be another thing.
 29          (.5)
 30   C1:    *(        ).* Having heard what Mr Wood said (.)
 31          that e:ven if he was negative. (.2) It wouldn't
 32          make him conduct his life any different. (.7) What-
 33          (.3) effect would that have: if:-
 34   W:     .hhhh
 35   C1:    I mean what are the things that it [would affect if=
 36   W:                                        [hhhhhhhh
 37   C1:    =he was positive.
 38   W:     gh hhhhh heh hh
 39   C1:    Umh:?
 40   W:     .hhhhhh I just don't know. (.4) I'm afraid, (.3)
 41          .hhh (2.0) I'm in a frame of mind- (.2) mind at the
 42          moment (.2) .hhh (3.0) that I'm not so (lots) of
```

```
43                   use: f(h)or hypothe(h)ti(h)cal things.=.hhh I'm not-
44                   (.2) err: (.3) very useful to you I mean.=Because
45                   (.2) .hh (.5) I feel that as if- (1.6) the things
46                   which are actually happening (.4) are as much as I
47                   can cope wi[th.
48      C1:                     [Yes:. That's- (.3) well- (2) I ag- I
49                   understand t[hat.
50      W:                       [.hhhhh (.2) gheh hhhh heh .hhh The
51                   world could fall apart. (.5) At the moment it isn't
52                   (tearing) (.) and [so- (.2) th- I just=
53      ( )                            [No.
54      W:           =have to say (.) well .hhh It has to get on with it.
55                   (.3)
56      C1:          But then let's take [ourselves- let's-]
57      W:                               [(        ) be ru]de
58                   but (.) I (.) just how [ I feel       ] at the moment.
59      C2:   ->                           [ DO THEY-]
60      C2:   ->     (           ) do they want to know the results, have
61                   they not been told the [result.
62      C1:                                 [Have you not been told.=
63      W:           =Yes we've been told we've been negative as far as
64                   I'm awa:re
65                   (.9)
66      C1:          Who's been negative y[ou::-
67      W:                                [I (.) I have (.) because I
68                   had (.2) ( [       ) another test done.
69      C1:                     [Yes I know?

(8)     (E4-72:111-67)
1       C1:          =Yeah but you've got a very good idea.=The virus
2                    cuts your immune system out and you haven't got the
3                    cells to fight the infection,=that's absolutely
4                    ri:ght. .hhh So you get infections that you can't
5                    fight off by yourself but many of them can be
6                    treated. (0.5) So it doesn't mean that because you
7                    can't fight them off you just (.) there's no point
8                    in treating you.
9                    (0.2)
10      P:           Yeah but [er what-
11      C1:                   [There are many things we can tre:at,=
12      P:           =What annoys [me about it is .hh that (0.2) if=
13      C1:                       [and-
14      P:           =I've got this infection now: .h what's stopping me
15                   from getting another one and another one, and then
16                   another [one.
17      C1:                  [I can't answer that.=There's nothing
```

18		to stop [you but there's nothing to stop us=
19	P:	[No it- it'd carry o:n.
20	C1:	=treating you.=And if we don't treat you what d'you
21		suppose will happen next.
22		(0.2)
23	P:	Well I suppose it won't get better.
24	C1:	No?
25	P:	er If I keep ca:lm it won't get worse:.
26		(0.5)
27	C1:	What will stop it getting worse?
28	P:	Well it's only when I get exer:tion. .hhh (0.2)
29		Exert myself and my breathing gets a bit shallow.
30		(.)
31	C1:	So how will you manage
32		(.)
33	P:	By keeping calm. .hhhh But okay it can never s-
34		I can't [( )
35	C1:	[But if your- if your chest gets worse and
36		worse and worse what will happen to you?
37	P:	I don't know:. .hhh=
38	C1:	=We:ll
39		(.)
40	(P):	((Coughs))
41	C1:	[have a gue:ss.
42	(P):	[( )
43		(0.6)
44	P:	Just [that-
45	C2: ->	[Who do you think Doctor Kaufman will
46		suffer most over the next few day:s if (0.2) Doug
47		goes home without the treatment that we know might
48		have a chance of helping him,=will it be hi:m? .h
49		Will it be Philip having to bring him agai:n?=Will it
50		be his mother?=His father?
51	P:	.hhhh=
52	C2:	=[( )
53	C1:	=[Who will have the worst Christmas if you (0.2) go
54		ho:me Dou:g?
55	P:	Well if I go ho:me (0.2) .hh and I do what I do:
56		(0.8) normally (0.5) it won't affect anybody. (.)
57		Because-

In both (7) and (8), the principal counsellors pursue an aggressive line of hypothetical questioning.[9] In (7), the questions concern the

---

[9] Hypothetical questions will be analysed more in chapters 6 and 7.

clients' choices in a hypothetical situation where P has tested positive. Through her questions, C1 observably aims to confront W (the patient's wife) with the possibility that her husband could be HIV positive. In (8), the principal counsellor's questions are about a hypothetical situation where P's chest infection is left untreated. Through her questions, C1 tries to persuade P to remain in hospital by demonstrating to him that if he refuses to have his current chest infection treated properly, this may result in a life-threatening situation. (Before beginning the questioning, C1 offered statements (lines 1–11, 17–20) where she emphasized how there are means available for the treatment of the infection.)

In neither of the cases above do the main counsellors manage to gain the clients' cooperation in their hypothetical questions and in the projects for which the questions are vehicles. In (7), W claims lack of knowledge and produces extensive accounts to avoid talk about AIDS. In particular, she claims her unwillingness to deal with 'hypothe(h)ti(h)cal things' (lines 40–7). In (8), P first gives evasive answers, and then claims lack of knowledge. In both extracts the counsellors, in spite of the clients' resistance, appear to pursue their questions: in (7), before being forcefully interrupted by W, C1 starts in line 56 a turn which appears to be built towards a new enquiry; and in (8), C1 asks P to guess (line 41) after he has claimed that he doesn't know. In sum: the principal counsellors have, prior to the interventions, made several consecutive attempts to get answers to their questions, and have failed to get an answer that they would have treated as adequate.[10]

In both (7) and (8), C2's interventions establish an alternative route towards the same direction that was unsuccessfully pursued by the main counsellors. In (7), C2's intervention dismantles the hypothetical frame of questioning. By asking whether the clients want to know or have been told the result, C2 preserves the clients' relation to the test result as the focal object – but approaches this in a less threatening way than C1's hypothetical questions did. C2's

---

[10] Technically, the co-counsellors' interventions in (7) and (8) occur in slightly different circumstances. In (7), by the time of initiation of C2's intervention (line 60), W is in the process of completing her account for not answering the questions. In (8), however, P is technically speaking in the process of beginning a turn of talk which has not yet revealed its character when C2 interrupts him (line 45).

intervention is, therefore, attentive to W's self-professed inability to deal with hypothetical issues.

In (8), C1's initial enquiries concern the medical consequences for P of not having his current chest infection treated properly. C2's intervention preserves the hypothetical pattern of questioning; it also continues the underlying project of pointing out the reasons for staying in hospital. However, C2's question approaches the possibility of not staying in hospital from another direction. Instead of the medical consequences for P himself, the intervention focuses on the negative social and personal consequences for P's family members.

The opening-up of alternative routes appears to involve two things. First, the co-counsellors offer the patients alternative questions to be answered instead of the ones that the patients have shown reluctance to deal with. By doing this, the co-counsellors contribute to finding a way out from an interactional deadlock. But second, these interventions also preserve the activity that was initially pursued by C1. In (7), the exploration of the implications of a positive test result is not abandoned through the co-counsellor's intervention; rather, the client is asked to proffer additional information which can serve as the background for such exploration in the further unfolding of the interaction. Equally in (8) the effort to persuade P not to go home is by no means given up; it takes different means as a result of C2's intervention and thereby is possibly even intensified.

In (7) and (8), the clients cooperate by answering the questions asked by the co-counsellors. The interactional deadlock is therefore broken. Just as it is suggested in the counsellors' theory, these interventions were successful in eliciting more cooperation and resolving 'an apparent impasse' (Cade and Cornell 1985: 50).

From the point of view of Conversation Analysis, however, it is important to ask a further question: what makes these interventions so effective? In extract (7) the co-counsellor's intervention was observably less threatening than the principal counsellor's questions that preceded it – but the same cannot be said about extract (8). Therefore, it may not be the degree of threat only that explains the success of the interventions.[11]

---

[11] Issues related to the degree of threat are discussed more thoroughly at the end of this chapter.

In the first place, the co-counsellors' interventions are to be seen in their specific sequential context. They are actions taking place just after the clients have demonstrated their inability/unwillingness to produce the conditionally relevant responses to the main counsellors' questions. By intervening, the co-counsellors offer a way out for the clients: the co-counsellors' questions bring to a halt the main counsellor's line of questioning, and also sequentially delete, or at least de-intensify, the conditional relevancy of the answers to the questions that the main counsellors already have spelled out. Therefore, the co-counsellors are demonstrably 'letting the client off the hook'.

Given this, it may be very difficult for the clients to turn down the co-counsellors' questions. Declining them would have made the client accountably 'doubly uncooperative': she/he would have been the one who first refused to answer to C1's questions, and then, when C2 offered him/her an alternative question, turned that down, too. Thus, it may be their quality of 'letting-the-client-off-the-hook' that makes C2's interventions likely to achieve the clients' cooperation. Thus, even though it might seem that the clients are offered a way out, they actually end up cooperating in C1's project. This is because, as we have pointed out above, C2's interventions preserve the activity that was initially pursued by C1.

Greatbatch (1992) has suggested that in broadcast news interviews with more than one interviewee, these are often inclined to escalate their disagreements in a manner that interlocutors of ordinary conversation would find inappropriate. In escalating their disagreements, the interviewees can orient to the fact that the disagreement sequence will be controlled and closed by the intervention of the interviewer, through his or her new question; and therefore, they do not need to mitigate or soften their disagreement. It may very well be that there is a comparable situation in AIDS counselling. The counsellors' awareness of the possibility of the co-counsellor's intervention may give the main counsellors confidence in pursuing an aggressive line of questioning. If a deadlock should appear, it is likely that the co-counsellor can help.

One of the contributions of Conversation Analysis is that it makes possible to examine in detail how the abstract principles of a therapeutic theory are worked through in the details of interaction. In the preceding pages, this kind of analysis has been done. We have seen how, in the AIDS counsellors' work, ideas based on Family Systems Theory about the advantages of live supervision have materialized in three different procedures.

However, there remains a number of cases where the co-counsellors do intervene, but where their questions do not seem to work in ways that are suggested in the Family Systems Theory texts. These are the cases from which we may seek the 'latent functions', or unacknowledged interactional uses of the co-counsellors' interventions; and we will now turn to them.

Interventions that transcend the theory

Apart from the interventions where the co-counsellors analysably display and trade off their meta-position, and those where the co-counsellors' questions operate to dissolve interactional deadlocks, there are others, which seem not to correspond to the statements in Family Systems Theory. In other words, there are co-counsellors' interventions which seem not to have such uses or functions as are described in the Family Systems Theory texts.

In principle, it is quite possible that the counsellors can use *in a routine way* the technique they once have adopted. It is possible that in many instances the application of the live open supervision format of questioning can be 'incidental', so that this questioning technique does not have any particular interactional pay-offs at that specific occasion.[12] There are, indeed, cases in my corpus in which the use of the live open supervision format of questioning seems to be 'non-functional' and 'unmotivated' in this sense.

However, on closer analysis, some of the interventions that do not correspond to the statements of Family Systems Theory do betray their specific character and function; even though that is not something that is discussed in the counsellors' theory. This 'unacknowledged' interactional function has to do with the way that the questions establish the relation between the two counsellors, *vis-à-vis* their client(s). To put it briefly, the live open supervision format of questioning makes it interactionally less

---

[12] As Durkheim (1964) had pointed out, there is no reason why a social arrangement could not live its own life by the strength of 'inertia of habit', in spite of the fact that it is not functional to a larger social whole.

problematic for the counsellors to deliver potentially threatening questions to the clients. We will examine this in the remaining part of the chapter.

Extracts (9)–(12) are examples of the use of the co-counsellor's questions in addressing potentially threatening issues.

```
(9)    (E4-46)
 1   C1:          And you can- (.2) I'll se[nd you a letter with=
 2   C2:                                   [letter
 3   C1:          an appointment a[nd then you can let=
 4   P:                           [Yeah
 5   C1:          =me know whether you want to [keep it (or not).
 6   P:                                        [(No well) I'll
 7                keep walking (.3) anyway (.2) (which will make
 8                me a) (      ).
 9   C2:    ->    Doctor Kaufman I'd like (0.3) to a::sk (1.7)
10                what (.) at the moment hh (.2) is Michael's
11                main concern.
```

```
(10)   (E4-41)
 1   P:           =We:ll (.3) as you said to me this morning (it might
 2                have meant) (.) (me agonize more)( ) (it might
 3                have put-) it would have put extra [pressure on.
 4   C2:                                             [So can I be
 5                clear because I need some questions clear in my
 6                mi:nd,=does (.) Mr Brown agree with his wife
 7                about that. That he would have had it anyway.
 8                (.3)
 9   P:           Ye:s
10   ( ):         ((Clears throat))
11   C2:          hh okay h
12                (1.6)
13   C2:    ->    I have one question more Doctor Jay and then (.)
14                perhaps then more questions need to be asked.=I'd
15                like to know: (1.8) wh-what Mr Brown thinks:
16                (.) Helena's greatest concern is having heard this
17                conversation toda:y?
```

```
(11)   (E4-46)
 1   C1:          I mean (.) clearly already there's a difference
 2                between you and Harry because Harry got ill
 3                when you were feeling well.
 4                (.)
 5   P:           Mm
 6   C2:    ->    Doctor Kaufman there's one other question that
 7                (0.2) Michael is (1.2) leading me to. .hh If
```

```
8                    Michael became ill: (0.7) how would he want us
9                    to treat him,
10                   (.4)
11      C2:   ->     That- .hhh say he became very ill (0.3) and we
12                   needed to do things (.) that you as doctors
13                   felt would be:: (0.6) life sustaining.=Keep his
14                   life [o:n, what's his view=
15      C1:          [Mm
16      C2:          =about that for himself.
```

```
(12)    (E4-46)
        ((This exchange takes place a few moments after the one in extract
        (9).))
1       C1:          Can I (s[ay) what's your greatest (0.6) fear=
2       C2:                   [(      )
3       C1:          =for th- what might happen.
4                    (0.3)
5       P:           My greatest fear:?
6       C1:          Mm
7                    (0.7)
8       P:           Uh::m (1.5) Well obviously at the moment I mean
9                    I don't (.) particularly want to get AIDS or
10                   nothing like that. (0.5) You know (.) but I
11                   still suppose there's- there is that on the
12                   back of your mind still. And I know I've got
13                   the er HIV, (.) but I don't know how far (0.5)
14                   into AIDS I a:m. (0.6) yet.=So:
15                   [I don't know. (I don't [like to be)
16      C2:          [Does-              [s-
17      C2:   ->     How much does (0.2) Michael want to know about
18                   (0.8) how far he's (in[to AIDS)
19      P:                              [Well I think I should
20                   know everything.=I think it's only- only right.
21                   (Isn't)    (it really).
22      C2:          [One other question first before we go into=
23      C1:          [Mm
24      C2:          =(what he might be doing) is that, .hhh (.7)
25            ->     What if he did get AIDS,=what does he think
26                   (0.7) will be: the (0.2) hardest thing for
27                   him.=What does he fear most.
```

The sequential location of the co-counsellors' interventions in (9)–
(12) is variable. Extracts (9) and (10) are examples of elicitation of a
fresh topic through C2's intervention. In extract (11) there is also an
intervention which introduces fresh thematic material; but in this
case, C2's enquiry does not constitute the beginning of a new

sequence in such a disjunctive way as the interventions in extracts (9) and (10) did. Finally, in extract (12), the co-counsellor's intervention, rather than adding new thematic material, only further develops a topic which has already been introduced.

The core of my argument regarding extracts like (9)–(12) is this: in cases which involve *potentially threatening and difficult topics*, counsellors can use the live supervision format of questioning, instead of 'direct' or unmediated questioning, as a strategic resource to alleviate the interactional complications involved in their questions. The mediated pattern of questioning makes it possible to *diffuse the interactional accountability* of the counsellors' actions.

Reducing the interactional accountability of asking a question

In (9)–(12), the co-counsellors' enquiries dealt with potentially threatening matters, which could be expected to be difficult for the clients to talk about. In (9) and (10), the enquiries involved the clients' biggest 'concerns'. As will be argued in the next chapter, asking about 'concerns' may involve indirect elicitation of fears and worries. In (11), the issue was 'life sustaining treatment' in case the patient got 'very ill'; and in (12), it was 'getting AIDS'. Using the live open supervision format of questioning renders enquiries about these issues interactionally less problematic.

The strategic advantage of the mediated pattern of questioning is built up step by step in the construction and delivery of the question. When using this pattern, the question is always initiated by the co-counsellor. However, she doesn't address the client (target of the question) but the main counsellor instead. How this is achieved was analysed in detail in the preceding chapter. It was also shown that when the clients comply with this participation framework, they do so by not aligning as addressees of C2s' turns (which in the first place is indicated by them withholding their answers before the question is relayed by C1s). Consequently, there is no mutual monitoring between C2 and P during the time that the question is first spelled out. A *social distance* is established, using local interactional means, between the questioner and the projected answerer. In terms of the immediate response, C2 is not accountable for her action to the client but rather to the other counsellor. As a result of all this, a question about potentially threatening matters, targeted to the client, has been spelled out at the end of the co-counsellor's initial turns, and *without* the client thus far having been directly asked that question. Or to put it in another way, C2 has 'asked the question without asking it'.

The following step, as we have seen, is that the main counsellor relays the question. If C2 was operating in the shield of de-intensified interactional accountability, does not the delivery of the question re-establish full accountability, now involving C1? That appears not to be the case, because *C1 is now doing something that was not initiated by herself*. C1 is indeed operating directly *vis-à-vis* the client and in that sense she is immediately accountable for her actions in relation to the client. But in the preceding chapter we saw how the main counsellors either relay the questions using non-verbal means, or design their turns with close reference to the co-counsellors' turns so as to show that they are renewing and redirecting the co-counsellors' questions. In either case, they are observably relaying the question initiated by someone else. The main counsellor commits herself to the question, but the question remains as something that the other counsellor initially asked; it remains 'somebody else's question'. So the main counsellor is accountably asking someone else's question, not her own.

As a result of all this, in the standard sequences employing mediated questioning a question is posed to the client collaboratively by the two counsellors, without either of them being fully and singly accountable for asking it. This has two important implications.

First, the issues raised in these questions may thereby be marked as 'delicate' issues (Schegloff 1980). More concretely, through the application of the mediated pattern of questioning, the subject-matter of the questions may be constituted as an issue or issues that are sensitive in this particular interaction. This is achieved via the very social distance that appears between the original deviser of the question and the projected answerer, and by the alignment of the two counsellors as questioners. The questions are something that neither of the counsellors chooses to present to the client(s) in a direct fashion. This structurally embedded 'expressive caution' (cf. Atkinson and Drew 1979) in delivering the question may imply on the one hand courtesy and deference for the clients' feelings and on the other an invitation for the client to treat the issues raised as real and serious matters that do concern him or her.[13]

The other implication for the counsellors' collaboration in delivering the question to the client involves the conditional relevance of the client's answer. The diffused accountability does not reduce the conditional relevance of the client's answer as the second part of the adjacency pair: the question is there, establishing fully an expectation for the answer to appear next. Even more, perhaps: two counsellors, instead of one, have now committed themselves to the question and the consequent conditional relevance of an answer.

When the live open supervision format of questioning is used for delivering questions about potentially threatening topics, these features intrinsic to the pattern are mobilized as powerful resources in eliciting the client's talk. In general terms, that was the case in extracts (9)–(12). However, these intrinsic resources of the live open supervision format of questioning can also be used in a more specific way to establish a particular differentiation of the local moral profiles of the two counsellors. In order to explore this, we will have to return to the data, and closely examine a few single cases.

Sweet and sour

The live open supervision form of questioning makes it possible for two counsellors to adjust and control the degree of threat involved in their questions. In this adjustment of threat, one of the counsellors can adopt a demanding profile, while the other can take a more cooperative position, asking questions that are less threatening or less demanding for the client. This may be an effective strategy in eliciting clients' talk.

It has to be emphasized, however, that not very many of my empirical cases demonstrably involve this kind of adjustment. But even those few cases suffice as evidence for the *possibility* of this kind of practice; and in those few cases, it seems that the counsellors skilfully make use of it.

---

[13] The accents of reality involved in the counsellors' questions will be examined more closely in chapter 7.

As was pointed out earlier in this chapter, in some cases the co-counsellor's intervention constitutes a way out from an interactional deadlock. In those cases, the co-counsellor's question can involve a more cooperative position *vis-à-vis* the client, in contrast with the position that the principal counsellor has adopted in the immediately preceding talk. That is what happened in extract (7), a part of which is shown below.

```
(13)  (Section of (7))
 1   C1:        *( ).* Having heard what Mr Wood said (.) that
 2               e:ven if he was negative. (.2) It wouldn't make him
 3               conduct his life any different. (.7) What- (3) effect
 4               would that have: if:-
 5   W:         .hhhh
 6   C1:        I mean what are the things that it [would affect if=
 7   W:                                            [hhhhhhhh
 8   C1:        =he was positive.
 9   W:         gh hhhhh heh hh
10   C1:        Umh:?
11   W:         .hhhhhh I just don't know. (.4) I'm afraid, (.3) .hhh
12               (2.0) I'm in a frame of mind- (.2) mind at the moment
13               (.2) .hhh (3.0) that I'm not so (lots) of use: f(h)or
14               hypothe(h)ti(h)cal things.=.hhh I'm not- (.2) err: (.3)
15               very useful to you I mean.=Because (.2) .hh (.5) I feel
16               that as if- (1.6) the things which are actually happening
17               (.4) are as much as I can cope wi[th.
18   C1:                                          [Yes:. That's- (.3)
19               well- (2) I ag- I understand t[hat.
20   W:                                        [.hhhhh (.2) gheh hhhh heh
21               .hhh The world could fall apart. (.5) At the moment it
22               isn't (tearful) (.) and [so- (.2) th- I just=
23   ( )                                 [No.
24   W:         =have to say (.) well .hhh It has to get on with it.
25               (.3)
26   C1:        But then let's take [ourselves- let's-]
27   W:                             [(      ) be ru]de
28               but (.) I (.) just how [ I feel      ] at the moment.
29   C2:   ->                          [ DO THEY-]
30   C2:   ->   (       ) do they want to know the results, have
31               they not been told the [result.
32   C1:                                [Have you not been told.=
33   W:         =Yes we've been told we've been negative as far as
34               I'm awa:re
```

As was pointed out earlier, in (13) the principal counsellor's aggressive line of questioning is responded to by the client's firm refusal to cooperate. By abandoning the hypothetical format of questioning, and by focusing away from the implications of the positive test result, C2 (lines 29–31) offers in her intervention a less threatening question for W to answer.[14] As a result, W begins to cooperate in answering. Thus, in (13), the local contingencies of the interaction (W's refusal to cooperate with C1's questions) prompted C2's adoption of a more cooperative profile in her intervention.

The differentiation of the two counsellors' interactional profiles can also operate in and through the two-step delivery of the co-counsellor's question. As was argued in chapter 4, when both counsellors produce their versions of the enquiry, there often occurs a slight transformation of the meaning of the question. In chapter 4, this transformation was described primarily as a 'side-product' of the counsellors' effort to avoid mechanical repetition and redundancy. However, the transformation of meaning can also be used as a strategic resource. In such usage, the principal counsellor can adopt a different position *vis-à-vis* the client from the one taken by C2. Depending on the contingencies of the interaction, this position can be more or less demanding towards the client.

Extract (14) is an example of the principal counsellor adopting a more demanding and tougher position when rephrasing the question. C1's version has more negative implications for the client: the choice of the temporal reference (substituting 'Christmas' for 'next few days'), C1 emphasizes the importance of the days that will be spoiled.

```
(14)   (Section of (8))
 1    C2:      Who do you think Doctor Kaufman will
 2             suffer most over the next few day:s if (0.2) Doug goes
 3             home without the treatment that we know might have
 4             a chance of helping him,=will it be hi:m? .h Will it be
 5             Philip having to bring him again?=Will it be his
```

---

[14] Remarkably, the way that C1 relays C2's question in line 32 (by choosing to relay the factual query and leaving aside the subjectively focused one) further de-intensifies the potential threat. The client's response (lines 33–4) is targeted to this de-intensified query: W describes the factual situation and does not tell whether they want to know. Therefore, the co-counsellor's intervention appears to initiate a two-stage de-intensification of the initially more aggressive questioning.

```
6              mother?=His father?
7    P:        .hhhh=
8    C2:       =[(                      )
9    C1:       =[Who will have the worst Christmas if you (0.2) go
10             ho:me Dou:g?
```

C1's tougher position is in line with and advancing the counsellors' effort to convince P to remain in hospital for treatment: by emphasizing the importance of the days that will be affected by P going home, C1 increases the pressure for P to stay in the hospital.[15]

P does not cooperate in dealing with the tougher version of the question. As the extension of extract (14) below indicates, P constructs his answer (arrow 1) so as to avoid any reference to 'Christmas'. After P's response, however, C1 renews the temporal reference to 'Christmas' in her follow-up question (arrow 2).

```
(14)  (Extension)
8     C1:            =[Who will have the worst Christmas if you (0.2)
9                    go ho:me Dou:g?
10    P:    (1) ->   Well if I go ho:me (0.8) .hh and I do what I do:
11                   (1.8) normally (1.0) it won't affect anybody. (.)
12                   Be[cause-
13    C1:   (2) ->      [But if you go home and you can't do what you
14                   do normally: and you get more breathless and you
15                   need everybody doing everything for you: (2.0)
16                   how will that be that Christmas for- for you: and
17                   for everybody else.
```

Perhaps more interesting, however, are the cases where the principal counsellor takes a more cooperative position through the way that she relays the co-counsellor's question. A single case study can most effectively demonstrate this possibility. Extract (15) below, which begins with the materials presented above in extract (9) and ends with materials from extract (12), is illustrative in this respect.

---

[15] It is notable that P produces an inbreath in line 7. It is possible to think that in producing the more aggressive version of the question, C1 orients to this inbreath. It is hearable as an indication of P's intention to begin a turn (cf. Jefferson 1981). Through his inbreath, P can be heard to display his preparedness to cooperate in responding to C2's question; and after having perceived P's preparedness to cooperate, C1 is in a position where she can produce the stronger version of the enquiry. The video, unfortunately, does not give any clear impression whether or not P's inbreath is an indication of his intention to begin a turn.

(15) (Extension of (9) and (12))
1   C1:   And you can- (.2) I'll se[nd you a letter with=
2   C2:   [letter
3   C1:   an appointment a[nd then you can let me know=
4   P: [Yeah
5   C1:   =whether you want to [keep it (or not).
6   P: [(No well) I'll keep walking
7   (.3) anyway (.2) (which will make me a) (   ).
8   C2:   Doctor Kaufman I'd like (0.3) to a::sk (1.7) what
9   (.) at the moment hh (.2) is Michael's main concern.
10   (0.2)
11 C1:   Yes.=Michael what's your main concern today.
12   (2.4)
13 P: It depends (o:n) I suppose what you (.) mean by
14   concer:n,=I'm not really uh:m
15   (0.4)
16 C2:   Or [what's top of his mi:nd.]
17 P: [worried about anything a]t the moment.
18   (0.6)
19 C1:   Wha- [what d'you most want from us today.
20 P: [Well er
21   (1.6)
22 P: Uh:m: (1.5) well it would be nice to sort of sort
23   me- me knees out (I think but er u-unless er)
24 C1:   Mm hm
25   (0.2)
26 C1:   [So that's one thing we can]
27 P: [S o r t that out (.2) y]eah.
28 C1:   look at ortho[paedically,=but what else?
29 P: [Yeah.
30   (1.0)
31 P: Uh:m (1.0) I'm not sure really I've never thought of
32   it (.4) anything.
33   (0.2)
34 C2:   [(Wh)-
35 P: [(But) you've been helping me all the (.) last
36   little while,
37   (0.2)
38 C2:   What- (0.2) I mean what (.) Michael mentioned at-
39   initially is that you know (0.2) he didn't have any
40   concerns but he's been feeling funny again,=is that
41   a worry to him or is it no problem to him that he
42   feels funny.
43   (0.3)
44 C1:   Mm=
45 P: =I don't know: I- I just go th- er through stages of

```
46                    uh:m (1.1) you know I mean I've had a really (0.2)
47                    sort of a quite a hectic weekend, quite a busy
48                    ti:me,=and it's not as though I've been sitting down
49                    moping again. (0.6) But you know it's just sort of
50                    like as though- as though it just clicks:. (0.5) And
51                    then I think it will all
52                    (     ) what's going to happen (wi:th) (.)
53                    (so and so) if you know what I mean.
54    C1:             Can I (s[ay) what's your greatest (0.6) fear for=
55    C2:                  [(          )
56    C1:             =th- what might happen.
57                    (0.3)
58    P:              My greatest fear:?
59    C1:             Mm
60                    (0.7)
61    P:              Uh::m (1.5) Well obviously at the moment I mean I
62                    don't (.) particularly want to get AIDS or nothing
63                    like that. (0.5) You know (.) but I still suppose
64                    there's- there is that on the back of your mind
65                    still. And I know I've got the er HIV, (.) but I
66                    don't know how far (0.5) into AIDS I a:m. (0.6)
67                    yet.=So: I don't know. (I don't like to be)
```

In (15) above, C2 initiates a series of enquiries in line 8 by her
question

> Doctor Kaufman I'd like (0.3) to a::sk (1.7) what (.) at the moment
> hh (.2) is Michael's main concern.

C1 relays this question by saying in line 11

> Yes.=Michael what's your main concern today.

C1's turn almost repeats C2's initial question. However, there is
some difference, which may not be insignificant. Most notably, the
choice of the words referring to time has changed: whereas C2
spoke about main concerns 'at the *moment*', C1 says 'to*day*'.

'To*day*' is the day when P comes to the clinic for his regular
medical checks and counselling; 'at the *moment*' points to his present existence in general, without a specifying frame. 'At the
moment' can thus be heard to refer to present concerns as they
appear to the patient beyond or prior to any instrumentalities,
whereas 'to*day*' can be heard to refer more specifically to the concerns as they can be presented to the clinicians. In other words, a
possible hearing of the transformation from 'at the *moment*' to

'today' is a shift from an enquiry aimed at disclosing P's inner fears and experience as they appear to the patient himself to an enquiry aimed at eliciting what P wants to present about himself to the clinicians in this particular context.

If there is indeed such a difference between C2's question and its reformulation by C1, then by implication the counsellors also adopt different roles *vis-à-vis* the patient. C2 more actively seeks the disclosure of P's inner experience, whereas C1 deals with him in a more instrumental frame. In the unfolding of the interaction, the questions and answers operating within the instrumental frame are treated as less demanding than those eliciting the client's disclosure of his inner experience.

As the interaction unfolds further, the differentiation between the two counsellors' roles is first solidified, and afterwards dissolved. The differentiation becomes apparent when both counsellors offer their clarifications of the initial enquiry, after the patient has claimed that the answer depends on what the counsellors mean by concern. C2's clarification of the question is in line 16:

> Or what's top of his mi:nd.

By referring to the 'top of P's mind', the clarification appears to indicate nicely C2's orientation to disclosure of P's experience. As was argued above, P's claim that he is not 'worried about anything at the moment' seems to work both as a completion of his response to the initial enquiry, and as an answer to C2's clarifying enquiry. A new clarification from C1 follows in line 19:

> Wha- what d'you most want from us today.

This spells out equally nicely C1's instrumental orientation: the time reference 'today' is now accompanying a question about what P wants from the counsellors (or from the whole medical team). Instead of disclosing his 'mind', P is asked to name what he wants from his co-interactants in this particular situation.

It is interesting that in his initial response, in lines 13–14 and 17, P had adopted the time reference 'at the moment', used initially by C2. Even more interestingly, this temporal reference was used in connection with the object 'worries', when P claimed that 'I'm not really (...) worried about anything at the moment.' So the patient appeared to use the time reference 'at the moment', first, in connection with a reluctant, less than fully cooperative response; and second, attached to an experiential, or mental object. In other words, in his reluctant response the patient seemed to orient to the initial formulation of the enquiry produced by C2 and seemed to interpret that as indeed concerning his mental states.

P's second response in lines 22–3 is still reluctant. It appears after a long gap (1.6 sec. in line 21 and 1.5 sec. in line 22), and is vaguely marked as uncertain, with the uncompleted qualification 'but er u-unless er'. However, in comparison to the initial response, this is more cooperative; now P does name an object to be dealt with.

> Uh:m: (1.5) well it would be nice to sort of sort me- me
> knees out (I think but er u-unless er)

Apparently, this utterance by P responds to *C1's* clarification of the initial question: it is about the 'things that the patient wants from the clinic today' (C1's version) rather than about the 'top of his mind' (C2's version).

In summary, then, the first cooperative response from the patient was elicited by re-focusing C2's initial enquiry from the experience of the patient to his wants regarding the services of the clinic today.

However, the first collaborative response then leads to new enquiries. In lines 26 and 28, C1 categorizes the 'knees' as a matter that can be looked at 'orthopaedically', and elicits something else, thus establishing the present interactional setting (i.e. the counselling session) as something designated for dealing with different kinds of matters. Turning down 'knees' as an appropriate topic, then, appears to trade off the distinction between psychological/social on one hand and medical on the other: the present setting is for the former rather than for the latter.

C1's action here is ambivalent in an interesting way. In her earlier utterance, she has invited the patient to name what he most wants from the counsellors/the clinic today. As was argued above, this establishes an instrumental frame for the discourse. But by turning down 'sorting out P's knees' as a relevant issue, C1 appears to distance herself from this instrumental orientation. If 'knees' is not an appropriate object to be talked about, but P is still asked to name 'what he wants today' (instead of being encouraged to disclose his mind), it may be indeed difficult for him to find an appropriate response.

Perhaps predictably, then, C1's enquiry 'but what else?' in line 28 turns out to be unsuccessful: in lines 31–2 and 35–6 P claims not having thought anything else, afterwards complimenting the counsellors for having helped him earlier.[16] At this point, then, the participants are in observable interactional difficulties: the client has not produced the kind of 'concerns' that the counsellors have been pursuing through their questions.

Afterwards, in lines 38–42, C2 makes a fresh start. In a manner discussed earlier in this chapter, her question opens up an alternative route for the participants to progress along. C2's question retrieves an object P has mentioned earlier during the session ('feeling funny'), and topicalizes that together with P's earlier statement about not having concerns (lines 13, 14 and 17).[17] It is noticeable that C2's fresh enquiry refocuses on the experiential sphere and 'disclosure' orientation: what it topicalizes are the funny feelings that the patient had mentioned earlier, inviting P to say whether they are a worry for him.

Normally (as here) using the live open supervision format of questioning for finding an alternative way leads to an instant success. In lines 45–53, P produces an extended answer, where he reports his 'moping'. At the end of his response, he makes an indirect reference to his fears concerning the future: 'what's going to *h*appen (wi:th) (.) (so and so) if you know what I mean.' This provides the main counsellor an opportunity to deliver a focused enquiry: in lines 54 and 56, she asks a question, focusing openly on P's fears of the future:[18]

Can I (say) what's your greatest (.6) fear for th- what might happen.

---

[16] This compliment appears to orient to the sensibilities of the interaction at this juncture. By complimenting the counsellors P shows that he appreciates their work, in spite of the fact that right now he is not offering them the kind of answers they are eliciting.

[17] This technique of eliciting P's talk will be discussed at somewhat greater length in chapter 6.

[18] The first part of C1's utterance 'Can I (say)' appears quite intriguing, given that C1 is the main counsellor whose task in the first place is the allocation of turns. Probably C1 has detected here C2's intention to produce a follow-up question for P – which intention is confirmed by C2's poorly recorded action, possibly turn-beginning, in line 55 – and uses the preface 'Can I (say)' as a device of politely turning down the co-counsellor's further action.

By the completion of this question, the main counsellor, who initially adopted a less demanding, instrumental orientation, has realigned herself to the elicitation of P's experience.

In summary, and with the risk of over-simplification, what happened in the course of the interaction in (15) can be summarized as a six-step procedure.

(1)   First C2 makes an enquiry eliciting a disclosure of P's feelings and worries. This is met by resistance from P.

(2)   The initial enquiry is transformed by C1 into an instrumentally oriented one. P cooperates in dealing with this.

(3)   C1 turns down P's offer of an 'instrumental' issue to be dealt with, and elicits something else. However, the renewed enquiry is so designed that its focal object is difficult to identify.

(4)   P fails to cooperate with this new enquiry.

(5)   C2 offers P a way out by a fresh enquiry. This re-establishes the initial orientation to disclosing the experience. P cooperates with this enquiry.

(6)   C1 aligns herself to a line of questioning oriented to the disclosure of experience.

In the course of this procedure, C1 temporarily adopted a less demanding position *vis-à-vis* the patient, transforming the enquiry initiated by C2 into one that turned out to be easier to handle for the patient. However, this less demanding position was only a temporary move, which secured P's first cooperation. After having obtained the first cooperation, the counsellors each made further moves which led to the establishment of the relevancies of the initial enquiry of C2.

Extract (16) below is another single case where the principal counsellor adopts a less demanding position.

```
(16)  (E4-46)
 1    C1:    I mean (.) clearly already there's a difference
 2            between you and Harry because Harry got ill when
 3            you were feeling well.
 4            (.)
 5    P:     Mm
 6    C2:    Doctor Kaufman there's one other question that (0.2)
 7            Michael is (1.2) leading me to. .hh If Michael
```

```
 8            became ill: (0.7) how would he want us to treat him,
 9            (.4)
10   C2:      That- .hhh say he became very ill (0.3) and we
11            needed to do things (.) that you as doctors felt
12            would be:: (0.6) life sustaining.=Keep his life
13            [o:n, what's his view about that for himself.
14   C1:      [Mm
15            (1.5)
16   P:       I think it depends how: (.3) really (I could-) how
17            ill I was I suppose in- (.2) [in the long run.
18   C1:                                  [Well supposing you
19            were too ill to make a decisio[n.
20   C2:                                    [Mm::
21            (1.5)
22   C1:      and it was- (.4) ulti[mately it- it is really down=
23   P:                           [Mm
24   C1:      =to the doctors in the end any[way to decide=
25   P:                                     [Mm
26   C1:      =whether to go on battling and battling .hh[h
27   P:                                                  [Mm
28   C1:      to save someone's life against all the odds when
29            it'[s- (.2) seems to be ( ) against them.=bu[t-
30   P:         [Mm                                       [Mm
31            (0.4)
32   C1:      supposing (0.5) ((Clears throat)) you were (0.7)
33            very ill and the doctors had to make that decision
34            it would obviously be helpful to them to know your
35            [views on the matter.
36   P:       [Mm
37            (0.2)
38   C1:      .hh Although people's view[s change.=they might=
39   P:                                [Mm
40   C1:      =not be the [same next week or next month as they=
41   P:                   [Mm
42   C1:      =are toda[y?=but
43   P:                [Mm
44            (.3)
45   C1:      what are they toda:y .hh (0.4) about if[:
46   P:                                             [Mm
47            (0.2)
48   C1:      you were very i:ll
49            (.)
50   P:       We[ll uh:m
51   C1:        [would you want them to do everything (.3)
52            absolutely possible [to save your li:fe.
53   P:                           [Hm
```

54	P:	Well if a <u>machine</u> is sort of keeping me going well
55		then obviously I would (1.0) probably would want-
56		want you to turn it off:.=if it was the machi:<u>ne</u>

In (16) above, the co-counsellor's question is about P's preferences concerning life-sustaining treatment (lines 6–8 and 10–13).[19] In his first response (lines 16–17) P, however, does not offer his preferences, but points out that his view depends on 'how ill' he would become. In response to this, the principal counsellor offers clarification of the question. It is delivered in three parts; after each part of the clarification, there is a slot where P could take the floor. In the course of the production of the clarification, C1 in various ways plays down the threat involved in the question.

The first part of C1's clarification is in lines 18 and 19. By describing P's hypothetical illness in terms of being unable to make a decision, C1 focuses away from the medical description of issues directly related to life and death ('life-sustaining things') that were mentioned in C2's initial question. By choosing the new description, C1 adopts a perspective that is attentive to P's point of view. Thereby, she takes a more cooperative position vis-à-vis the client. P however, does not give his answer after this first clarification: he only produces a continuer, and after a gap of 1.5 sec., C1 continues with more clarification.

C1's second clarification is in a long stretch of talk in lines 22–35. This stretch of talk is built from several turn-construction units; but it is designed so as to forestall P's response before the end of the clarification. In this second clarification, C1 emphasizes how the decision regarding the treatment belongs ultimately to the doctors. Thereby, she mitigates the consequentiality of the client's answer. It is notable that in this part of the clarification, C1 returns to the

---

[19] C2's question is offered in two parts, the latter elaborating the first. The first version of C2's question is hearably incomplete for two reasons. First, its semantic content is unclear in this institutional context. An HIV-positive haemophilic patient can hardly be expected to be able to tell the members of a medical team how he would want to be treated if he became ill: the question needs to be specified. Second, the slightly rising intonation at the end of the first version of C2's question (line 8) makes it also hearable as incomplete. C1 treats it accordingly: she does not begin to relay the question by turning to P or by rephrasing it, but remains silent and oriented to C2. In other words, C1 remains aligned as a recipient of C2's talk, and accordingly C2 produces a more specific version of her question in lines 10–13.

descriptions of a life-and-death situation. These descriptions are, however, presented in the third person ('whether to go on battling and battling (...) to save someone's *l*ife against all the odds when it's- (.2) seems to be ( ) against them') and thereby only indirectly focused on P. In connection to P himself, C1 only refers to 'that decision' (line 33).

After the completion of line 34, the client would have had another chance for proffering his view. In the absence of P's immediate response, however, C1 continues her clarification. The consequentiality of P's answer is mitigated once again, now by the counsellor pointing out that people's views may change. This implies that P is not expected to proffer his final and conclusive words about the matter. After C1 has returned to the hypothetical question format in lines 45 and 48 (thus possibly projecting the renewal of the initial question) P begins a turn by 'Well' (line 50). At this point, then, P has finally given signs of cooperativeness (even though the 'Well' projects a dispreferred answer) after all the clarifications by the principal counsellor.

The counsellor, however, does not give space for the client's response yet. In lines 51–2, she completes her question. Now she returns explicitly to life-and-death-related description ('would you *w*ant them to do everything (.3) absolutely possible to save your li:fe.'). This description, however, is now framed so as to preserve P's 'agency'. It is not a description of a hypothetical situation which P is in, but a description of a choice that he can make. It is also notable that C1 becomes this explicit only after the client has displayed his willingness to answer through the turn beginning in line 50.

Again, with the risk of over-simplification, the interaction in (16) can be described as follows.

1.   Co-counsellor delivers a threatening question.
2.   The client asks for clarification.
3.   Principal counsellor produces a series of clarifications which play down the demanding and threatening aspects of the question.
4.   Client produces his answer.

The single-case analyses presented above have not brought forward any unified pattern in the counsellors' adjustment of the degree of threat involved in their questions. Whether or not the the counsellors move between the demanding and cooperative versions of their questions, and what direction this movement takes, is dependent on the local contingencies of the interaction. It is crucial, however, that the apparatus of 'live open supervision' provides an *operating space* for the counsellors, which *makes it possible* for them to move between different versions of delicate, potentially threatening enquiries. Such a space would probably not be as unproblematically available if the counsellors were to use only unmediated questioning, even with two counsellors in the same room. This operating space appears to be one of the resources available for the counsellors in eliciting patients' talk about issues that they initially may be reluctant to talk about.

Multiplicity of interactional uses

In this chapter, we have examined some interactional uses that the mediated pattern of questioning may have in AIDS counselling sessions. The chapter has had an explorative character: its results are more like hypotheses than firmly grounded conclusions.

Preliminary as they are, the observations made in this chapter nevertheless give rise to three further comments. First, they confirm the assumption raised at the end of the preceding chapter: the interactional uses of the technique of live open supervision seem not to be limited to those discussed in the Family Systems Theory textbooks. Even if this chapter has not specified all the unacknowledged or 'latent' functions, it has demonstrated some directions where they can be found.

Second, the observations in this chapter also show that there appears not to be a single overarching function of the live open supervision format of questioning. As with any other interactional device, the systematic manipulation of the participation framework involved in this type of questioning can serve a multiplicity of purposes, depending on the local circumstances and, in the last analysis, the choices that the speakers make in those circumstances.

Third, on a more general level of analysis these results suggest that an interactional technique can have a 'life of its own', as it were. By this I mean that as soon as the counsellors have established a pattern of interaction that can be routinely enacted (such as the live open supervision format of questioning), this interaction pattern is available for them as a vehicle for many kinds of purposes. The data analysis in this chapter has shown that not all these purposes need to be related to the original, intended purpose that the technique was consciously created for. In AIDS counselling, the management of the talk about potentially threatening and delicate issues is a persistent challenge for the professionals (and clients as well). It is not surprising, therefore, that the live open supervison format of questioning has been successfully used as a vehicle for this.

This chapter closes the part of the book where 'participation framework' has been the key analytical concept. Chapters 3, 4 and 5 have demonstrated the analytical potential of this concept in the investigation of institutional talk. In substantial terms, the examination of the participation frameworks related to 'circular questioning' and 'live open supervision' has shown in detail *where* the power of these practices based on Family Systems Theory resides. In this respect, the (Conversation Analytical) study of participation frameworks has been able to complement the self-understanding of Family Systems Theory.

The remaining two full chapters of the book will concentrate on the organization of talk about a single, potentially delicate issue, central for AIDS counselling: the patients' future. However, we will not look at the matter from the point of view of participation frameworks, but instead from the point of view of the task-oriented features of sequence organization and turn design.

6

Addressing 'dreaded issues'

One of the central tasks of AIDS counsellors – regardless of their theoretical orientation – is to help clients to come to terms with the uncertainty of their future. In pre-test counselling, counsellors have to prepare the clients for a possible positive test result; and in counselling with HIV-positive patients, they have to help the clients to live with the knowledge of prospective illnesses and a shortened life-span.

Counsellors at the Royal Free Hospital have particularly emphasized the importance of this aspect of their work. They have pointed out that AIDS counsellors face three therapeutic options in dealing with the clients' fears and worries concerning their future (Bor and Miller 1988). One of these is to reassure the client that everything will be all right with him or her. In that case, the counsellor will probably collude with the patient's denial of the severity of the problem. The second option is to wait until the patient has developed symptoms related to AIDS and counsel him or her at that point. In such situation, however, the patient and those close to him or her can be unprepared for the 'bad news'. They are likely to be 'resistant' to any intervention by the counsellor. The third option, favoured by the counsellors at the Royal Free Hospital, is to 'use hypothetical and future-oriented questions at the right moment with patients while they are still relatively well' (Bor and Miller 1988: 401).

A central part of AIDS counselling based on Family Systems Theory is to facilitate talk about the clients' fears concerning their future. Counsellors want to encourage their clients to talk about issues like illness, deterioration, pain, separation and death well in advance of their possible occurrence in the patients' lives. By addressing these 'dreaded issues' in advance, counsellors in this clinic try to help the patients to prepare themselves so that they have better chances of coping when the situation is at hand (see Miller and Bor 1988; Bor and Miller 1988).

In the Family Systems approach, 'hypothetical future-oriented questions' constitute a central tool in management of the talk about the clients' future. The paradigmatic form of these questions can be paraphrased as 'If so-and-so happened, what would this-and-that aspect of your life be like.'

Naturally occurring examples will be analysed below (see e.g. extracts 29–31 in this chapter, and many more in the following chapter). According to the counsellors' theory, this type of question can help clients to talk openly about their fears concerning 'dreaded issues' such as loss, disfigurement, death and dying. The hypothetical questions also indicate to the clients that the counsellor 'is not afraid to address these issues with the patient' (Miller and Bor 1988: 17).

But other kinds of questions also have to be asked when talking about the clients' future. These other questions are not very much discussed in the counsellors' own theory. As will be shown in the data analysis, these are often needed in order to prepare an adequate conversational environment for hypothetical questions.

In this chapter and chapter 7, the counsellors' task of 'addressing dreaded issues' (Bor and Miller 1988) will give direction to the analysis of data. We will examine how the potentially delicate talk about the future is managed. Certain features of turn design and sequence organization will be found to be of crucial strategic importance in the counsellors' work of helping the clients to talk about their future.

By virtue of focusing on particular questioning techniques, these chapters will resemble closely chapters 3–5, where 'circular questions' and 'live open supervision' were examined. However, the analytical tools by which we will approach the questioning involved in talk about the future will be different from the tools that were used in the preceding chapters.

As we have seen, the specific character of live open supervision and circular questioning arises from the particular relations that these techniques establish between speakers, hearers, and the words spoken. These relations were most fruitfully analysable using the concept of the 'participation framework'. 'Hypothetical future-oriented questions' and other questioning techniques involved in talk about the clients' future do not, however, specify the speakers' or hearers' relation to the words spoken. Consequently, various different participation frameworks can be activated in these questions,[1] and therefore, the specific features of these questions are better analysable from a different theoretical perspective.

In what follows, this perspective will first be outlined, after which we will turn to the data analysis again.

Turn design and sequence organization in informal settings

We will examine the the the questioning involved in 'future talk' from the point of view of *turn design* and *sequence organization*.

Drew and Heritage (1992; also Heritage and Greatbatch 1991) point out the complexity of the analytical tasks in examining interaction in informal institutional settings. In these, it is not likely that 'a single recursive procedure (such as is found in special turn-taking procedures) can be found that would pinpoint the participants' turn-by-turn instantiations of institutional role-based identities as a single stroke' (Drew and Heritage 1992: 28). In other words, in informal settings – of which counselling is one – the participants' orientation to their institutional identities is likely to be found in various aspects of talk, and not in just one single organizing principle such as turn-taking. Moreover, the multiple interactional events that may incorporate the institutional identities are possibly of a non-recurrent type, i.e. they may be located in individual sequences of talk rather than being continuously present throughout the encounter.

Drew and Heritage suggest that the institutional character of talk in informal settings can be found in *various aspects of turn design and sequence organization*. 'Systematic aspects of the organization of sequences (and of turn design within sequences) having to do

---

[1] This is to say that 'future-oriented hypothetical questions' and other questioning techniques involved in talk about the clients' future can be embedded in the 'circular questioning' format, as well as in the 'live open supervision' format. We will see below some extracts in which all the three techniques are used simultaneously.

with such matters as the opening and closing of encounters, with the ways in which information is requested, delivered, and received, with the design of referring expressions etc. are now beginning to emerge as facets of the ways in which the "institutionality" of such encounters are managed' (1992: 28).

Turn design and sequence organization could be described as 'umbrella' concepts, which cover a very wide range of phenomena. The management of the participation framework involves one aspect of 'turn design' and 'sequence organization': different participation roles are assumed and ascribed by the participants through designing their turns and connecting successive turns in specific ways. However, there are infinitely many *other* aspects of turn design and sequence organization which also may, in a close analysis, turn out to incorporate the specific, institutional character of counselling.

Which aspects of sequence organization and turn design operate as vehicles of institutional talk in a given setting is in the first place an empirical question. The earlier CA research, however, provides some key findings which can be used as signposts to possible directions for new studies.

Sequence organization and institutional tasks

By *sequence organization* the CA practitioners refer to patterns and structures controlling the relation between successive turns (and successive activities accomplished through turns) in talk-in-interaction. Whatever activities are done by the participants of an interaction, their accomplishment involves organization of sequences (Drew and Heritage 1992: 37–42). Questions, requests, offers, blaming, etc. – any activity in talk-in-interaction – are made possible by virtue of the participants' orientation to sequential patterns which control the relation of successive utterances. Questioning is possible by virtue of the participants' orientation to the structural relation between questions and answers; blaming is possible by virtue of the participants' orientation to the structural relation between blame and rebuttal/admittance, and so on. The activities arising from the participants' institutional roles and tasks are no exception here: they also are made possible by the sequence organization.

Two examples, arising from empirical CA research, of sequences that serve as vehicles of institutional activities are presented below.

Maynard (1991a; 1991b; 1992) has studied the ways in which clinicians give negative diagnostic news to the parents of children who have been found to be mentally retarded. His key observation is that medical professionals, before giving the bad news, often first elicit the parents' view. After the parents have given their view, the clinicians proffer the diagnosis. Maynard argues that this three-step sequence, which he calls a 'perspective display series', accommodates the participants' institutional tasks and roles in several ways. Most importantly, perhaps, it makes it possible for the clinicians to proffer the distressing diagnostic news in a manner that 'confirms and co-implicates recipient's perspective' (Maynard 1992: 352). Thereby, the possibilities of open disagreement are minimized. Secondly, the 'perspective display series' also incorporates the difference between the parents' 'lay' knowledge and the clinicians' 'expert' knowledge, as the parents' knowledge is systematically framed as tentative, and the clinicians occupy the position where they can confirm, elaborate or correct the parents' views (Maynard 1991b).

Another sequence frequently used in client–professional interaction was studied by Wowk (1989). Her data were from counselling interviews with patients who were due to undergo, or who had recently undergone, surgery for the removal of breast cancer. Wowk argued that a key aspect of the counsellors' work during a session was to facilitate the translation of general emotional terms (such as anxious, worried, or depressed) into a more specific sense related to the occasion of its use and its meaning to each individual patient. This unpacking was regularly done through the counsellors producing what Wowk called *candidate elaborations*: the counsellor suggests a detailed sense of what the anxiety/worry/depression might mean for this individual patient, who in turn is in the position of being able to accept or reject the candidate elaboration.

In an interesting way, the institutionally specific sequences briefly described above originate from *ordinary conversation*. Maynard (1991b: 167–8; 1992: 334) points out that the 'perspective display series' resembles closely various 'pre-sequences' often used in conversation; and according to Wowk (1989), the operation that the 'candidate elaboration' does is a variation of the generic activity called 'unpacking of a gloss', a conversational practice analysed originally by Jefferson (1985a). The sequential patterns that have their home-base in ordinary conversation can thus be systematically applied in institutional settings, so as to perform institutionally specific tasks.[2]

Turn design and institutional tasks

Turn design involves the details of the verbal construction through which the turn's activity is accomplished[3] (Drew and Heritage 1992: 32–3). Drew and Heritage put it this way: 'because there is always a range of alternative ways of saying something, a speaker's selection of a particular formulation will, unavoidably, tend to be heard as "motivated" and perhaps chosen' (1992: 36). Different ways of saying something (and of doing something) involve issues such as syntactic, lexical and prosodic selections. By choosing certain words instead of others, by employing certain syntactic constructions and in uttering words and sentences in certain ways, speakers may orient to their institutional tasks and roles. In short, the turn design may be a central vehicle for accomplishing institutional tasks.

Illustrative examples of institutionally relevant features of turn design are provided by the studies on courtroom interaction[4] and psychiatric intake interviews. Atkinson and Drew (1979; cf. Drew 1992) pointed out how in the context of the cross-examination of a

---

[2] Another aspect of the sequence organization in institutional settings involves *the absence of what would be relevant in ordinary conversation*. For example, Atkinson (1982) discusses the absence of 'newsmark tokens', 'second assessments' and 'second stories' in small claim courts and other institutional settings. Jefferson and Lee (1981) have commented upon the absence of 'announcement receipts' and displays of affiliation in response to the announcement of problems in 'service encounters'; and Heath (1989) has pointed out how the patients' expressions of pain do not occasion sympathy or appreciation by the doctors conducting diagnostic examinations. These kinds of systematic absences are relevant in many informal institutional settings; but I have not analysed the AIDS counselling data from this point of view.

[3] Drew and Heritage actually include also *the choice of activity that the turn is designed to accomplish*, in the notion of turn design. In this context, however, I will concentrate only on details of the verbal construction.

[4] The cross-examination is a typical example of a *formal* institutional setting. The specific turn-taking procedures in a formal setting, however, are not alone

policeman giving evidence to a tribunal, accusations were constructed through a skilful *selection of descriptions* in counsel's questions. In Atkinson and Drew's data, counsel systematically sought
to describe the events (riots and related police action in Northern
Ireland) so as to indicate that the witnessing policeman had acted in
an inappropriate manner. These accusations were built up progressively during the course of several questions and answers, so that
the upshot of the accusation was spelled out only after long preparation. Moreover, the witness oriented to this build-up, which is
indicated by his producing answers which sought to forestall the
blame. To do this, the witness selected descriptions which implied
the *adequacy* of his conduct given the circumstances. In short, then,
both parties' selection of descriptions was informed by orientation
to their institutional roles as counsel and defendant.

Bergmann (1992) examined how psychiatrists conducting intake
interviews in mental hospitals formulate their prior knowledge
about the patient. He observed that the practitioners frequently
used expressions which pointed out the *derivative and uncertain
character* of the speaker's knowledge: for example, they reported
what they had been told by the referring doctor, and conveyed that
they were not sure what the situation really was. Moreover, when
telling the patient what they knew about the patient's 'disturbed'
behaviour, the psychiatrists recurrently used litotes formulations,
i.e. understatements by negation of the opposite. Bergmann argued
that the use of these techniques amounts to an indirect invitation for
the patient to deliver the first-hand, authentic and unmitigated version of his situation and behaviour. Eliciting such confession from
the patient is, Bergmann argues, a central task of psychiatrists conducting an intake interview.

In sum, the way that the speakers assemble their utterances –
their choice of descriptive terms and syntactic constructions, and
even their prosodical choices – can be informed by their orientation
to their (and their interlocutors') institutional tasks and roles.
Moreover, these very choices can be vehicles for the accomplishment of those tasks.

---

sufficient to accommodate all the aspects of the participants' institutional tasks and
identities. Also needed are other layers of the organization of talk-in-interaction to
accomplish the institution's activity: and one of these is turn design.

Sequence organization and turn design in 'addressing dreaded issues'

In the empirical analyses that will follow, we will examine counsellors' and their clients' discussions concerning the clients' future. To put it broadly, the purpose of the ensuing data analyses is to explore which aspects of the sequence organization and turn design involved in the 'future talk' demonstrably accommodate the counsellors' institutional tasks.

For this analysis, I collected all the fragments of future-oriented talk in our work. By examining them in detail, I wanted to find out exactly how the task of 'addressing dreaded issues' is accomplished by counsellors, and how clients cooperate in this.

In this chapter we will examine how counsellors, during the course of the session, *introduce* and *constitute as sensitive* future-related issues such as illness and death. In chapter 7, we will concentrate solely on hypothetical future-oriented questions and their interactional features.

Building a possible world

If any two or more persons talk about the possible illness or death of somebody who at the moment is alive and well, they are creating a possible world, an alternative reality, by linguistic means. They are not talking about the world as it appears at the moment around them, but about the world as it can be imagined.

In any talk-in-interaction, the participants put their 'minds together by building a world to co-inhabit' (Moerman 1988: 119). This holds true for what we call 'objective' realities as well as for those which we call 'fantasy'. By noticing the objects around us through conversational means, Moerman argues, we orient ourselves and our co-conversationalists towards them. By talking about our fantasies we invoke them as an intersubjective reality which we can invite others to coinhabit.

Focusing the intersubjective attention to any object, even the most mundane and unproblematic, requires an appropriate sequential environment. To put it in the biblical terms suggested by Erickson and Shultz (1982: 72–5), any focusing of attention on something requires its specific *kairos* moment, its *right time*. This is most clearly seen in the context of the activity that can be called 'noticing'. Regarding visible physical objects to which we often draw our co-interactants' attention (such as 'nice weather', 'fine car', or 'your new blazer'), Moerman (1988: 107) tells us that '[t]he moment of perception is not the moment of public noticing'. Whether or not, and when, and how, we 'notice' something is in reciprocal relation with the other activities that we are engaged in. The *kairos* of noticing arises from the progression of the overall activity that the noticing is part of.

In AIDS counselling, talking about the patient's illness and death when she or he is not very ill and certainly not dead, entails the invocation of a potentially delicate, hostile world. To bring an untoward reality such as this into the shared focus of attention can be a very complicated interactional task. In her analyses of 'troubles telling' in ordinary conversation, Jefferson (1980; 1985a; 1988) has shown how the interactants in a very careful, stepwise manner move from attention to 'business-as-usual' towards attending to the problem. Before the problem is announced, a series of fine-grained interactional moves usually takes place. Regarding the treatment of untoward realities *in institutional talk*, Maynard's work, cited earlier in this chapter, is of great relevance. One of the functions of the 'perspective display series' is to establish the participants' – clinicians' and parents' – mutual alignment in relation to the idea of the child having a problem, before the actual delivery of bad diagnostic news takes place. Thus, earlier CA research suggests that invoking untoward realities usually cannot take place in a straightforward fashion, but needs to be preceded by the careful preparation of an appropriate interactional environment. The right time (*kairos*) is preceded by 'long and indefinite stretches of not-yet-right time' (Erickson and Shultz 1982: 72).

In this chapter we examine the resources that the counsellors (and their clients) have available for invoking the potentially hostile world of the clients' future. I will argue that the core of these resources consists of four types of question, each of which will be presented shortly. Moreover, I will argue that these four types of question are *ordered* roughly in relation to one another: taken together, they make up a potential strategy, beginning with less coercive techniques and ending up with much more coercive ones, which almost compel the client to talk about his or her perception of the future.

The relative ordering of the four questioning types does *not* mean, however, that all four techniques are consecutively used in each individual case when the client's future is talked about. Rather, it means that the earlier stages in the sequence *create possibilities*, in terms of a favourable conversational environment, for the latter to occur. The latter stages may, then, occur or not occur, depending on the 'results' achieved in the application of the techniques earlier in the sequence. Moreover, the favourable environment for the latter stages may appear through other ways, 'spontaneously' as it were, for example as a result of the client volunteering some key information.[5]

The counsellor's set of tools for 'addressing dreaded issues' consists of the following four types of question. *First*, the counsellor may offer the patient an opportunity to name any issues he might want to raise during the session. We will call these questions topic elicitations. In response to such questions, in some cases the client produces a description of his or her fears concerning a possible distressing future situation. *Second*, the counsellor's question may retrieve potentially worry-related themes that were mentioned in, or were absent from, the client's earlier talk. *Third*, the counsellor may topicalize a worry-indicative theme that appeared in the patient's prior turn; and in response the patient may explicate his worry in terms of a fearful future situation. Finally, the *fourth* type of question used in invoking a world of illness and death involves what the counsellors call 'hypothetical questions'.

As will be argued at the end of this chapter, the first three question types can be used, in different combinations, to create possibilities for the fourth to occur.

---

[5] Jefferson's (1980; 1988) analysis of the sequential structure of 'troubles talk', consisting of a number of relatively ordered elements, is a paradigmatic example of the examination of a socially organized 'big package' of interaction. Jefferson also clearly indicates and discusses the *difficulties* that the CA approach may face when being applied to stretches of talk that are longer than a few utterances. The 'big packages' can be described as 'ideal typical' constructions: they do not occur as clean cases in the data, but are constructed by the researcher. Jefferson's analysis, along with the comments of John Heritage, has been a central source of inspiration for me in trying to understand the relative ordering of the different question types that are used in discussing the client's future in AIDS counselling.

Question type 1: topic elicitations

One of the most obvious ways in which many forms of institutional talk differ from ordinary conversation is in the manner of topic change. In ordinary conversation, the topics often (but not always) flow from one to another, without any boundary between them (Jefferson 1984a; Button and Casey 1985; Sacks 1987). In various forms of institutional talk, the topics change in a 'marked' fashion, so that successive topics are segmented from one another. AIDS counselling is one of the institutional environments where this kind of topic disjuncture is often seen.

At the beginning of a counselling session, or after having completed the discussion of a topic, the participants have to find something new to talk about.[6] If the counsellors want to generate talk about the clients' fears and worries concerning their future, an obvious location where the talk can be so directed is, of course, in these topical junctures. In AIDS counselling, the new topics are usually generated in an orderly and cooperative fashion, through a question–answer sequence, whereby the counsellors elicit the new topics from the clients. Now we will examine some features of counsellors' questions and clients' answers in this topic elicitation.

The general pattern of topic elicitations in counselling sessions can be described as a three-step procedure:

(1)   The counsellor elicits a topic from the client(s) through a question.
(2)   The client proffers a candidate topic in the answer.
(3)   The counsellor topicalizes the answer through a follow-up question.

This pattern does not exclusively belong to 'counselling', or to 'institutional talk'. It is a *generic* procedure, which also can be used in everyday conversation – even though it most probably is much more infrequent there. Button and Casey (1984; see also 1985) have analysed its dynamics in detail; one of their examples is reproduced in extract (1). In Button's and Casey's (1984: 167)

---

[6] A possible completion of a topic is also a possible place for starting the closure of the encounter (Schegloff and Sacks 1973).

terms, arrow 1 points to a 'topic initial elicitor', arrow 2 to a 'newsworthy event-report' and arrow 3 to a 'topicalizer'.

```
(1)   (Button and Casey 1984)
 1    N:            You'll come abou:t (.) eight. Right?=
 2    H:            Yea::h,=
 3    N:            Okay
 4                  (.2)
 5    N: (1) ->     Anything else to report,
 6                  (.3)
 7    H:            Uh:::::: m:::,
 8                  (.4)
 9    H: (2) ->     Getting my hair cut tihmorrow,=
10    N: (3) ->     =Oh rilly?
                    ((Continues on topic))
```

In everyday conversation, of course, the roles of the participants in the application of this procedure (as 'topic-solicitor' and 'topic-provider') are not pre-specified. In AIDS counselling, however, the counsellor regularly is the one who asks the the client to proffer new topics, and not vice versa.

In what follows, we will examine how this three-step procedure of topic generation operates in AIDS counselling. There is space for a considerable amount of variation within the pattern. As regards one of the central tasks of the counsellors, which is to help clients come terms with the uncertainty of their futures, trajectories that the topic elicitations may follow can be divided into three different types. These are retrospective elicitations, open elicitations and distress-relevant elicitations.

The *retrospective topic elicitation* is so formulated that it makes relevant a description of the past events or the present state of life of the client as an answer. Therefore, these elicitations are the least effective as regards the generation of talk about the clients' future. Extracts (2)–(4) are examples of retrospective topic elicitations.

```
(2)   (N-19)
      ((W = P's wife Mrs Davies))
      ((Beginning of a session))
 1    C1:            ((receives the consent form of videorecording from
```

```
2                    the clients)) [Thank you. hhh very much. hh
3    (W):                        [(            )
4                    (1.0)
5    C1:             Well, hh (1.4) it's not so: long since I saw you
6                    las:t an:d today is your- (1.2) six monthly review,=
7    (W):            =(    )
8                    (1.3)
9    C1:   ->        How do you see thing[s::: (.) how thing-=
10   W:                                 [hhhhhh
11   C1:             = how'v[e things been over the last few=
12   W:                   [hh(   )hh
13   C1:             =months.=Mrs Davie:s.
```

```
(3)  (E3-58)
     ((Beginning of a session))
1    C1:             Let's: (.) let's see where are we.
2    P:              er: (.) [(                  )
3    C1:                    [It's about a month since we saw you.
4                    (.)
5    P:              Yeah.
6                    (.)
7    C1:   ->        Liza how: would you describe things as being
8                    now:.=For John:.
```

```
(4)  (N-24)
     (C1 and W are about to complete a sequence of talk where they
     arrange how C1 will write a letter to a community-based occupa-
     tional therapist)

1    C1:             Well if you give me the name: (.2) and address:: (.)
2                    when I have a moment I'll do that.
3    W:              Mm::
4                    (.6)
5    C1:             Okay,
6    W:              Yes.
7                    (.2)
8    C1:   ->        Ho[:w have::- (.8) the health issues been Mrs=
9    (W):             [(   )
10   C1:             =Davies do you think- (.2) for your husband.
```

These topic elicitations have a retrospective character: the counsellors elicit clients' reports of something that has happened or has
been experienced before the counselling session. In (2) and (3),
which are from the beginning of two sessions, the retrospective
orientation is strengthened by the formulations that precede the

queries: the counsellors' first remarks concern the time that has elapsed since the participants' previous meeting.

Retrospective queries usually generate retrospective answers. The candidate topics that the clients bring forward may be worry-oriented, and thereby relevant for counselling; but they nevertheless involve description of past or present, not future, states of affairs. Extract (5) below, which is an extension of (2) may serve as an example. The topic elicitation is marked with arrow 1, the client's first response with arrow 2, and the counsellor's turn whereby she topicalizes the issues brought forward by the client, with arrow 3.

```
(5)    (Extension of (2))
 1    C1:   (1) ->   How do you see thing[s::: (.) how thing- =
 2    W:                        [hhhhhh
 3    C1:             =how'v[e things been over the last few=
 4    W:                   [hh(     )hh
 5                    =months.=Mi[ssis Davie:s.
 6    W:    (2) ->                [Hectic to be quite ( ).=
 7    C1:   (3) ->   What's been [hectic.
 8    (W):                       [.hhh
 9    W:             Erm::
10                   (.8)
11    P:             ( [     ) (Molly) (.hh[hh)
12    W:               [Well.           [The good news first of all.
13                   (.3)
14  - W:             Our [daughter was got into the: (.3) high-school
15    C1:                [Mm:
16                   (.2)
17    W:             gover[nment assisted place.
18    C1:                [Mm:
19    C1:             Mm:
20    W:             That's the good news. hh .hhh heh heh .hhh
```

The open-topic elicitations do not specify the temporal (or any other) character of the sought-after matter. In this sub-type of topic elicitation, the counsellors plainly give the patients an opportunity to name a fresh issue or fresh issues. to be addressed, without focusing the enquiry at all. This type of elicitation makes it possible for clients to name their worries concerning the future as the subject-matter for the discussion; but the relevance here is of a very unspecified nature, as worries about the future is only one subject among a very wide range of subjects that are 'talk-about-able' in a counselling session. Extracts

(6)–(9) are examples of open-topic elicitations. The counsellors' 'first turns' are marked with arrows.

(6)   (E3-3 /N-47)
      ((Opening of a session.))
      C1:   Any rate hh
                  (2.5)
      C1:   ->   Well,=in coming today::hh (.6) Heather what- (.5)
                  m:os:t- (.5) would you now like- (.5) to disc̲uss.

(7)   (E4-12)
      ((W = P's wife))
      C1:   What are the practical close at home rea[sons.
      W: [Money heh
                  heh [heh heh [heh heh .hhhhh heh heh heh heh=
      P: [([   )
      C1:   [Money.
      W: =heh heh [heh heh .hhh
      C1:   [Fine.
                  (1.0)
      C1:   ->   So Graham I mean in si̲tting today: is there anything
                  you particularly would̄ like (.8) to use:: the rest
                  of our time to disc̲uss,

(8)   (N-8)
      ((W = P's wife))
      ((C1 has been showing a sample of condoms to the clients.))
      W: Y(h)e(h)s that's right yes .hhhhh (yes.)
                  (.2)
      C1:   ->   Graham [are there a̲ny i̲ssues you'd like to discuss:.
      P: [(Mm)
      P: Err:: hhh (let me t[hink)
      C1:   [that you ha̲ven't said so far,

(9)   (N-45)
      ((W = Liza, P's wife; D = P's and W's daughter, 1.5 years old.))
      C2:   Erm: (.2) Mrs Heller (   )[(   )
      C1:   ->   [Yes I'm, .hhhh Liza
                  I [wanted to s:ay: erm (.3) is there
      C2:   [(   )
                  (1.2)
      (D):   (Uh-huu)
      C1:   anything that [we haven't had the chance to talk=
      D: [oh wee?
      C1:   =about today, that you('ve) (.2) h̲oped to discuss.

Nominally at least, the discursive space created by the open-topic elicitations provides an opportunity for the clients to name any kind of issues to be discussed during the session. In most cases, however, the clients respond in one of two alternative ways. One is to offer subjects with a certain specific character: in one way or another, 'problematic' topics. The other common client response is to claim that there is nothing they want to talk about.

In extract (10) below, which is an extension of (7) shown above, the client produces, as a response to the counsellor's enquiry (arrow 1), a description of an anxiety that he might contract 'some kind of dementia' (arrow 2).

```
(10)   (Extension of (7))
1      C1:   (1) ->   So Graham I mean in sitting today: is there
2                     anything you particularly would like (.8) to
3                     use:: the rest of our time to dis[cuss,
4      P:                                              [Erm:
5                     (2.8)
6      P:    (2) ->   .hh I think that the things that (.) th (.2)
7                     that worry me about (2.1) myself
8      C1:            umh
9      P:             and: (.) by implication that of (.)
10                    o[f course means as (       )
11     C1:             [um:
12                    (.5)
13     P:             for us as as: as family >as well< .hh are::
14                    (.8) I get very: sca:red about (.4) this thing
15                    that people keep on (dangling round) about .hh
16                    even if you don't contract AIDS: a lot of people
17                    can end up crac- (.5) contracting some kind of
18                    dementia.
```

This response of the patient in turn provides the counsellor with material that she can begin to examine in detail in the subsequent talk. With clients' responses like the one in extract (10), the conversation smoothly and easily progresses into the kind of area that the counsellors regard as the essential subject-matter of AIDS counselling: clients' fears concerning their future.

Extract (11), which is the continuation of (8) shown above, is an example of a response where the client produces a less intensive future-related worry:

```
(11)   (Extension of (8))
 1    C1:    (1) ->    Michael [are there any issues you'd like to=
 2    P:                     [(Mm)
 3    C1:               =discuss:.
 4    P:                Err:: hhh (let me t[hink)
 5    C1:                               [that you haven't said so far,
 6                      (2.5)
 7    P:                Err::
 8                      (2.0)
 9    P:                I ↑don't think so,
10                      (.7)
11    P:     (2) ->    Err .hh- (.4) Yea- I (me- only) thing:s like:
12                     wh::ich (.3) it will happen on: (.2) sort of a- (.2)
13                     of beginning to apply for (.8) training courses and
14                     stuff so if I'm getting problems with- (.2) with
15                     that at the time I will-.hhh
16    C1:              Ho[w would you handle it Michael.
17    P:                 [(                    )
18    P:                Well I mean ((continues with the answer))
```

In (11), the client responds by naming possible problems with 'training courses' as a topic to be discussed. Interestingly, the client first declines the offer to name any issues (line 9). The new topic is only entered into after some interactional movements: the counsellor remains silent in line 10 after the client's first negative response, and after a gap of 0.7 sec. the client offers his concern about the 'training courses'.[7]

Finally, in (12) below, the client claims that there are no more issues she would hope to discuss. In response, the counsellor gives up the topic elicitation.[8] C's elicitation is marked with arrow 1, W's response with arrow 2, and the counsellor's turn which amounts to 'giving up' the elicitation with arrow 3.

---

[7] In remaining silent, the counsellor may have been informed by the relative delay (in lines 6-8) of the client's first response, by his use of the qualification 'I don't think', and by the rising intonation at the end of his reply (line 9). These are hearable as indications of the client having less than a firm position in claiming that he has not got any more issues to discuss.

[8] There are cases, however, where counsellors do not give up the topic elicitation after the client's first negative response. Extract (6) is an example of this: its continuation is given in extract (19) in chapter 3. In that case, the counsellor pursues the elicitation until the clients finally name an issue to be addressed. The counsellors' decision whether to give up or to pursue the elicitation is obviously related to the location of the elicitation within the overall structure of

(12) (Extension of (9))
```
1    C2:              Erm: (.2) Mrs Heller (      )[ (      )
2    C1:   (1) ->                            [Yes I'm, .hhhh Liza
3                     I [wanted to s:ay: erm (.3) is there
4    C2:                [(           )
5                     (1.2)
6    (I):             (Uh-huu)
7    C1:              anything that [we haven't had the chance to talk=
8    I:                            [oh wee?
9    C1:              =about today, that you('ve) (.2) hoped to discuss.
10   W:               Hhhhhhh
11                    (.5)
12   W:               .hh
13                    (2.2)
14   W:(2) ->         N:::::::o:: because the:: (.) the situation has .hh
15                    (.3) calmed down (.3) so (.) c[onsiderably since=
16   C1:                                           [Mm:
17   W:               =last week that there isn't anything
18                    (.2)
19   C1:   (3) ->     Okay [(you've) nothing m[ore.
20   W:                    [pressing (      ) [Ye::
21   W:               I don't [(think so)
22   C1:                      [John
23   P:               Well: nothing nothing mo:re. ((continues))
```

As noted above, open-topic elicitations do *not* overtly specify the type of subject that clients are asked to bring forward; they only create a space for the clients to name 'discussable' issues that arise from their own perspective. However, clients regularly respond with particular kinds of topic: if they name anything at all, the clients name issues that are *problematic* for them.

This 'client-centred' interactional procedure leading into the realm of problems and worries holds an obvious advantage. If a client names a distressing issue (future-oriented or not) in response to an open-topic elicitation – like the clients in extracts (10) and (11) did – then the participants have entered a space of 'problem-talking' in full agreement, through a genuinely shared initiative.

---

the counselling session. In (9), shown above, the elicitation was designed so as to exhibit its location at the end of the session, whereas the elicitation in (6) is constructed as a part of the opening sequence. To give up an elicitation that is part of the closure (i.e. elicitation of 'any more topics') does not create problems for the overall management of the session, whereas giving up an elicitation which is part of opening does.

Their orientation to 'problems' is therefore more strongly established than it would have been if the counsellor had been more active in naming the problems. But the analytical question that we have here is this: why don't the clients bring forward trivial or positive or funny or bizarre issues, in sum, any kinds of issue other than problematic ones?

Two considerations are relevant here. First, by responding with problem-oriented topic namings, the clients display their orientation to the institutional context of the talk as 'counselling'. This orientation is documented in all extracts discussed above. The orientation to the context operates in and through the inferences the clients make out of the counsellors' enquiries.

For example, in (10), when given the chance to name any topic for discussion, P begins with a reference to 'the things that (...) worry me'. By this transformation of the verbal shape of the object of attention – from the counsellor's elicitation concerning 'anything you particularly would like (.8) to use:: the rest of our time to dis*cuss*?' into 'things that (...) worry me' – the patient displays his orientation to the counselling session as something where talk about worries is relevant.

Even in extract (12), where the client did not bring forward any new topic nevertheless she displayed the same kind of orientation. W coupled her declination with an account:

'N:::::::o:: because the:: (.) situation has (...) calmed down (...) so (...) considerably since last week that there isn't anything'

By using the report about the 'calming down of the situation' as an account for the absence of any new topics, W displays her interpretation of the counsellor's elicitation. In this interpretation, the counsellor's preceding utterance is treated as an act which aimed at bringing forward aspects of the clients' life that are something other than 'calm', i.e. distressing and problematic issues.

In sum, then, the participants display their orientation to the specific context of 'counselling' through these inferential procedures which facilitate talk that involves problems and distressing issues.

Another aspect that accounts for the counsellors' obvious success in the open-topic elicitations relates to the optional quality of the use of this device. The counsellors do have a long acquaintanceship with most of the clients. As a result of this, they can be expected to know which of the clients are 'cooperative' enough to be offered an 'open' possibility for topic-naming. They do not use this pattern of topic elicitation with all the clients; and it can be expected that the decision whether or not to use this pattern is informed by all the relevant knowledge about the client's history in counselling as well as the impression the counsellors have about the client's cooperativeness in the current session (cf. Maynard 1992). If counsellors feel that the client's response could possibly be inadequate regarding the aims of the counselling session (as the counsellors see them), they can use different procedures, such as retrospective topic elicitation (described in the beginning of this section) or distress-relevant topic elicitation, to which we will now turn.

The distress-relevant topic elicitation conveys indirectly to the client an invitation to disclose his or her fears and worries. This is done by formulating the experiential quality of the sought-after discussable matter. Most typically, instead of plainly eliciting anything to discuss, the counsellors focus on primary 'concerns'.[9]

(13) (E3-20)
    C: If [I was to ask you Mr Wood (.)=
    P: [(   )-
    C: =[sort of what is your main concern=
    P: [Mm hm
    C: =at the moment what would that be.

(14) (E4-16)
    C: Can I just ask you what are your greatest
          conce:rns:: (.) Liz.

(15) (E4-65)
    C: So if I was to ask what's your main concern today
          Mike what is it.

Eliciting primary 'concerns' seems to attend to the sensitivities of the counselling encounter in a very subtle way. 'Concern' may include very different kinds of issue. Mathematicians may be concerned about the proofs they are trying to develop for a new

---

[9] A further focusing involves eliciting 'concerns about something', such as 'concerns about health', 'concern about the test result'. Due to limitations of time and space, we have to leave aside an examination of these forms of focusing.

formula, a motorist may be concerned about a new car and a dog-owner shopping for his pet's dinner may be concerned about different brands of dogfood: depending on the person and context, 'concern' may refer to a wide variety of objects.[10] But on the other hand, 'concern' does also have a special connotation with 'serious' issues. We may be concerned about our illnesses, weaknesses, or failures. We are not concerned about things that are of minor significance to us. In other words, 'concern' seems potentially to have a rather ambiguous meaning. I wish to argue that this ambiguity is preserved and exploited when this term is used in topic elicitations.

By eliciting 'concerns' and drawing upon the 'serious' connotation of the term, counsellors may provide space for the disclosure of the patients' fears. But because 'concern' also has its inclusive aspects, counsellors may also avoid *overtly asking* the patient to disclose their troubles. So eliciting 'concerns' seems to create a space that can be filled with descriptions of worries and fears, but without overtly naming that space as one reserved for worries and fears. The space is provided, but indirectly, or 'off record' (cf. Brown and Levinson 1987). Or to put it another way, space is created for the client nominally to *volunteer* his or her fears. By using the ambiguous term 'concerns' in topic nomination, the counsellors leave it to the patients to move into more unambiguous terms in naming the topic (cf. Bergmann 1992).[11]

---

[10] I wish to thank Paul Drew for drawing my attention to this 'inclusiveness' of many usages of the word 'concern'.

[11] Some additional evidence for this function of the use of 'concerns' can be obtained from a rare case, where the counsellor *overtly* elicits patient's troubles.

> C: So s- at the the moment Nick what do you think are the hardest things around for you. (I mea:n) (0.6) we agreed to talk today if we've got enough ti::me (0.5) I mean what are the things that (0.2) which it would be helpful to: kind of (0.5) turn round a bit.

In the extract above, the counsellor first openly elicits 'the hardest things around for you'. This formulation lacks the inclusiveness and ambiguity of 'concerns'. Interestingly, C herself seems to orient to her elicitation as something in need of a repair, or at least of an account. After the initial elicitation she produces 'a reason for the enquiry' by emphasizing that P has agreed to talk with the counsellor, followed by an alternative formulation of the elicitation. The rephrasing is less explicit about the quality of the topic. Thus, in the extract above the counsellor herself treats the 'explicit' elicitation of 'the hardest things around for you' as problematic.

Details of how the enquiry is delivered may also convey to the patient that here is a possibility for disclosing fears and anxieties. The counsellors may not ask bluntly 'what are your greatest concerns', but often use additional linguistic devices along with the delivery of the question. In (13), C's utterance is begun with a question projection, 'If I was to ask you Mr Wood', followed by the hedge 'sort of'. Only thereafter does the question itself appear. Equally in (14) and (15), question projections are used.

It has been argued previously that such projections and hedges typically occur in connection with 'delicate' (Schegloff 1980) or 'face-threatening' (Brown and Levinson 1987) talk. These features often anticipate utterances relating to sensitive topics or utterances accomplishing speech acts that threaten the hearers' public self-image. Now these linguistic features accompany a topic elicitation. There they may have a very special and important function: by marking the elicitation as they do, they may convey to the hearer that something face-threatening or delicate is under way alongside the mere topic elicitation. Or, to put it another way, they may convey to the patient that the space that the counsellor's elicitation creates for the patient to fill is indeed designed to accommodate something that the patient may initially be reluctant to talk about.

But again, this qualification of the space provided is done by using indirect means. The question projections and hedges do not *overtly* claim the counsellor's wish that the patient should name delicate issues. The indirectness allows a possibility for the patient not to pay attention to these cues, and thereby to fill the space provided with less delicate matters.

After the counsellor has delivered the topic elicitation, the next conversational move is allocated to the client. In most of the cases, the clients bring forward fresh issues, either having to do with their current problems or their fears about the future. By returning to the clients' problem-oriented responses, the counsellors typically produce follow-up questions which topicalize the materials brought forward by the clients.

In extract (16), the patient produces a current anxiety as a response to the counsellor's elicitation. Arrow 1 stands for the elicitation, arrow 2 for the response and arrow 3 for the topicalization of that response.

(16) (Extension of (11))
```
1    C:    (1) ->   So if I was to ask what's your main concern today
2                   Mike what is it.
3                   (1.0)
4    P:    (2) ->   Uh::m: (1.0) Nothing really. (0.2) I'm feeling a bit
5                   depressed lately but
6    C:    (3) ->   About what.=
7    P:             =Uh:m Over that bike accident I had.
```

In extract (17) the client produces a future-related worry in response to the distress-relevant topic elicitation. The first arrow stands for the initial topic elicitation, the second arrow for the beginning of the future-oriented response, and the third for the counsellor's turn where she topicalizes a core element of this response.

(17) (Extension of (14))
```
1    C:    (1) ->   Can I just ask you what are your greatest
2                   conce:rns:: (.) Liz.
3    P:             [Liza
4    C:             [Liza: I ca:n't get it [(        )
5    W:                               [((coughing))
6    C:             Liza about- .hh (.4) at this mo:ment in ti:me. (.)
7                   can you s:ay alou:d.
8                   (3.0)
9    W:    (2) ->   Erm:: (.) the uncertainty[:?
10   C:                                  [mmh:
11                  (1.5)
12   W:             obviously:?
13                  (.6)
14   W:             an::d (3.0) trying to get John to cope with it (.2)
15                  an:d-(.3) lead as normal a life as possible (.) I'd
16                  (.) I don't see .hhh (1.0) I don't really see any
17                  f::easible r:ealistic alterna:tive.=
18   C:             =mm:h
19                  (.5)
20   W:             than (.) (both) to carry on:: (.3) as (.) as
21                  no:r[mal.
22   C:                 [ mmh
23                  (1.6)
24   Baby:          gjuu
25                  (.7)
26   W:             an::d (1.6) what would happen to me:?
27   C:             mmh
28   W:             and the children (2.1) if he did
```

29			devel̲[op (.3) something?
30	C:		⎡mmh
31			(.2)
32	C:		mmh
33			(.6)
34	C:	(3) –>	What's your greatest fe̲:ar about that.
35			(2.0)
36	C:		([ ) (.2) ( )
37	W:		⎡ T:here is̲n't anything (.2) speci̲fic (.) I mean
38			it's just a ge̲neral abstra:ct:hh

In (17) above, the client produces first a gloss, 'the uncertainty', as a response to the counsellor's elicitation. The counsellor encourages her to produce more through her continuers and silence. A long narrative by W ensues, ending up with the delivery of the description of a distressing future situation 'what would happen to me:? (...) and the *children* (...) if he did *develop* something?' This description is then topicalized by the counsellor through her question in line 34.

It is emphasized above that, as means for inviting clients' talk about their fears and worries, the distress-relevant elicitation operates mainly in an indirect, 'off-the-record' way. Therefore, this type of elicitation also gives the client an opportunity to name something other than fresh, problem-oriented issues to be talked about. This happens in case (18) shown below. The client does not reveal any troubles of his, but instead refers first to an issue that had been extensively dealt with earlier in the session (data not shown). The counsellor, in turn, turns aside this candidate topic and renews the elicitation; but even this does not bring up particularly troubles-relevant issues.

The stages of the interaction are indicated with arrows as follows. The first arrow stands for the initial topic elicitation, and the second for the client's first response. The third arrow points at the renewed elicitation, the fourth for the beginning of the client's new response, and the fifth for the counsellor's turn where she finally topicalizes some of the other-than-problem-oriented matters brought forward by the client.

(18)	(Extension of (13))		
1	C:	(1) –>	If [I wa̲s to ask you Mr Wood (.)=
2	P:		[(̄)-
3	C:		=[sort of wh̲at is your main conce̲rn=

```
 4   P:              [Mm hm
 5   C:              =at the moment what would that be.
 6                   (1.0)
 7   P:    (2) ->    Well I suppose the main concer:n er: w- w- would
 8                   be the house settling.
 9                   (.)
10   C:    (3) ->    [So getting out of the [house:.=And=
11   P:              [(set)- (set)-           [Yes:.
12   C:              =what comes after that.
13                   (1.0)
14   P:              Uh:m hhh
15                   (0.5)
16   P:    (4) ->    Well of course as er as (Anna er says) the- the- the
17                   good news of er Tina.=She's all right.
18   C1:             Mm:
19                   (.)
20   P:              [Uh:m
21   C1:             [( )
22                   (1.4)
23   P:              I suppose really: er that- that's the
24                   main thing:.=I'm settled down with the little job
25                   that I ha:ve,=
26   C1:   (5) ->    =What is the lit[tle job you've got.
27   P:                              [and that is in- in: in
28                   (Woki:ng),
```

The course of interaction in (18) shows that although it is up to the
patient to decide what kind of topic he introduces, after the introduction of the first 'candidate' topic the counsellor has another
opportunity to exert her influence. The counsellor can 'close' the
initial topic proposed by the patient, and try to see whether another
elicitation would produce something else. But even then, the client is
free to produce the kind of topic he or she chooses.

The variety of patients' responses to all types of topic elicitation
shows that the topic elicitation alone may be rather ineffective in
invoking descriptions of hostile future worlds. They may bring forth
many different kinds of concern that the counsellors may or may
not find useful to talk about with their clients. Descriptions of fears
concerning the future are among those types of concern; but
obviously there are many other kinds of issue that come to the
surface in this way. In order to get further into the hostile future
world, the counsellors usually have to ask other kinds of questions,
too.

Question type 2: retrieving themes that were mentioned or absent in clients' earlier talk

Apart from the topic-elicitation procedures described above, the counsellors can use another type of question to begin a sequence which may lead to talk about a hostile future. This second question type is typically available in the middle parts of the session (not in the beginning or at the end). In this second question type, the counsellor retrieves a potentially worry-indicative theme that was mentioned in, or absent from, the client's earlier talk, and elicits a further account of his or her possible worries related to that. In response to this, the client can disclose more about his or her fears related to the future, or about other anxieties.

As implied above, these enquiries constitute *fresh first acts* in the sense that they are not directly responsive to the preceding turn. In that respect, they have much in common with the topic-elicitation procedures described earlier in this chapter. However, the questions which retrieve themes that were mentioned or absent from earlier talk are different in two important aspects: (1) unlike the topic elicitations, they use as a resource the earlier talk (not the immediately preceding turn but a longer section of talk) in the same encounter, and (2) in this form of questioning, the counsellor, while using the client's talk as a resource, is more active in defining the new topic.

There are two different sub-types of these enquiries: (1) the worry-indicative theme may have appeared earlier in P's talk, and the counsellor retrieves it later, or (2) the counsellor can make the client accountable for the absence of certain themes in his or her earlier talk.

Extracts (19) and (20) are examples of the first type of procedure that retrieves a worry-indicative theme.

```
(19)  (E4-46)
  1    C1:      [So that's one thing we can]
  2    P:       [S o r t that out (.2)      y]eah.
  3    C1:      look at ortho[paedically,=but what else?
  4    P:                    [Yeah.
  5             (1.0)
  6    P:       Uh:m (1.0) I'm not sure really I've never
  7             thought of it (.4) anything.
  8             (0.2)
```

```
  9  C2:        [(Wh)-
 10  P:         [(But) you've been helping me all the (.) last
 11             little while,
 12             (0.2)
 13  C2:   ->   What- (0.2) I mean what (.) Michael mentioned
 14             at- initially is that you know (0.2) he didn't
 15             have any concerns but he's been feeling funny
 16             again,=is that a worry to him or is it no
 17             problem to him that he feels funny.
 18             (0.3)
 19  (C1):      Mm=
 20  P:         =I don't know: I- I just go th- er through
 21             stages of uh:m (1.1) you know I mean I've had a
 22             really (0.2) sort of a quite a hectic weekend,
 23             quite a busy ti:me,=and it's not as though I've
 24             been sitting down moping again.
 25             (0.6)
 26  P:         But you know it's just sort of like as though-
 27             as though it just clicks:.
 28             (0.5)
 29  P:         And then I think it will all (            )
 30             what's going to happen (wi:th) (.) (so and so) if
 31             you know what I mean.
```

(20) (N-21)
((C1 is just closing a sequence of talk with W about a letter that she is
going to send to an occupational therapist))

```
  1  C1:        I think we'll leave that till-
  2  ( ):       (    ) it's very (    )
  3  W:         Yes,
  4  C1:   ->   just afterwards. .hhh What else has been
  5             hec- what else do you think
  6             [your wife's referring to as being hectic.
  7  (W):       [hhhh heh heh
  8             (1.0)
  9  P:         Ts .hh Erm: hhhhh (1.2) Well I think there have been
 10             the: err:m the main things real[ly.
 11  C1:                                        [Mm::
 12  P:         Erm:: hhh (1.0) An:d I:: I suppose that hhhh where
 13             we: are the present moment,
 14  C1:        Mm:=
 15  P:         =It err:: mm er er (1.2) this is a:ll (.3) an:d it
 16             has helped. .hh (there are) things have sort of been
 17             getting on (.6) err:: one another's nerves in:
 18             certain respects.
 19             (.3)
```

```
20   P:        So I thin[k-
21   C1:                 [Which are the things t[hat have been=
22   P:                                         [Because of-
23   C1:        =getting on one another's n[erves.
24   P:                                     [Well it's:: it's:: err::
25              I suppose (.) m: (.2) living with:: in-laws: you
26              know?
```

In extract (19), C2 refers to something that the patient has said
earlier, afterwards enquiring whether what the patient talked
about earlier is a 'worry' to him or not. The patient responds
with a description of his recent states of mind, alluding to his worries concerning the future. Following the same pattern, in (20) the
counsellor brings up the patient's wife's earlier description that
things have been 'hectic' (see extract (5) on p. 245 above). Before
this segment in the session, the wife had already described a number
of 'hectic' matters (the sequence that began in extract (5) shown
earlier in this chapter); now the counsellor returns once again to this
theme, asking *the patient* to name more 'hectic' things. After some
search and pursuit, the patient tells the counsellor that living with
in-laws is getting on the couple's nerves.

So in (19), retrieving a worry-indicative theme led to an indirect
disclosure of future-related worries, whereas in (20), the use of the
same device led to an explication of the clients' current worries. In
both cases, the counsellor first produced a formulation of the client's prior talk. By producing the formulation, the counsellors
emphasized the continuity between their current enquiry and
what the clients had said earlier. They thus revealed that they
were pursuing further something that the clients themselves had
initially raised. By carefully preserving the sense of mutual cooperation, the counsellors show their appreciation of the clients' talk and
also make it less likely that the clients will resist their enquiries.

When using clients' earlier talk as a point of departure for enquiries eliciting fears concerning the future, counsellors could be
assumed to be dependent on the clients having first inserted at
least potentially worry-related items in their turns. However,
there is a way around this: the counsellors can also topicalize *absent*
themes in the clients' talk. That is the case in extracts (21), (22) and
(23).

(21)   (N-48)
```
 1    P:              ((...)) I can d- I can deal
 2                    wit[h that in any case you k(h)now(h) .hh
 3    C1:                 [Of what side are you most concerned with.
 4                    (1.2)
 5    P:              So it's:: it's it's mainly the:: er: (.2) erm I
 6                    would think (of) th:: the knee joints:.
 7    C1:             Uh[m.
 8    P:                [and the:: and the ankles.=( ) my elbows and
 9                    (.) general health I=
10    C1:             Mm:
11    P:              I feel okay, I [feel ↑ fine.
12    C1:                            [Mmh
13                    (.8)
14    P:              ([     )
15    C1:    (1) ->   [You haven't mentioned AIDS as a concern today.=How
16                    much of a conc[ern (now [it is).
17    W:     (2) ->             [(     ) [I've got so many other
18                    worries really t[hat that has to take a back [seat.
19    C1:                          [Uhm:                    [Uhm:
20    P:              Mm:
21    W:              Hhh heh heh .hhh h[eh ( )hhh
22    C1:    (3) ->                  [WOULD YOU SAY:
                      that you're less
23                    concerned than were?
24    W:              I'm less concerned than I was when- (.4) before we
25                    ((continues))
```

(22)   (E4-74)
```
 1    C1:    (1) ->   You say the rest of your work is fi:ne .hh your
 2                    health is fi:ne uh:m .hh have you had any worries
 3                    about HIV at all?
 4                    (0.5)
 5    P:     (2) ->   Uh:m Not really no:.
 6                    (0.6)
 7    P:              er:
 8                    (.3)
 9    P:              I understand fully (.4) what it i:s and
10    C1:             Mm[:
11    P:                [as much can be done is being done as possible.
12    C1:             Mm:
13                    (0.6)
14    C1:    (3) ->   What is being done as far [as you see:?
15    P:                                       [Uh:m
```

(23) (E4-48)
1   C1:   Ha[ve you any concerns about that?
2   P: [(   )
3   (0.5)
4   P: (I don't know) (.2) not really.
5   (0.6)
6   C1: (1) ->   And what about (.3) you (.2) mentioned the blee:ds and
7   you mentioned your (.5) concern about transport
8   and things .hhh uhm (.2) how about the HIV: (.)
9   business.
10   P: (3) ->   I mean that's (0.7) (   )
11   (0.5) further from my memory than- sort of mind at
12   the moment really.=I'm more concerned (of my leg) my
13   joints for example it's
14   not [something I can
15   C1:   [Mm:
16   (1.0)
17   C1: (3) ->   Is there anything (.3) that if you were to bring in
                  to your mi:nd, you'd want to ask about that.

In (21), the counsellor formulates the absence of AIDS in the clients'[12] talk during the session; in (22) and (23) the counsellor reiterates two items that P has talked about, and contrasts these with a third item, HIV, which P has not mentioned before. In all three cases, the absence of a key object (HIV/AIDS) is locally constituted as noticeable and accountable. Therefore, the counsellors create an expectation that the clients would account for the absence – which is what they do in the next turns (marked with arrows numbered 2). These accounts, in turn, provide the counsellors with an opportunity to generate follow-up questions, whereby the initially absent themes have been topicalized (arrows numbered 3).

In retrieving worry-indicative themes which have appeared earlier in P's talk, and in rendering accountable the absence of potentially problematic topics, counsellors are explicitly narrowing down the realm of relevant objects that can be focused on in the clients' responses. Therefore, in spite of the sense of continuity that is established between the clients' earlier talk and the current enquiry, these queries have a more *coercive* character than the topic elicitations discussed earlier in this chapter. Now the counsellors are

[12] It is not exactly clear to whom the 'you' in C1's turn in line 15 refers. The preceding dialogue is between P and C1; but the one who responds to C1's formulation is W.

explicitly eliciting clients' reports of something that can be related
to their worries concerning the future.

Question type 3: topicalizing worry-related themes in clients' prior turns

The third tool that the counsellors use in generating talk about the
clients' fears and worries concerning the future is the follow-up
question focusing on a potentially worry-related theme that has
occurred in P's prior turn. Unlike the two types of question discussed earlier, these queries are not fresh first acts, but observably
responsive to a preceding turn by the client. Therefore, they constitute a continuation of a sequence. The sequence that these queries
are located in may be (but does not need to be) initiated by question
types 1 or 2, discussed earlier in this chapter.

    Some of the follow-up questions operate in a 'neutral' way, as it
were: they simply topicalize what the client has brought forward in
his or her preceding turn. Extract (24) below is an example of that.

```
(24)  (Extension of (10))
      ((P = Graham; W = his wife.))
 1    P:      (...) I get very: sca:red about (.4) this thing
 2            that people keep on (dangling round) about .hh
 3            even if you don't contract AIDS: a lot of people
 4            can end up crac- (.5) contracting some kind of
 5            dementia.
 6    W:      *(          [        )*
 7    P:                  [I really don't like that so
 8            ( [   ).
 9    C1:       [Mm
10    P:      I suppose because .hhh having g[ot used=
11    C1:                                    [(    )
12    P:      =to the fact that (.) that (.3) my body isn't
13            always as good as it should
14            [be or done the things [that it ought to:.
15    C1:     [Mm                    [Mm
16    P:      .hh[h I've got (so I'm) quite fond of my=
17    C1:        [Mm
18    P:      =mi:nd and my bra:in an:d (.) the tho[ught
19    C1:                                          [Mm::
20    P:      =of (.5) >of anything happening to tha:t< I
21            actually fi[nd really quite (.4) quite=
22    C1:                [Mm
```

```
23   P:        =th[reatening.
24   C1:          [Mm-m
25             (.8)
26   P:        Err::
27             (.4)
28   C1:  ->   Do you both share that?
29             (3.0)
30   W:        I don't think about that as much as
31             Gra[ham.=But I suppose [because it isn't=
32   C1:          [Mm              [Mm.
33   W:        =me I (can't) think about it much more
34             ((continues on topic))
```

By asking W whether they both share 'that', the counsellor topicalizes P's description of his fear concerning that something could happen to his 'mind and brain'. Even though C1's follow-up question is addressed to F (instead of P who gave the target description), it can be characterized as neutral because it focuses on a theme that was *prominent* in P's prior turn. C1 responds to the issues that P observably brought forward as the upshot of his turn. The simple design of C1's question is a vehicle of this neutrality: in referring to 'that', she allows P's description of his worry remain self-explanatory.

In many cases, however, the counsellors' follow-up questions have a more complicated relation to the preceding turns. They can be designed so as to *pick up* specifically the worry indicative objects in the preceding turns (cf. Jefferson 1984a); or alternatively, they can *upgrade* the problem relevance of those referents. Extracts (25) and (26) provide examples of the first sub-type.

```
(25)  (E4-50)
      ((P has pointed out earlier that HIV is 'further' from his memory))
 1    C1:       How would it uhm: affect (.) your:: (0.8) uh- your
 2              current view: of- of (HIV) bei:ng further from your
 3              mi:nd. If you [were on a- this drug tri:al.
 4    P:                      [(It's)- (It's)-
 5              (2.2)
 6    P:        I mean ( ) I mean perhaps that's wrong when I've
 7              said it's far fr[om my mind,=it's not.=
 8    C1:                       [Mm
 9    P:        =[(Far fr-)
10    C1:        =[Would you say further.
11    P:        Yeah sort [of
12    C1:                 [Yes.
```

```
13   P:              you know [further or far- farther from my=
14   C1:                     [Mm
15   P:    (1) ->    =[mind but (.) I do think about it [but at the=
16   C1:             [Mm                               [Mm
17   P:              =moment it's not (.) you know it'[s not sort=
18   C1:                                             [Mm
19   P:              =of (0.4) to me it's pointless to think about
20                   it,=[(if I) consider everyday well what=
21   C1:                 [Mm
22   P:              =shall I[:
23   C1:   (2) ->            [When you do think about it what do you
24                   think about it.
25                   (0.7)
26   P:              Uh::m
27                   (1.1)
28   C1:             What ki[nd (of)-
29   P:    (3) ->           [Well I think sometimes for example if I'm
30                   you know: I'm trying to sort out a business for
31                   myself and do all this wo[rk a:nd (.) perhaps=
32   C1:                                     [Mm:
33   P:              =you know (.) I mean I could die or some[thing=
34   C1:                                                    [Mm
35   P:              =but (0.4) I mean the thought (        ) of
36                   fleetingly through my mi:n[d but it's not=
37   C1:                                      [Mm:
38   P:              =something I you know dwell o:n.
```

In (25), the counsellor links her follow-up question with the part of
P's earlier turn where he admitted that 'I *do th*ink about it' (arrow
1). The client's multi-unit turn in lines 11–22 is not designed so as
to offer this statement as its upshot; rather, it is offered as a subsidiary theme leading towards the assertion 'to me it's pointless to
think about it' and its continuation (lines 19–22). Due to the subsidiary status and the remote sequential location of the target assertion, the counsellor has to do specific work to contextualize her
follow-up question. This is done by the counsellor repeating '*do*
think about it' in the beginning of her turn. Through this selective
focusing, she achieves a position where she can ask what P thinks
about HIV; and in his response, P discloses his concern about dying
(arrow 3).[13]

---

[13] Note, however, how P in his response also mitigates the significance of this fear.

In extract (26), the counsellor's follow-up question equally topicalizes materials that are subsidiary rather than central in the client's earlier turn:

```
(26)  (Extension of (22))
 1   C1:            You say the rest of your work is fi:ne .hh your
 2                  health is fi:ne uh:m .hh have you had any
 3                  worries about HIV at all?
 4                  (0.5)
 5   P:             Uh:m Not really no:.
 6                  (0.6)
 7   P:             er:
 8                  (.3)
 9   P:             I understand fully (.4) what it i:s and
10   C1:            Mm[:
11   P:     (1) ->     [as much as can be done is being done as
12                  possible.
13   C1:            Mm:
14                  (0.6)
15   C1:   (2) ->   What is being done as far [as you see:?
16   P:                                       [Uh:m
17                  (0.7)
18   P:     (3) ->  Well as far as what I know: there's (.2)
19                  there're countries all pulling together (.2) to
20                  try and fi:nd (1.0) er: (1.0) something (.4) to
21                  either hold it or cure it [within ti:me.
22   C1:                                      [Mm
23                  (0.8)
24   P:             So it's just a ma:tter reall[y of waiting [to=
25   C1:                                         [Mm          [Mm
26   P:             =see.
```

In (22), the client produces the statement 'as much as can be done is being done as possible' as a final part of an expansion of his initial statement where he asserts that he does not have worries about HIV (line 5). The expansion is prompted by the counsellor's silence after the initial statement (line 6) and by her continuer after the first part of the expansion (line 10). Due to its sequential location and semantic content, the expansion has a subsidiary status in the client's prior turn: it works as an account for the patient having no worries. The counsellor's follow-up question, however, rather than focusing on the patient's 'no worries' statement, focuses on this account. The follow-up question exhibits its connection with the account through the repetition of the phrase 'is being done' (lines 11 and 15). By this selective focusing, the counsellor manages to preserve HIV in the topical focus in spite of P's initial claim that he hasn't got any worries about it, without having to violate the sense of mutual cooperation in the topical development.

In extracts(25) and (26) above, the counsellors' follow-up questions operate through selective focusing on aspects in clients' talk that were built as subsidiary. In the two examples shown below, that is not the case: the follow-up questions focus on themes that are observably prominent in the clients' earlier turns. In these cases, however, the follow-up questions upgrade the problem-relevance of their referents.

```
(27)  (E4-41)
  1   C2:              Well what does he think just mig[ht be top of]=
  2   ( ):                                          [(          )]=
  3   C2:              =[her mi:nd just
  4   ( ):             =[(       )
  5   P:               .hh We:[ll-
  6   C2:                     [now thinking it through.
  7                    (0.9)
  8   P:     (1) ->    On the top of her mi:nd?=Well I think she's probably
  9                    affected by:: (1.0) the idea that I move from one
 10                    stage to another:,
 11   C2:    (2) ->    Bu[t what about that-
 12   P:                 [and that might be a bit of a sho:ck.
 13   C2:    (2') ->   What about that (.) might she be most concerned
 14                    about.
 15                    (2.0)
 16   P:               I don't quite understand the question.=
 17                    =[I mean ang:- [anxiety about-
 18   C2:    (2") ->    [Well wha-    [wha- what is her greatest fear at
 19                    the moment. D'you think.
 20                    (1.2)
 21   P:     (3) ->    Well that I would go on to develop (.7) sort of
 22                    further symptoms I suppo:se. (.9) An:d (.2) a-
 23                    anxiety about the future.=(I can't- I cu-)=
```

Through her follow-up question, which is first started in line 11 (arrow 2), then aborted, and thereafter restarted and completed in lines 13–14 (arrow 2'), C2 elicits a specification for P's initial non-specific statement that his wife is 'affected' by the idea that P might 'move from one stage to another' (arrow 1).[14] The follow-up question is designed so as to upgrade the problem-relevance of its referent, as it elicits P's description of what his wife is 'most concerned' about in this respect. After P has claimed that he does not understand the question, C2 produces an alternative version of it (arrow 2″), where she simply focuses on P's wife's 'greatest fear'. In response, P produces a more specific description where he refers to further symptoms and anxiety about the future (arrow 3).

In extract (28) below, there is another example of a follow-up question that upgrades the problem-relevance of its referent.

```
(28)   (Extension of (19))
1    C2:            What- (0.2) I mean what (.) Michael mentioned
2                   at- initially is that you know (0.2) he didn't
3                   have any concerns but he's been feeling funny
4                   again,=is that a worry to him or is it no problem   5
                    to him that he feels funny.
6                   (0.3)
7    (C1):          Mm=
1    P:             =I don't know: I- I just go th- er through
2                   stages of uh:m (1.1) you know I mean I've had a
3                   really (0.2) sort of a quite a hectic weekend,
4                   quite a busy ti:me,=and it's not as though I've
5                   been sitting down moping again. (0.6) But you
6                   know it's just sort of like as though- as
7                   though it just clicks:. (0.5) And then I think
8          (1) ->   it will all (              ) what's going
9                   to happen (wi:th) (.) (so and so) if you know
10                  what I mean.
11   C1:   (2) ->   Can I (s[ay) what's your greatest (0.6) fear=
12   C2:                    [(        )
13   C1:             =for th- what might happen.
14                   (0.3)
15   P:              My greatest fear:?
16   C1:             Mm
17                   (0.7)
18   P:    (3) ->    Uh::m (1.5) Well obviously at the moment I mean
19                   I don't (.) particularly want to get AIDS or
20                   nothing like that. (0.5) You know (.) but I
```

[14] Note, however, how P adds a more specific worry-related description 'and that might be a bit of a sho:ck' in his continuation of his turn in line 12. However, in referring to his wife's 'shock', P still leaves unspecified the reason for the shock (P moving 'from one stage to another').

```
21                    still suppose there's- there is that on the
22                    back of your mind still. And I know I've got
23                    the er HIV, (.) but I don't know how far (0.5)
24                    into AIDS I a:m. (0.6) yet.=So: I don't know.
25                    (I don't like to be)
```

By her enquiry concerning P's fears for 'what might happen' (arrow 2), C1 responds to allusions to worries concerning the future in P's preceding turn (arrow 1). Notably, C1 repeats P's word 'happen', thus displaying the connection between her enquiry and P's prior turn. C1's question topically stabilizes the theme of the future that vaguely appeared in the patient's response.

Apart from topically stabilizing 'what might happen', C1's enquiry also upgrades the problem-relevance of this issue. The enquiry concerns P's *fears* of 'what might happen'. Through this lexical choice, the counsellor reframes the focal object in the context of P's fears. This new enquiry is indeed successful, as the patient ends up naming his concern about progression towards AIDS (arrow 3).[15]

Follow-up questions are a most generic conversational device: in ordinary conversation and in numerous institutional environments (though not in every institutional environment: recall Sacks' remarks on presidential press conferences, referred to above in fn. 5 to chapter 2) the participants can be requested to make more specific an answer that they have just given. To ask a follow-up question involves inevitably some choice regarding the focus and direction of the specification. The questioner has to explicate what kind of specification he or she wants.

In AIDS counselling, this generic device is recurrently used in a particular way for a particular institutional purpose. The counsellors' hearing of the clients' talk and response to it is often selective in a special, institutionally relevant way. A central task of the counsellors is to help the clients to talk about their fears and worries related to their future as people affected by HIV/AIDS. Often, the counsellors hear and respond to the clients' talk accordingly. To use a visual metaphor, it is as if the counsellors' perception could *high-*

---

[15] Note, however, that P doesn't explicitly collaborate in disclosing *fears*. He says that he *doesn't want to get AIDS*, instead of saying that he is afraid of getting AIDS.

light[16] those parts in the clients' turns that can possibly allude to, or cover, HIV-related fears and worries; and their responses often aim at uncovering and specifying these.

The *coerciveness* of the follow-up questions that focus on worry-related themes that have occurred in the clients' prior turns can vary. It depends in each individual case on *how* subsidiary the theme is that the follow-up question picks up, or *how* radically it upgrades the problem-relevance of its referents. Because of this variability, the degree of coerciveness of these questions cannot easily be compared on a general level with the degree of coerciveness involved in the other question types.

In spite of their variable coercive character, these questions nevertheless always have their cooperative aspects. In the first place, the counsellors are dependent on the clients having inserted at least latently worry-related descriptions into their turns. The follow-up questions are designed so as to display their connectedness to the clients' prior turns. Therefore, in spite of the selective focusing and the upgraded problem-relevance, these questions exhibit their referents as something that the clients initially brought into the focus of shared attention.

Question type 4: hypothetical questions

The fourth questioning technique counsellors regularly use in invoking a possible hostile future world is to produce the initial description of a hypothetical future situation, and then to invite the patient to discuss it. The counsellors' own theory emphasizes the importance of these 'hypothetical future-oriented questions'. They are exemplified in extracts (29)–(31).

```
(29)  (E4-10)
  1   C1:    A:nd (1.6) from what you know: of Ga:ry I mean:
  2           (2.0) if it was to be positive what d'you think his
  3           main concern would be?
  4           (1.4)
  5   C1:    [Or how d'you think- (.3) how would you see him=
  6   (P):   [(   )-
  7   C1:    =coping.
```

---

[16] On the practice of 'highlighting', see Goodwin and Goodwin (1992).

(30) (E4-51)
```
1   C1:        s::Say:: (.2) we can't say and you can't say,
2   P:         Ye[ah
3   C1:            [but say you did begin to get i:ll (0.8) or say
4                  you got so ill that you couldn't kind of (0.2) make
5                  decisions for yourself.=who would (.4) you have to
6                  make them for you:.
7                  (.3)
8   C1:        Who do you: (.2) consider your:
```

(31) (E4-61)
```
1   C:         .hhhh If Harry die:d (1.0) in the next=
2   P:         =Mm
3   C:         few months
4   P:         M[m
5   C:           [I'm not saying he's going to but if he did.=how
6              would that change your life.
```

In (29), the clients are a gay couple. The counsellor elicits the view
of one partner (who has just been diagnosed as HIV positive) about
the concerns and coping of the other, should he also turn out to be
positive. In (30), the counsellor asks the patient who he would like
to make decisions on his behalf if he became so ill that he couldn't
make them himself. Finally, in (31), the counsellor asks the patient
how his life would change if his brother should die (both the patient
and his brother are HIV-positive haemophiliacs).

All these turns follow the typical pattern of hypothetical questions: a description of a possible hostile future situation is followed
by a question orienting to the client's fears or ways of coping in this
particular situation. The perspective on the future established by
these enquiries is very special: the objects of the patients' fears are
assumed to have been realized. The counsellors invite the patients to
examine their (or their relations') life in the hypothetical world at
some future point where the dreaded crisis is either taking place, or
has already taken place.[17]

---

[17] The hypothetical question is probably a generic conversational device, which is
available in various different types of talk in interaction, and can be used for
various different purposes. Even in AIDS counselling, hypothetical questions can
also be used for purposes other than generating clients' talk about the future. The
extract below is an example: W has asked the counsellor to write a letter to the local
council, in order to help the clients have their council flat renovated.

Hypothetical questions are *the most coercive question type* that the counsellors use in eliciting clients' talk about their future. Other question types examined above create opportunities *for the clients to name* the objects of their fears and worries. With hypothetical questions, however, the *counsellor* spells out the core description of the 'hostile world'. Only after the delivery of this description does the counsellor invite the client to examine his or her life in that world.

In spite of this coerciveness, the counsellors carefully maintain the sense of mutual cooperation with the clients, when delivering hypothetical questions. This is achieved through the careful location of these questions: they are produced only in specific conversational environments. The careful selection of environment also displays the counsellors' orientation to the issues raised in the hypothetical questions as delicate matters.

The adequate environment for hypothetical questions

Counsellors never produce hypothetical questions involving descriptions of distressing future situations 'out of the blue'. Only when the participants' prior talk has provided a proper environment can these questions be delivered. A proper environment is one where the possible future situation has already been hinted at, but has not yet been made explicit. Extracts (29)–(31) were each preceded by such hints; we will first examine the environment of (29) which is shown in extract (32) below.

```
W:      S:[:o-
C1:        [I'm not quite clear about this letter to the
           building ( ) department.=.hhh[h what would you-
W:                                       [Well-
           (.3)
C1:   -> If you were writing it what would you be saying.
W:       Ts Erm:: (.2) the: (.2) alterations which Mr and
           Mrs Davies pro[pose .hhh (.) are:: ((continues))
```

The counsellor's question employs the same format as the other hypothetical questions shown above. However, in the extract above this type of question is used in eliciting the details of a client's view about a current practical matter, and not in generating talk about the future.

(32)   (Extension of (29))
```
 1   C1:    What d'you think at the moment Gary's main concerns
 2          are.
 3          (1.5)
 4   P:     hhhhh (1.0) Of course he's very concerned about my
 5          health.
 6   C1:    Mm:
 7          (0.6)
 8   P:     You know (and what-) (.4) what I'm going through:,
 9          (.2) Of course he has to be concerned about
10          himself.=Worrying .hhhh
11   C1:    Have=
12   P:     =about the test for him[self of course,
13   C1:                           [umh
14   C1:    M[m:
15   P:      [A:nd the doubts he may have:, er[:
16   C1:                                      [Have you just had
17          the tes[t Gary?
18   BF:           [Yes I have.
19   P:     Uhm
20          (.3)
21   C1:    A:nd (1.6) from what you know: of Ga:ry I mean:
22          (2.0) if it was to be positive what d'you think his
23          main concern would be?
```

In (32), P is first asked to describe his boy-friend's (BF's) main concerns. As we can see, the counsellor uses the topic-elicitation procedure analysed above. In the course of his response, P (who has recently tested positive) first asserts that BF is very likely to be concerned about his own test (lines 9–10; 12). In response to this, the counsellor first checks with BF whether he has just had the test (lines 16–17); and after he has confirmed this (line 18), the counsellor produces her turn where she nominates the stressful possible future situation: '*if* it was to be positive' (lines 21–3). The counsellor prefaces her turn with 'An:d', which emphasizes the continuity between the preceding talk (probably the factual enquiry in lines 16–17) and the forthcoming question (cf. Sorjonen and Heritage 1991).

Thus, in (32) the patient first asserted that his boyfriend is most likely to be worried about the test. Only thereafter did the counsellor nominate a possible future situation involving a positive test result. The counsellor seems only to have spelled out what was already implied by the patient; or to put it in Jefferson's (1985a) terminology, the counsellor *unpacked* the *gloss* that the patient had initially produced.

A similar movement from clients' hints to the explicit nomination of the possible future situation by the counsellor can be seen in extracts (33) and (34).

```
(33)  (Extension of (30))
 1    P:     (Can you-) (.) what are the main uhm symptom- (0.5)
 2           what actually does pneumonia (.3) do to you?
 3           (.4)
 4    P:     Once it's (      ) (within your system).
 5    C2:    It gives you a cough,
 6    P:     Yeah.
 7    C2:    breathlessness
 8           (3.5)
 9    C1:    Are these things you've thought about before or not
10           really.
11           (2.0)
12    P:     Uh::m (.2) Sorry what d'you mean- what
13           (lik[e the-)
14    C1:        [All these this discussion we're having
15           about.=Symptoms and things.
16           (0.4)
17    P:     Yeah I had (.2) I have thought about
18           them,=[(as I said) I thought before: mo:re=
19    C1:          [Mm
20    P:     =so [that (.2) err: (1.0) ( ) that I am=
21    C1:        [Mm
22    P:     =thinking more- (.4) about them more now because
23           (.6) I'm a little bit more settled in this
24           work (.) [job. And if it's (you sort of)=
25    C1:             [Right.
26    P:     =(                    ) (so now: I've got more) time
27           (I) will be-
28    C1:    (    [   )
29    P:         [(actually) taking a [leave (so)-
30    C1:                             [s : : S a y : : (.2) we
31           can't say and you can't say,
32    P:     Ye[ah
33    C1:      [but say you did begin to get i:ll (0.8) or say
34           you got so ill that you couldn't kind of (0.2) make
35           decisions for yourself.=who would (.4) you have to
36           make them for you:.
37           (.3)
38    C1:    Who do you: (.2) consider your:
```

```
(34)   (Extension of (31))
 1    C:        .hh Now last ti[me you came to the orthopaedic=
 2    P:                       [Mm
 3    C:        =clinic (0.5) you wanted to [have your: (.3) knee=
 4    P:                                    [Mm:
 5    C:        =done. [What d'you feel about that now.
 6    P:               [Mm:
 7              (.3)
 8    C:        Because that means being in hospital for weeks,
 9              (0.6)
10    P:        Yeah I know: I don- I don't know: I just don't know
11              what to do.=I mean if Harry's ou:t I mean er (0.5) I
12              ju- I just don't know:.
13              (0.8)
14    P:        To be honest I really don't know.
15              (2.6)
16    P:        er: And things are getting a bit (.) complicated
17              with- because he- he s- he seems to me to be getting
18              much worse.
19              (1.2)
20    P:        Especially er er- medically anyway. A:nd you know
21              it's very hard to know what to do:,
22    C:        .hhhh If Harry die:d (1.0) in the next=
23    P:        =Mm
24    C:        few months
25    P:        M[m
26    C:         [I'm not saying he's going to but if he did.=how
27              would that change your life.
```

In (33), the patient first asks the counsellor about pneumonia[18] (lines 1–3). After giving a short answer, the counsellor asks him whether he has thought about these kind of things before or not (lines 9–10). The patient responds by asserting that he is now thinking about them more than he did before (from line 17 onward). After that assertion, the counsellor produces her description of the possible future situation, where the patient would be too ill to make decisions about himself (lines 30–1; 33–7). Thus the counsellor produced the description of the hostile future, not only following

---

[18] 'Pneumonia' appears to be an object loaded with meaning in HIV-related conversation. It seems to be treated as a 'paradigmatic' indication of the collapse of the patient's immunity and, therefore, of 'full-blown AIDS'. So talking about 'pneumonia' may convey much more in an HIV-related context than in other medical contexts.

the patient's questions involving the symptoms he could have if he got ill, but also after the patient had asserted that he is nowadays, more than before, thinking about 'symptoms and things'. The sense that the counsellor is only making explicit what the patient has already implied is further emphasized by the counsellor through the use of 'did' in line 33: 'Say you did begin to get i:ll' conveys that the theme has actually been touched upon earlier.[19]

In (34), the counsellor's initial question involves the patient's feelings about having his 'knee done', in an operation which would mean a long stay in hospital. (The patient, as with many haemophiliacs, has persistent trouble with his knee joints.) The patient responds (from line 10 onwards) by expressing his current doubts about what to do, after which he produces the reason for his doubt: his brother's health is getting much worse.[20] Thus the gloomy prospects involving Harry were initially hinted at by the patient; only after such hints did the counsellor produce her explication of the situation. In her turn, she unpacks the patient's gloss 'He- he s- he seems to me to be getting much worse (...) especially er er- *med*ically anyway' with the conditional but explicit assertion 'If Harry *die*:d'.

In summary, the counsellors ask hypothetical future-oriented questions only when the fearful situation has been elliptically or vaguely hinted at in the preceding talk. The *kairos* moment for a hypothetical question is thus anticipated and prepared for. The preceding hints may have appeared as a response to the counsellor's prior enquiries that created space for such talk to be made (as in extracts (32) and (33)[21]), or they may have appeared more or less voluntarily in the client's talk (as in extract (34)). In other words,

---

[19] The contrast would be the counsellor saying 'Say you began to get ill'. That appears to nominate a future possibility without reference backwards in the talk. On the contrary, the use of 'did' in 'Say you did begin to get i:ll' seems to present 'getting ill' as a fulfilment of something referred to earlier.

[20] Exactly how his brother's medical condition accounts for the patient's difficulties in deciding whether to have his knees done or not remains somewhat unclear here. Possibly the patient implies that he should not spend a long period in hospital while his brother's state of health is deteriorating, and he would be needed in taking care of his brother.

[21] In (33), the patient's question in lines 1–3 followed a long information delivery triggered off by the patient's earlier question about possible treatments if his immunity deteriorated as a result of HIV. This earlier question by P appeared as a response to the counsellor's topic elicitation. (Data not shown.)

the counsellor can intentionally pursue a suitable environment, or it may appear spontaneously. In any case, the counsellors design the turns where they nominate the distressing future situations as turns which unpack something that has already been referred to by the patient, but only incompletely.

What do the counsellors *achieve* by locating their turns here rather than elsewhere? By portraying the nominations of distressing future situations as unpacking the patients' prior vague hints, the counsellors show their attention to patients' prior talk and avoid the impression of unilaterally imposing upon the patients an expectation to talk about difficult themes. By emphasizing the continuity, they locally constitute the topics involved in their enquiries as something that has to be approached and talked about carefully (cf. Bergmann 1992). On the other hand, they also make it more difficult for the patients to turn down the questions, because it now appears that the patients themselves actually have initiated the themes.

Clients' responses to hypothetical questions

A closer examination of the sequences generated by the hypothetical questions reveals more about the coerciveness of these queries.

First recall the general structure of hypothetical questions: a description of a possible hostile future situation is followed by a question orienting to the client's fears or ways of coping in this particular situation. The questions that occur after the descriptions would not make sense alone: the questions presuppose the description. And further on, the answers that the questions project also presuppose the descriptions. Or to put it another way, both the question (uttered by the counsellor) and the answer (elicited from the patient) have as their *horizon* the description initially given by the counsellor.

Re-examination of the first three extracts may further illustrate the point. In (29), the extension of which is shown below in extract (35), the counsellor's question about Gary's main concerns presupposes that he is HIV positive; in other words, the question appears on the horizon of Gary being positive. By producing his answer, the patient maintains this presupposition and horizon:

```
(35)  (Extension of (29))
 1    C1:        A:nd (1.6) from what you know: of Ga:ry I mean:
 2               (2.0) if it was to be positive what d'you think
 3               his main concern would be?
 4               (1.4)
 5    C1:        [Or how d'you think- (.3) how would you see=
 6    (P):       [( )-
 7    C1:        = him coping.
 8               (2.3)
 9    P:    ->   I (don't) think he'd cope we:ll,=because we
10               have discussed it over the weeke:nd, (.) uh:m
11               (0.6) (And just) (1.6) er: hhh uh- (.2)
12               following up on it. Being very careful about
13               everything.
```

By asserting that Gary would possibly not cope well, and by referring to the idea of 'following up on it being very careful about
everything', P effectively maintains the hypothetical assumption
that 'Gary is positive' as the horizon of his talk.

In (36) below, the question of who the patient would like to
make decisions on his behalf presupposes that he would get so ill
that he could not make the decisions himself. The question is
designed to provide for an answer preserving this hypothetical
state of affairs as the horizon of discourse:

```
(36)  (Extension of (30))
 1    C1:        s::Say:: (.2) we can't say and you can't say,
 2    P:         Ye[ah
 3    C1:          [but say you did begin to get i:ll (0.8) or
 4               say you got so ill that you couldn't kind of
 5               (0.2) make decisions for yourself.=who would
 6               (.4) you have to make them for you:. (.3) Who
 7               do you: (.2) consider your:
 8               (3.8)
 9    P:    ->   I think I'd probably (get) one of my say
10               closest friends (0.5) uh:m (.4) a friend of
11               mine called Anselm (the one) I lived with
12               because he's sort of (.3) ehh
13               (1.0)
14    C1:        Anselm?
15    P:         Yeah:.=
```

By naming Anselm as the person he would like to make the decisions on his behalf, the patient preserves the assumption of getting

so ill that he couldn't make decisions for himself as the horizon of the discourse.

Equally, in (37) the patient's answer preserves the horizon set up by the counsellor:

```
(37)  (Extension of (31))
  1   C:           .hhhh If Harry die:d (1.0) in the next=
  2   P:           =Mm
  3   C:           few months
  4   P:           M[m
  5   C:             [I'm not saying he's going to but if he
  6                did.=how would that change your life.
  7                (2.5)
  8   P:    ->     I don't know:.
  9                (.)
 10   P:           Uh:m:
 11                (1.2)
 12   P:    ->     I don't think it would change it that much to
 13                be honest.
 14   P:           (0.8)
 15   P:           We've drifted very far apart over the las::t
 16                sort of er few: (2.4) *(well)*
 17                (0.8)
 18   C:           But would it make your [life easier then.
 19   P:                                  [(            )
 20                (1.8)
 21   P:           I think possibly it- (.4) it might do.=but
 22                uh::m (0.6) what (I'm)- what I'm really- (0.5)
 23                thinking about is er:: (0.9) doing or saying
 24                something that I would er feel guilty about
 25                should it happen. ((continues))
```

Here the horizon is the assumption 'Harry die:d (...) in the next (...) few months', which the patient's answer preserves. After saying that his life wouldn't change much in the event of Harry's death, P produces the statement 'We've drifted very far apart over the las::t sort of er few:', as an account for the first part of the answer. Even though this focuses on past events instead of the future, it serves as an explanation of something that the patient says about the future. Accordingly, the counsellor's following turn 'But would it make your life easier then.' maintains the initial horizon.

The 'hypothetical future-oriented questions' seem to be very cleverly designed. Almost *any* answer that the patient could possibly give to them would *equally* preserve the initial description as the horizon of the discourse. So in (35), if P had said that Gary would cope well, or if he had named any particular problems of his coping, he would equally have treated '*if* it was to be positive' as the horizon. Or in (36), by naming anybody at all as the person whom he would like to make the decisions, the patient would also have maintained the assumption of himself as being too ill to make them as the horizon. And in (37), naming any change, or reporting that nothing would change, would equally have maintained the initial horizon.

Most notably, the client need not repeat or rephrase the hypothetical description: it is routinely preserved as a presupposition. Only in very rare cases do the clients actually rephrase the description; and, most interestingly, these cases seem to involve some kind of resistance towards the question. Extract (38) is an example:

```
(38)  (E4-4)
 1    C:        ↑Okay (.) say you were sick
 2    P:        Umh
 3    C:        What do you see yourself as doing.
 4              (1.2)
 5    C:        How would your life change? Would your job
 6              change?=Would your friends change?
 7              (.)
 8    C:        I'm wondering,=what would be different.
 9              (2.0)
10    P:  ->    If I was sick ((background noise)) (2.0) If I was
11              sick I've got to be in hospital (1.2) ( )=
12    C:        =well:: say (.) you (ain't have to be) in hospital
13              but say you were at home (.3) you you you're not=
14              ((continues))
```

In (38) above, the client does not describe changes in his life in the terms suggested by the counsellor. Instead, he offers a different kind of description of being sick. This less than fully collaborative response is prefaced by the client rephrasing the hypothetical description. But cases like this are very rare; normally the clients' responses preserve the hypothetical description as a horizon, without rephrasing it at all.[22]

---

[22] I wish to thank John Heritage for drawing my attention to the (lack of) repetition of the hypothetical description in clients' responses.

Therefore, the hypothetical questions can justly be considered as the *most coercive and effective tool* that the counsellors have available in addressing future related 'dreaded issues' with their clients. They constitute a most powerful invitation for clients to consider their life in a dreaded future situation; an invitation that is difficult to resist once it has been spelled out.

A stepwise strategy

In this chapter, I have examined four types of questions which can be used in the invocation of the world of untoward future realities in counselling sessions. Even though the dynamics entailed in each are different, there are at least two common features in all of them: first, by invoking the world of the future counsellors carefully maintain the cooperative work of both patient and counsellor. Unilateral moves openly imposing potentially dreadful future-related themes are avoided. Second, in preparing the way for explicit descriptions of possible future situations, the participants regularly use indirect and vague expressions.

These two features – careful maintenance of cooperation and movement from vague descriptions towards more explicit ones - constitute the clients' future as a very special topic in AIDS counselling. It is treated as a *delicate matter*: as something that in this context has to be talked about with special care. By their descriptive caution, the counsellors on the one hand approach the clients' possible fears and worries in an empathizing, sensitive way. And on the other hand, through very descriptive caution, the counsellors also indirectly suggest to the clients that in their future, something troublesome may indeed reside.

As already indicated, the four question techniques can be compared as regards their coerciveness, i.e. the degree that the counsellor's action controls the client's response.[23] In this respect, 'hypothetical questions' are the *most coercive* technique: when the counsellor has asked this kind of question, there is almost no way

---

[23] I am not talking about a 'general' or 'absolute' control. By the degree of coercion here I mean each question type's potential in directing the client's talk to worrying issues related to his or her future. Any question of course controls the addressee's conduct in numerous other ways, too: for example, by creating a conditional relevance for *some kind of* answer.

for the client to escape addressing his/her views concerning the future. The topic elicitation questions are obviously the *least coercive* technique, as they give the clients a relatively weakly controlled opportunity to choose what kind of topic (if any) they proffer. The other two question types – questions that retrieve themes that were mentioned in, or were absent from, the clients' earlier talk, and the questions that topicalize worry-indicative themes in the clients' prior turns – can be located between these two. They give more freedom to the client than hypothetical questions, but are more constraining than topic elicitations.

Each type of question described here can be applied individually, without the application of other question types. An appropriate situation for a given type of question may arise and the counsellors may choose to make use of that situation. On the other hand, the application of any question type may be unsuccessful, and further steps towards building a hostile world are not taken.

However, the four question types are also ordered roughly in relation to one another. As was argued at the beginning of this chapter, this ordering does not mean that the four techniques are all used in a consecutive order in each individual case, or even in the majority of them. Rather, it means that every type of question, considered in the order that they have been presented in this chapter, can *create a favourable conversational environment for the next type to occur.* The *kairos* – the right time – for each question type can be achieved through using another question type. In general terms, then, the less coercive questions can be used to create an appropriate environment for the more coercive ones to appear. To be more precise, this 'order of possibility' can be described figuratively.

- -
Relative ordering of question types in
'addressing dreaded issues'
- -

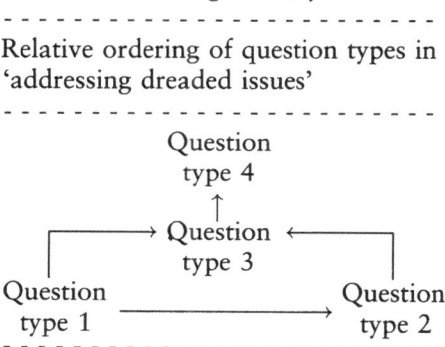

- -

By suggesting this relative ordering, I want to give direction to future work rather than proclaim any final truth.[24] The four question types, in their relative ordering, set up a potential strategy that the counsellors can use in eliciting the clients' talk about their fears concerning their future.

The first step can be taken through topic elicitation (question type 1). In response, the counsellors sometimes obtain answers that can be traded off in generating talk about the clients' future. Even if the answers do not directly refer to any fears, they possibly contain something that can be used as a point of departure for further enquiries, either in the very next turn, or somewhere later in the conversation.

The second step in the strategy is optional. If the discussion that follows topic elicitation does not lead to future-related topics, the counsellors can retrieve something potentially future- and/or worry-related that has nevertheless been said, or they can point out something that the client has not mentioned, and generate more talk about that (question type 2).

The core of the third step of the strategy consists of the topicalization of worry-indicative and/or future-relevant themes in clients' talk (question type 3). Through their follow-up questions, the counsellors invite more thorough talk about such themes. The follow-up questions can be specifically designed so as to transform subsidiary themes into prominence, or they can upgrade the problem relevance of the clients' initial descriptions.

Through the topical stablization of the worry-indicative themes, an appropriate environment for the delivery of hypothetical questions can be achieved. When the patient has begun to talk about his distress concerning the future, the counsellors can move to the

---

[24] It is an interesting challenge for future studies to find out whether this kind of 'order of possibility' can also prevail in other 'big packages' of talk. In many institutional environments the interaction seems to be divided into different phases. Doctor–patient interaction is an example. The relative ordering of the different stages of the medical consultation has been discussed by e.g. Byrne and Long (1976) and ten Have (1989). It is possible to think that each stage – such as the delivery of the complaint, the anamnestic interview or the delivery of the diagnosis – creates possibilities for the next to occur. The analytical difficulty with the idea of the order of possibility is, of course, that because it does not require and predict any strict empirical regularity in the actual cases, it is very difficult to empirically confirm or falsify.

fourth stage of the strategy. Through the hypothetical questions (question type 4), the distressful future situation is explicitly spelled out by the counsellor, and the patient is invited to share that as the horizon of the forthcoming discourse. The object of the patient's fear is hypothetically treated as part of the reality, and the patient is invited to examine his life in the world shaped by it.

In a number of cases, all three or four stages are passed through. Extract (39) is an example of this. This is an extension of extract (19) shown above in this chapter; the same segment was analysed from a different point of view in chapter 5. In spite of the length of the transcript, I have decided to present it here in its entirety as a conclusive illustration of the argument developed in this chapter.

```
(39)  (E4-46)
      C1:     And you can- (.2) I'll se[nd you a letter with=
      C2:                             [letter
      C1:     an appointment a[nd then you can let me know=
      P:                      [Yeah
      C1:     =whether you want to [keep it (or not).
      P:                           [(No well) I'll keep walking
              (.3) anyway (.2) (which will make me a) (     ).
```

```
((Question type 1))
      C2:     Doctor Kaufman I'd like (0.3) to a::sk (1.7) what
              (.) at the moment hh (.2) is Michael's main concern.
              (0.2)
      C1:     Yes.=Michael what's your main concern today.
              (2.4)
      P:      It depends (o:n) I suppose what you (.) mean by
              concer:n,=I'm not really uh:m
              (0.4)
      C2:     Or [what's top of his mi:nd.  ]
      P:         [worried about anything a]t the moment.
              (0.6)
      C1:     Wha- [what d'you most want from us today.
      P:           [Well er
              (1.6)
      P:      Uh:m: (1.5) well it would be nice to sort of sort
              me- me knees out (I think but er u-unless er)
      C1:     Mm hm
              (0.2)
      C1:     [So that's one thing we can]
      P:      [S o r t that out (.2)      y]eah.
      C1:     look at ortho[paedically,=but what else?
```

P: [Yeah.
          (1.0)
P: Uh:m (1.0) I'm not sure really I've never thought of
          it (.4) anything.
          (0.2)
C2:   [(Wh)-
P: [(But) you've been helping me all the (.) last
          little while,
          (0.2)

((Question type 2))
C2:   What- (0.2) I mean what (.) Michael mentioned at-
          initially is that you know (0.2) he didn't have any
          concerns but he's been feeling funny again,=is that
          a worry to him or is it no problem to him that he
          feels funny.
          (0.3)
C1:   Mm=
P: =I don't know: I- I just go th- er through stages of
          uh:m (1.1) you know I mean I've had a really (0.2)
          sort of a quite a hectic weekend, quite a busy
          ti:me,=and it's not as though I've been sitting down
          moping again.
          (0.6)
P: But you know it's just sort of
          like as though- as though it just clicks:.
          (0.5)
P: And then I think it will all (   )
          what's going to happen (wi:th) (.) (so and so) if
          you know what I mean.

((Question type 3))
C1:   Can I (s[ay) what's your greatest (0.6) fear for=
C2:   [(   )
C1:   =th- what might happen.
          (0.3)
P: My greatest fear:?
C1:   Mm
          (0.7)
P: Uh::m (1.5) Well obviously at the moment I mean I
          don't (.) particularly want to get AIDS or nothing
          like that.
          (0.5)

P: You know (.) but I still suppose there's- there is
        that on the back of your mind still. And I know I've
        got the er HIV, (.) but I don't know how far (0.5)
        into AIDS I a:m.
        (0.6)
P: yet.=So: [I don't know. (I don't [like to be)
C2:   [Does-   [s-
C2:   How much does (0.2 Michael want to know about
        (0.8) how far he's (in[to AIDS)
P: [Well I think I should know
        everything.=I think it's only- only right. (Isn't)
        (it really).

((Question type 4))
C2:   [One other question first before we go into (what=
C1:   [Mm
C2:   =he might be doing) is that,.hhh (.7) What if he did
        get AIDS,=what does he think (0.7) will be: the
        (0.2) hardest thing for him.=What does he fear most.
        (1.0)
P: I think (.3) accepting it I suppose.
        (.)
P: That's going to be quite- and I know I've accepted
        it this far.

In (39), the counsellors use consecutively all four questioning techniques in eliciting talk about the patient's distressing future (the
sections where the different types of questioning are used are separated in their own 'boxes'). Also, the optional second question type
is used as a consequence of the application of the first type being
unsuccessful. Through the consecutive application of all the question types, the counsellors overcame the patient's apparent initial
reluctance to speak, and soon ended up talking about a hypothetical
situation where the patient has AIDS.

As a three- or four-step strategy available to counsellors, the
questioning techniques presented in this chapter constitute a powerful device for eliciting the clients' talk about the future. The design
of the counsellors' questions, the organization of question–answer
sequences and the organization of the successive question–answer
pairs are all involved in the progressive build-up of the *kairos*
(Erickson and Schultz 1982) for 'addressing dreaded issues'.

The questioning techniques analysed in this chapter complement the other interactional techniques analysed in chapters 3–5, that also can be used to elicit the clients' talk about matters that initially they are reluctant to discuss. When consistently used, all these different questioning patterns and practices form a comprehensive set of tools which is very difficult to resist.

7

The interactional power of hypothetical questions

In the preceding chapter we examined four types of question that the counsellors use in introducing the topic of the future during counselling sessions. It was concluded that the four questioning techniques together set up a potential strategy whereby the participants can move from vague hints into explicit questions and answers about the clients' fears and beliefs. The fourth method, involving the use of what the counsellors call 'hypothetical future-oriented questions', is the final stage of that strategy.

In this chapter we will continue the examination of 'hypothetical future-oriented questions'. In terms of the progression of the talk about the future, as it were, we start from the point that we reached in the preceding chapter: now we take for granted that the interlocutors have achieved the interactional environment where hypothetical, future-oriented questions *can* be asked. We will examine what is done through asking and answering these questions.

In the Family Systems Theory literature, the therapeutic importance of hypothetical questions is pointed out (e.g. Penn 1985; Miller and Bor 1988) but the interactional dynamics related to their use is not thoroughly discussed. The goal of this chapter is, therefore, to use the analytical machinery of Conversation Analysis to examine how these questions work. What follows is an examination of the properties of hypothetical questions and of the methods of their use in generating talk about the clients' future.

The structure of hypothetical questions

We will begin with a brief re-examination of the examples of hypothetical questions presented in chapter 6.

(1)   (E4-10)
 1   C1:   A:nd (1.6) from what you know: of Ga:ry I mean:
 2   (2.0) if it was to be positive what d'you think
 3   his main concern would be?
 4   (1.4)
 5   C1:   [Or how d'you think- (.3) how would you see=
 6   (P):   [( )-
 7   C1:   =him coping.
 8   (2.3)
 9   P: I (don't) think he'd cope we:ll,=because we
10   have discussed it over the weeke:nd, (.) uh:m
11   (0.6) (And just) (1.6) er: hhh uh- (.2)
12   following up on it. Being very careful about
13   everything.

(2)   (E4-51)
 1   C1:   s::Say:: (.2) we can't say and you can't say,
 2   P: Ye[ah
 3   C1:   [but say you did begin to get i:ll (0.8) or
 4   say you got so ill that you couldn't kind of
 5   (0.2) make decisions for yourself.=who would
 6   (.4) you have to make them for you:. (.3) Who
 7   do you: (.2) consider your:
 8   (3.8)
 9   P: I think I'd probably (get) one of my say
10   closest friends (0.5) uh:m (.4) a friend of
11   mine called Anselm (the one) I lived with
12   because he's sort of (.3) ehh

(3)   (E4-61)
 1   C: .hhhh If Harry die:d (1.0) in the next=
 2   P: =Mm
 3   C: few months
 4   P: M[m
 5   C: [I'm not saying he's going to but if he
 6   did.=how would that change your life.
 7   (2.5)
 8   P: I don't know:. (.) Uh:m: (1.2) I don't think it
 9   would change it that much to be honest.

Each of the counsellor's utterances above has two parts, the coupling of which is a key feature of hypothetical questions. First, they all contain *a description of a hypothetical state of affairs*. Thus, in (1), this initial description is '*if it was to be positive*'; in (2), *say you did begin to get i:ll (0.8) or say you got so ill that you couldn't kind* of (0.2) *m*ake decisions for yourself; and in (3) 'If Harry *die*:d (1.0) in the next few months'.

Along with these descriptions, in each extract there is an enquiry where the client is invited to report something – a concern, a course of activity or the like – related to the hypothetical situation. As was argued in chapter 6, these enquiries treat the initial descriptions as their presuppositions, or as their horizons. To put it in another way, the latter part of the hypothetical question suggests a specific set of issues which can be treated as relevant to the state of affairs named in the initial description: in (1), this set of issues is Gary's main concerns and his coping; in (2), it is P's choice of person to make decisions for him; and in (3), the changes in P's life. For the purposes of this chapter, we might call these sets of issues *the project-ables*. The hypothetical questions operate by inviting the clients to produce mental predicates or action descriptions concerning the hypothetical states of affairs named in the first parts of the enquiries.

Hypothetical questions are extensively and recurrently asked by the counsellors when discussing the clients' future during counselling sessions. As we argued in chapter 6, much of the counsellors' strategy appears to be geared to achieve a state of talk where it is interactionally appropriate to ask hypothetical questions. That is one of the reasons why it is interesting to examine the details of their functioning.

The power of hypothetical questions: some preliminary considerations

The extensive use of future-oriented hypothetical questions suggests that they enable the counsellors to accomplish their institutionally ascribed task of 'preparing' the patients for distressing things which might happen in their future. Hypothetical questions may have at least three advantages in generating talk about the future.

(1) As argued in the preceding chapter, hypothetical questions establish a hypothetical description as a presupposition of the unfolding discourse. Establishing the hypothetical description as a presupposition of a question and the projected answer implies a 'sequential enclave', or protection, for it. Most of the possible

answers that the patients can give to hypothetical questions preserve the description as the horizon.

In analytical terms, hypothetical questions mobilize the resources of the powerful conversational rules related to questions and answers, to the work of establishing a future-related horizon for the discourse. Like any other question, a hypothetical question also creates the conditional relevancy for the answer. But because a hypothetical question preserves the description of a hypothetical state of affairs as the horizon of the discourse, and projects an answer which does the same, the adjacency-pair structure ends up being exploited in setting up this horizon for the discourse. This makes hypothetical questions applicable in facilitating talk about future-related matters that are potentially difficult to address.

(2) The counsellors' institutional task entails a dual challenge. On the one hand, they should be *indirective*, i.e. they should allow the clients to express *their* concerns and ideas about the future. In order for the counselling to be effective, however, the counsellors should also be able to *control* and *direct* the talk about the future, so that the clients can be helped to find new ways of thinking and coping. Now it appears that the hypothetical questions can accommodate in a subtle way these conflicting expectations. They are indirective, as they leave it up to the clients to name their fears, ideas or ways of coping. But this indirectiveness is embedded in a structure controlled by the counsellor. She formulates the description of a hypothetical state of affairs which is to operate as the horizon of the discourse. And, most importantly, the counsellor chooses the 'projectables' (the issues, relevant to the hypothetical future situation, that the client is asked to describe) whereby she can influence very much the thematic direction of the conversation. As we will see later, the counsellors' theoretical orientation can make her/him choose particular kinds of projectables.

(3) Finally, from the client's point of view, hypothetical questions allow for a manageable way to talk about the potentially threatening issues related to the future. When it comes to the terms of the discourse, the client can remain on a responsive footing. By naming the issues that the client is asked to describe, the counsellor in effect suggests a specific vocabulary for the client to use in talking about the future. It is left to the client only to 'fill in

the gaps' in the structure; and this, indeed, may be as much as many clients are able to say about their future.

Extract (4) below can, as a contrasting case, illustrate the inherent functionality of hypothetical questioning. Here an observer in a counselling session asks the patient a future-related question. Perhaps due to her inexperience, however, she *does not* use the hypothetical format. The patient's response shows how easily this kind of non-hypothetical enquiry can be turned down.

```
(4)   (E4-22)
      (O = Liz, the Observer)
 1    C:           Liz, (.5) any issues you wanted to raise today.
 2                 (2.5)
 3    O:    (1) -> .hhh (2.0) well I think- (.3) one of the things
 4                 I was- (.2) thinking about was:: (2.1) had- had
 5                 you (.2) you and Sue ever thought if things:
 6                 (1.6) got worse (.) how are you going to cope
 7                 o:r
 8                 (.4)
 9    P:           .hhhhhhhh[hhhhh
10    O:                    [>I mean has< (.) has that come
11                 [to your mind (.) at all?
12    P:    (2) -> [hhhhhhhhhhhh heh heh heh heh .hhhh (it must
13                 have gone through) our minds but erm: (1.4) .hh
14                 not particularly worried. .hh
```

In spite of its future orientation, O's question in (4) above does not employ the hypothetical structure. Elements which are like the description of a hypothetical state of affairs ('things: (1.6) got *wor*se') and naming the 'projectable' ('how are you going to cope') are included in O's question – but they are embedded in retrospective enquiry about P's and Sue's (P's wife) thoughts and worries about these kinds of matters (lines 4–5, 10–11). Consequently, the question allows for a 'no worries' type of answer, which, in turn, makes it difficult to continue to address the theme in the subsequent talk.

The inherent strength and functionality of hypothetical questions is not, however, automatic. Through the details of their careful turn design, counsellors recurrently activate and mobilize this strength. Therefore, in what follows we will examine the turn design of hypothetical questions.

The epistemological framework of hypothetical descriptions

One of the most interesting turn-design features in hypothetical questions is the counsellors' way of formulating the epistemological status of the hypothetical descriptions. Not only do they use the standard conditional forms of English, but they regularly 'upgrade' the conditionality of their assertions. Alternatively, they can emphasize the universal character of the described state of affairs as something that anybody could one day find him- or herself in. The likelihood of the use of these devices for the management of the epistemological framework seems to increase the more the counsellor's description departs from what the client has described as the objects of his fears earlier in the discourse.

There are two means available for upgrading the conditionality of the descriptions of the hypothetical future situations. One involves use of formulations along with the delivery of the description. That was done in extracts (2) and (3). In (2), the counsellor began her question this way:

> C: s::Say:: we can't say and you can't say,
> P: Yeah

Here the counsellor formulates her own epistemological position *vis-à-vis* the assertions about the patient's future: neither of them can say what will really happen. Interestingly, the patient produces an affirmative response token after the formulation, thus probably agreeing with the characterization of their epistemological position.

In extract (3), the counsellor adds to the description of a future state of affairs ('If Harry *d*ie:d (.5) in the next few months') a characterization of the limited force that she intends her words to have:

> C: I'm not saying he's going to but if he did

Normally, the use of the conditional form in itself is enough to convey that the speaker is not committed to the truth of the expressed proposition in the same way as in the case of ordinary 'representatives'. Here, however, the counsellor decided to emphasize the limited force of her words.

The formulations of the counsellors' statement's epistemological status and the force of their words recurrently accompany the counsellors' descriptions of the possible future states of affairs. Three further examples:

```
(5)    (E4-12)
1      C:              .hh I mean taking things to their worst (...) I
2                      mean as far as I understand if one- (.7)
3            ->        I'm not saying this can happen but taking it to
4                      its very worst (.) if .hh you did begin to
5                      ((continues))

(6)    (E4-41)
1      C:              (...) Say he did (.2) get AI:DS and (.2) the
2                      worst did happen, .hhh what (.5) does he think
3                      (1.0) is (.2) Helena's greatest fear.
4                      (.2)
5      C:    ->        How: (.3) what- what- what (1.3) just let's
6                      take it o:n (and ifs) this is all hypothetical,
7                      but I'd just like to know: ((continues))

(7)    (E4-55)
1      C:    ->        If you: if you- supposing I mean this is just
2                      supposing,=supposing you: (.2) had got infected
3                      (.) or were to get infected
```

In (5), the counsellor spells out the limited force of her words ('I'm not saying this can happen'), along with characterizing the motivation for the assertion ('taking it to its very worst'). In (6) and (7) the counsellors formulate the special character of the assertions: 'this is all hypothetical' and 'this is just supposing'.

In Extracts (2), (3) and (5–7) shown above, the counsellors' formulations are accompanied by pauses and self-repairs. Both the 'content' of the formulations and the perturbations surrounding them seem to have a 'pre-delicate' character. The counsellors hearably propose that the matters involved in the descriptions may be sensitive and delicate for the patients (cf. Schegloff 1980; Silverman and Peräkylä 1990).

There are cases, however, where no formulation of the epistemic status of the statements or the force of the utterance was given. Extract (1) above was. one of those cases.

```
(1)    (Section)
1      C:    A:nd (1.6) from what you know: of Ga:ry I mean:
2            (2.0) if it was to be positive what d'you think his
3            main concern would be?
```

However, the conditionality of the description of the future situation is maintained here as well, but differently. The counsellor does not ask simply 'if it is positive', nor even 'if it were positive', but uses a more complicated formula '*if* it was to be positive'. By substituting 'was to be' for 'is', and by prosodically emphasizing 'if' she upgrades the conditional character of the description.

A similar kind of technique of upgrading conditionality is used in a number of other cases. Extract (8) provides another example.

```
(8)    (E4-74)
1    C:        (...) You've come up .hh here and in your
2              review: (0.6) a number of tests are done.=Do
3              you know anything about the tests that are
4              done?=
5    P:        =Uh:m no not really.=As far as I know it's just
6              a blood test. Uh:m

              ((13 lines of discussion about the patient's willingness to
              be told about the results of the test omitted))

20   C1:  ->   What would happen say if Doctor Kaufma:n (0.6)
21             did these tests and thought that your immune
22             system wasn't quite as good as she (0.2) would
23             want it to be.=What should she do with that
24             information then.
```

In (8), after having talked about the tests that are routine in the clinic, the counsellor shifts into a conditional form when she addresses the possibility of troublesome test results. Instead of saying something like 'If Doctor Kaufman's tests show that your immune system isn't quite as good...', the counsellor says 'What would happen say if Doctor Kaufma:n (.6) *d*id these tests and thought that your immune system wasn't quite as good...'. Again, the conditionality of the description of the possible future situation is upgraded by using the more complicated formula. Using 'say' in the beginning of the utterance; referring to the tests that factually *are* done in the conditional 'If Dr Kaufma:n (0.6) *d*id these tests', referring to the doctor's observation through tentative formulation 'Doctor Kaufma:n (...) thought that your immune system ...'; and saying 'your immune system wasn't quite as good' instead of 'isn't as good', the counsellor recurrently emphasizes the hypothetical character of her assertion.

Apart from the formulations of the speaker's epistemological status and the force of the utterances, and the use of a 'compound conditional', there is a third strategy available in the management of the epistemic status of the descriptions of a possible distressing future. The descriptions can be 'over-generalized' to include everybody, not only the patient(s) attending the session. This strategy is applied in extract (9).

```
(9)   (E4-41)
1   C:          Say (.2) say Mr Brown did die what would be
2       ->      the hardest thing for Helena (0.5) any of us
3       ->      can die in crashes or anything but just let's
4               talk it out what would be the hardest thing for
5               Helena
```

'Dying' is here presented as something that can happen to anyone 'in *crashes* or anything', not as something that would be relevant exclusively for Mr Brown. Equally, in extract (10), the possibility of a threatening future is portrayed as a general rule.

```
(10)  (E4-46)
1   C1:         Mrs Walker is there anythi[ng (more- (.2) issues)
2   C2:                                   [(Well there- I don't)
3   C1:         =that you wanted to pursue:.
4   C2:         We:ll (.2) [it's not as though we have a s::]=
5   C1:                    [In the short time we have le:ft ]=
6   C2:         =[s:::::::::::::::    ]subject to pursue=
7   C1:         =[was there anything]
8   C2:         =but (.2) we (.3) always try to nowada:ys (0.7) do
9               what's best for individual patients and what's right
10              for Michael (.2) may not be right for Harry.=And one
11              of the things .hh that we know we're sort of
12      ->      faced with sometimes when people get very ill and
13              even die: is .hhh (0.9) of course views about
14      ->      postmortems in general and I just would like to
15              know what Michael feels about that just in gene[ral.
16  C1:                                                        [Mm
17  C2:         I mean (0.2) how would he feel about it if he was
18              asked (to say on) (0.7) Harry and if m-Michael was
19              asked for hi:m,=and just his views.
```

In (10), after the initial mitigation 'it's not (...) a *sub*ject to pur*sue* but', C2 begins her intervention in an 'individualizing' framework: she emphasizes that the clinic tries to follow each patient's individual wishes, and what is good for Michael may not be good for

Harry. Michael and Harry are the two haemophilic brothers with the HIV virus. When she speaks about Michael and Harry in this individual way, however, she has not yet revealed what she is aiming at: the claim thus far is that the clinic wants to do things that are best for Michael and Harry as individuals.

After this C2 starts a stepwise production of the description of possible future situations. She switches into a 'universalistic' approach and she also adopts an 'institution-centred' perspective, designing the question so as to be motivated by the professionals' needs. She describes the general situation faced by the staff sometimes 'when people get very ill and even *die:*', thus focusing away from the possibility of this individual patient or his brother getting ill or dying. The institution-centred perspective brings in the questions that 'we', i.e. the medical staff, face in such situation, instead of the problems that this patient or his family might face; and the questions are about postmortems 'in general'. Finally, when the counsellor spells out the first version of the question (lines 14–15) to the patient, she still elicits his feelings 'just in general'. Only afterwards does she become more specific, ending up eliciting Michael's views about Harry's postmortem and vice versa. This stepwise progression involves that the patient is *first* brought into a world 'in general' where people die and postmortems are done; and only thereafter is he asked to locate *himself* into that world.

In (10), then, the issue of postmortem examination is presented after an extraordinary amount of 'pre-delicate' work (cf. Schegloff 1980). Through this work, the issue is constituted as one which may be extremely sensitive for the patient.[1]

---

[1] Extract (10) appears to be an exceptional case because the description of a distressing future situation is here delivered by the counsellor without a preceding hint by the client. However, this 'abruptness' is softened in at least three ways by the participants. (1) Even if 'postmortems' appears here to be a fresh topic, its 'newness' is hearably counter-balanced by its connectedness with the immediately preceding topic, which was P's views about *preparing wills.* (Data not shown.) 'Will' and 'postmortem' are both matters relevant in the time after one's death. (2) By her formulation 'it's not as though we have a s::::::::::::::::::*subj*ect to pur*sue*' (lines 4 and 6), C2 seems to explicitly downgrade the 'newness' of the matters she is bringing in. (3) C2's key turn is produced after C1's invitation for her to name new issues; therefore, C2 is not just suddenly and unilaterally bringing in the question about postmortems; she is bringing in that question *as a response to* C1's invitation.

In summary, the recurrent patterns of the management of the epistemological framework of the counsellors' descriptions of the clients' future seems to display the counsellors' orientation to such descriptions as sensitive and delicate matters. By mitigating the accuracy of their descriptions (by upgrading the conditional) or by generalizing their applicability (by presenting their descriptions as general rules concerning everybody), the counsellors overtly *minimize the threat* that the descriptions constitute to the patients. However, what overtly appears as a plain minimization of threat may have other, more subtle, functions, too. In the following, we will try to take one step further in analysing the *local, sequentially specific* functions of the linguistic devices described above.

Securing the clients' cooperation

Apart from the interactants' general interest towards limiting threat, we can find a more specific and local function that the use of the three devices for the management of the epistemological framework may have. In order to identify it, we must first recall the sequential context in which these descriptions appear. The descriptions are followed by questions seeking to elicit the patients' fears or ways of coping given that the threatening situation would arise. So the descriptions lead to questions, and the questions naturally elicit answers. Both the questions and the projected answers presuppose the description.

In this particular context, the specific management of the epistemological framework appears to be geared towards securing the clients' cooperation in building up the hypothetical reality. By applying the various techniques of the management of the epistemological framework the counsellors publicly minimize their commitment to the accuracy of these descriptions, as predictions concerning this particular patient. The world that the counsellors invite the patients to cooperate in building up is thus marked as a hypothetical one, or as a *fantasy world*.

Through this marking, counsellors seem to be conveying to their patients that they can answer the questions without having to think that those things really will happen to them. The patient is not openly required to make any more epistemic commitments than the counsellor does. Or, to put it in another way, marking the world as a hypothetical one, the counsellors make it very difficult for the patients to find valid accounts for refusing to cooperate in building up this world. For example, it is difficult for the patient to refuse to answer since he doesn't think this will happen, because, after all, it *is* only hypothetical.[2]

Additional support for this analysis can be drawn from deviant cases where there is little or no management of the epistemic framework. Indeed, if a central task of this management is to secure the clients' cooperation in building up the hypothetical world, then the *absence* of this management can be understood as an indication of the counsellors' perception of the clients' *likely willingness to cooperate* in any case.

As was mentioned earlier, in some of the cases where the clients have quite directly spelled out hypothetical future possibility, the counsellors often do not take any measures for the management of the hypothetical framework. Extract (11) provides an example of this:

```
(11)  (E4-46)
1    P:              Uh::m (1.5) Well obviously at the moment I mean I
2         (1) ->     don't (.) particularly want to get AIDS or nothing
3                    like that.
4                    (0.5)
5    P:              You know (.) but I still suppose
6         (1) ->     there's- there is that on the back of your mind
7                    still. And I know I've got the er HIV, (.) but I
8         (1) ->     don't know how far (0.5) into AIDS I a:m.
9                    (0.6)
```

---

[2] In the extract below, the patient first declines to answer and claims that the future situation presupposed in the question is unrealistic. The counsellor's response indicates how the hypothetical character of the question can be used as a resource to circumvent the client's reluctance.

```
        C1:         But [supposing you can't get up to the loo:=
        P:              [So-
        C1:         =and s- you're too short of breath (0.2) to sit
                    up in bed and have a drink (0.6) and you become
                    so short of breath that it's all you can do to
                    just lie there (0.5) what's- what's everybody
                    else going to be doing while you do that?
        P:          Well it won't be as bad as tha:t.
                    (0.6)
        C1:  ->     But I'm saying supposi:ng
```

```
10   P:                 Yet.=So: [I don't know. (I don't [like to be)
11   C2:                         [Does-              [s-
12   C2:                How much does (0.2 Michael want to know about (0.8)
13         (1) ->       how far he's (in[to AIDS)
14   P:    (1) ->                   [Well I think I should know
15                      everything.=I think it's only- only right. (Isn't)
16                      (it really).
17   C2:                [One other question first before we go into (what=
18   C1:                [M̲m
19   C2:   (2) ->       =he might be doing) is that,.hhh (.7) What if he
20                      did get AIDS,=what does he think (0.7) will be: the
21                      (0.2) h̲ardest thing for him.=What does he fear most.
```

In (11) the co-counsellor's turn where her description of the hypothetical state of affairs is spelled out is marked with arrow number 2. 'Getting AIDS' is here delivered in a relatively straightforward fashion. In the earlier talk, the hypothetical future possibility (getting AIDS) has been touched upon several times by the client and the counsellor (arrows numbered 1). Through his cooperation in this earlier talk, it can be argued, the client has already displayed his readiness to talk about 'getting AIDS'. Therefore, the counsellor does not need to take any extra measures for securing this result. (See extract (13) below for another example of a straightforward formulation of the hypothetical future situation.)[3]

The paradox of marking questions as hypothetical

A world once marked as hypothetical by the counsellors may not be meant to be treated only as hypothetical. I would like to argue that

---

[3] When there is no threatening material in the query, no extra measures are needed in the management of a hypothetical future state. See the extract for an example:

```
1   C1:            I'm not quite clear about this letter to the building
2        ->        ( ) department.=.hhh[h what would you- (.3) if you=
3   W:                                  [Well-
4   C1:  ->        =were writing it what would you be saying.
5   W:             Ts Erm:: (.2) the: (2) alterations which Mr and
6                  Mrs Davies pro̲pose .hhh (.) are:: (.2) because
7                  ((continues))
```

Here the hypothetical description contains no threatening material, and the counsellor can trust in the client's cooperation. Therefore she takes no measures for the management of the epistemic framework.

this world, which manifestly is marked as a hypothetical one, in an unacknowledged manner will be treated as a *possible* world.

If the counselling sessions where hypothetical questions are asked and answered are to carry out successfully the task of preparing the patients for their future, however threatening that may be, then the world overtly marked as hypothetical must be treated as *more* than mere fantasy. In a paradoxical way, the very marking of the discursive space may also suggest this for the clients. In playing the 'desert island games' we ask directly 'If you were alone on a desert island, which book would you like to have with you?' No management of the epistemological framework is needed, because it is obvious to everyone that the likelihood of such a situation is extremely small. But by saying 'I'm not saying he's *going to*' die, the counsellor may be saying indirectly that he indeed *may* die.

Therefore, the emphasized hypothetical character of questions may serve a double function. On a manifest interactional level it makes it easier for the participants to talk about the future situation; and on a non-manifest, unacknowledged level it marks the likelihood that this future situation may take place. The 'accent of reality' (Schutz and Luckmann 1974) which is overtly tuned down, may be brought back and consolidated through these indirect means. Correspondingly, by cooperating in the invocation of the untoward reality, the patients may be agreeing to treat the objects invoked as something that may in the future be true in their lives. And that, indeed, is what the counselling aims at.

Managing the counsellors' role conflict

Marking the future world as hypothetical may also have another advantage, related to the counsellors' professional role. There is a potential tension between the two opposing poles of the counsellors' role: their speciality in social and mental issues on one hand, and their membership of the medical team on the other. As 'mental' and 'social' professionals the counsellors are expected to generate talk about the patients' fears and their conceptions of the future, even if the patients currently are fine and their medium-term prospects good. But because the counsellors also are members of the medical team, their words are easily heard as implying a prognosis.

In any serious illness, giving a prognosis is an extremely sensitive issue. Doctors are expected to tell their patients beforehand if something dreadful is going to happen – but they easily lose their credibility if they issue warnings about something that actually turns out not to be serious (cf. Sudnow 1967; Peräkylä 1991). With HIV this problem is particularly acute because the course of the illness is very unpredictable.

Inviting patients to talk about a markedly hypothetical world provides for a means of navigating between these rocks. The counsellors create a space where their words markedly *do not* imply a prognosis. In that space, pursuing the patients' fears and fantasies is possible, even when some of the counsellors are medical doctors. It also enables those members of the team who do not have a formal medical authority (social workers, nurses, psychologists) to address the issues related to the patients' future without needing to worry about saying something that they, as non-medics, would not have the authority to say.

To summarize, then, the counsellors' technique of questioning, applied along with the management of the epistemological framework, provides for a means to create discursive space where the clients' talk about the details of their distressing future is highly relevant. This space, however, is created without the counsellors themselves needing to go on record for asserting almost anything about this future.

Variety of projection domains

Naming the projectables is another central element of hypothetical questions. Tentatively, it was argued in the beginning of this chapter that a key aspect of the counsellors' professional conduct is to choose the projectables, i.e. the issues (relevant to the hypothetical state of affairs) that the patient is asked to report on. By examining what kinds of issues are chosen as projectables, we can gain access to cultural themes and symbolism by which matters like 'illness' or 'death' – matters involved in the descriptions of hypothetical states of affairs – are managed in counselling interviews.

As a crude classification, projectables fall into three categories: (1) feelings, (2) practical conduct of life, and (3) coping strategies.

However, this classification is an analyst's construct: in actual talk the different types of projectables often get mixed up.

(1) The client can be asked to report his or her feelings related to the hypothetical description. That is the case in extract (11) above, a fragment of which is reproduced below.

```
(11)   (Section)
1     C2:       What if he did get AIDS,=what does he think (0.7)
3               will be: the (0.2) hardest thing for him.=What does
3               he fear most.
```

The latter part of the question especially sets up a 'feeling'-centred projectable, as the issue is P's fears.[4] Similarly, in extract (12), taken from pre-test counselling, the projectable has a component of feelings, as the counsellor's question is about P's 'concerns' – even though, as argued in the preceding chapter, 'concerns' is a rather ambiguous class of objects.

```
(12)   (E4-4:1-38)
1     C:     Right (0.5) Just think: too, erm eh (.) what if
2            it's: (2) positive.
3     P:     Uh-hum.
4            (4.0)
5     C:     What for you: would be your greatest conce:rn,=do
6            you think about that test result?
7            (2.5)
8     P:     (The) thought that I would develop AI:DS?
```

(2) Sometimes the client is invited to report issues having to do with the 'practical conduct of life'. This is the case in extracts (13) and (14), where the counsellor asks the patient what would be different if there were medical problems:

```
(13)   (E4-4)
1     C:     ↑Okay (.) say you were sick
2     P:     Umh
3     C:     What do you see yourself as doing.
4            (1.2)
```

---

[4] Interestingly, the counsellor here uses the present tense: the question is 'what does he fear most' and not 'what *would* he fear most' or 'what *will* he fear most'. Even though the initial descriptions regularly apply the future or the conditional tense , the projection invitation is often in the present tense, as here. Among other things this appears to give 'permission' for the patient to express his or her *current* fears about the future.

```
 5   C:   How would your life change? Would your job
 6        change?=Would your friends change?
 7        (.)
 8   C:   I'm wondering,=what would be different.
 9        (2.0)
10   P:   If I was sick ((background noise)) (2.0) If I
11        was sick I've got to be in hospital
```

```
(14)  (N-13)
 1   C:   What if one was- (2.0) I mean- (.5) I'm not saying
 2        it but if I was to turn (round) to say: and say to
 3        you .hhh (1.3) from where things are your immune
 4        system is having a struggle .hhh I mean what
 5        difference would that make to how you're carrying on
 6        now?
```

(3) Finally, the client can be invited to report his or her ways of coping in the hypothetical situation. This is the case in extracts (15) and (16) below:

```
(15)  (E4-12)
 1   C:   I mean as far as I understand if one- (.7) I'm
 2        not saying this can happen,=but taking it to
 3        its very worst, (.) if .hh you did begin to
 4        fi:nd it difficult to make decisions and all
 5        that,=↑who would you want to make them for you?
 6        (.2) Who would you want to help you?
```

```
(16)  (E4-46/5)
 1   C1:  To get back to wi:lls if (0.2) one of you die:d
 2   P:   Mm hm
 3        (0.5)
 4   C1:  Would either of you want (0.3) the other one to
 5        have everything that was left, or would you
 6        want your mother to [have a share:.
 7   P:                       [Mm
 8        (0.6)
 9   P:   Well the way I figured it uh:m last night was
10        er:: (0.7) I'd give everything to Ba:rry
11        ((continues))
```

In (15), the description of a hypothetical state of affairs involves P beginning to find it difficult to make decisions, which refers to fears of contracting dementia that P earlier disclosed (see extract (10) in chapter 6). In (16), the hypothetical situation involves the death of one of the two haemophilic, HIV-positive brothers. In both cases, the counsellor names a projectable related to the clients' ways of coping in these situations.

The three different types of projectables set up three different locally constructed identities of the clients (cf. Strong 1979; Silverman 1987; Peräkylä 1989). When the projectables involve feelings then the clients are treated as 'emotional subjects' whose experience may be affected by the possible future state of affairs. When the projectables involve the practical conduct of life the patient is constructed as an 'acting subject' whose conduct is impeded by the future situation. Finally, when the projectables involve coping strategies then the client is also portrayed as an 'acting subject', but now as one making his or her active choices in the hypothetical future situation.

However, as stated above, this classification of projectables is an analyst's construction. In the actual interaction, the parties may produce mixtures of these classes. This happens in extract (17), where the co-counsellor, using the live open supervision format of questioning, first produces an enquiry involving a 'feelings' domain (arrow 1), and thereafter, prompted by the delay of the main counsellor's or the patient's response, delivers two more enquiries which bring in a 'coping' domain and that of 'practical conduct of life' (arrows 2 and 3 respectively).[5]

```
(17)   (E4-41/1)
1      C2:              Doctor Jay what does Mr Brown think.=Say he
2                       did (.2) get AI:DS and (.2) the worst did
3           (1) ->      happen, .hhh what (0.5) does he think (1.0) is
4                       (.2) Helena's greatest fear.
5                       (.2)
6      C2:              How: (.3) what- what- what (1.3) just let's
7                       take it o:n (and ifs) this is all hypothetical,
8                       but I'd just like to know: what (.5) it might
9                       be:-
10                      (1.4)
11     C2:   (2) ->     How she'd handle it.=How does he think she'd
```

[5] We could speculate here about the different degrees of threat, implied by different projection domains. Naming 'Helena's fears' is potentially more delicate and threatening than describing how she would 'handle' AIDS or have 'difficulties', especially given that Helena herself is present in the conversation. The counsellor could then be seen as moving towards a less problematic alternative as the patient fails to respond.

12   handle it.
13   (1.8)
14   C2:   (3) ->   would be the greatest difficulty for her.

There is, however, one important aspect where the participants obviously orient to the 'classification' of the projectables. That is related to the *closing* of the talk about the future: the environment favourable for closing is regularly established by the counsellors choosing *coping*-centred projectables. Closings will be discussed at the end of this chapter.

The social scope of the projection domain

Extract (17) is indicative of another possible quality of the projectables. The description of the hypothetical state of affairs in (17) concerns the answerer of the questions, Mr Brown: his possible AIDS. However, the projectables here involve not primarily Mr Brown but his wife, Helena. The counsellor's choice of the projectable, then, transforms Mr Brown's possible AIDS into a shared family matter.

In a different way, people other than the addressed client himself were involved also in extract (15) above, where the patient was invited to name those persons whom he would want to make decisions for him and to help him, and in (16), where the hypothetical death of a client is discussed in terms of deciding who would have his property. People other than the patient are also included in (18) below, as P is questioned about his *sister*'s worries should it turn out that he had 'full-blown AIDS':

(18)   (E4-24)
1   C: If she- if (.2) if you did have full-blown AIDS what
2   would she be most wo:rried about (.) do you think?
3   (.8)
4   P: Er::: my health?
5   C: Uh-hum.
6   P: Probably (my morale and)- (.3) probably not me
7   passing it on to: (.2) anyone.

To put it in general terms, hypothetical questions give the counsellors the opportunity to *expand* the social scope of the discourse beyond those subjects who in the first place 'bear' the circumstances named in the initial description of a hypothetical state of affairs. Other people are brought in through the choice of the projectable. Any subjects who can be thought of as relating to the clients can be involved in this. Family members', partners' and friends' feelings, conduct of life or coping can be explored; as well as these subjects, possible help or influence in the patients' life. In counselling based on Family Systems Theory, such expansion is actively sought: any future circumstances involved in the hypothetical description can thus be treated in the context of the family and the other relevant 'systems'.

Deeper penetration into the client's perception of the future

Hypothetical questions do not occur as isolated events during the counselling sessions. In chapter 6 we saw how much interactional work can be done to achieve a state of talk where it is interactionally appropriate to ask a hypothetical question. But also the talk *after* (the first occurrence of) a hypothetical question is distinctively influenced by the relevancies created by this device. Therefore, in what follows we will examine briefly the dynamics involved in the longer stretches of talk triggered by hypothetical questions. Through follow-up questions, it will be argued, the participants achieve a deeper penetration into the clients' perception of their future.

A recurrent way to a deeper penetration into the client's perspective of his/her future is through the elaboration of the client's initial response to the hypothetical question. Quite simply, the counsellor can elicit a specification of the initial response and through this, a more detailed discourse about the future is achieved. That is what is happening in extracts (19)–(21): the clients' initial responses are marked by arrows numbered 1, the counsellors' follow-up questions by arrows numbered 2, and the clients' elaborations of their responses by arrows numbered 3.

(19) (E4-46:75-)
1   C2:   [One other question first before we go into=
2   C1:   [Mm
3   C2:   =(what he might be doing) is that,.hhh (.7) What
4   if he did get AIDS,=what does he think (0.7) will

```
 5                       be: the (0.2) hardest thing for him.=What does he
 6                       fear most.
 7                       (1.0)
 8   P:     (1) ->       I think (.3) accepting it I suppose.
 9                       (.)
10   P:                  That's going to be quite- and I know I've
11                       accepted it this far.
12                       (0.7)
13   C1:    (2) ->       Is thi[s accepting (.2) AI:DS or=
14   P:                       [Mm
15   C1:                 =the- (.2) outcome of AIDS.=Is it (0.9) the
16                       [things that might happen to you like=
17   P:                  [Mm
18   C1:                 =happened to Harry (.) or (.) is it
19                       [dying in the en:d.
20   P:                  [Mm
21   P:     (3) ->       I think probably a bit of both really.=I mean
22                       I've s- (.) I've seen what Harry's gone through
23                       and going through.
24                       (1.1)
25   P:                  You know uhm (1.0) the way he's er (1.0) going
26                       on all these different trials and things
27                       ((continues))
```

```
(20)  (E4-4)
 1   C:                  Right (0.5) Just think: too, erm eh (.) what if
 2                       it's: (2) positive.
 3   P:                  Uh-hum.
 4                       (4.0)
 5   C:                  What for you: would be your greatest
 6                       conce:rn,=do you think about that test result?
 7                       (2.5)
 8   P:     (1) ->       Thought that I would develop AI:DS?
 9                       (.3)
10   C:                  Right=
11   P:                  =Of course.
12   C:     (2) ->       What about AIDS:: in particular (.3) bothers
13                       you
14                       (2.8)
15   P:     (3) ->       Erm:: (1.8) Dying I suppose.
16                       (2.0)
17   P:                  Ermh ((bleep somewhere in the room))
18                       (3.0)
19   P:                  Because there can't be anything more
20                       fundamental than that.
```

```
(21)  (N-26)
  1  C1:              I [want [to have one more (.3) hard=
  2  W:                  [An:d [So there hh heh .hhhh heh heh
  3  C1:              =question (.2) which .hhh I'm going to- (.8) ask you
  4                   Mr Davies.=S[ay: and this is hypothetical=
  5  (P):                         [(Mm)
  6  C1:              =and (in) just to finish on the AIDS business .hhh
  7                   if anyone in the housing department: (.) or
  8                   anywhere should say to you: .hhh Mr Davies, (.5)
  9                   all is fi:ne but I'm worrried I can get AIDS from
 10                   you >What how< would you answer that.
 11                   (2.0)
 12  P:    (1) ->    .hhhh Erm:: hh I would think that err: (.2) I would
 13                  try: if I could .hh err: to reassure them[::.
 14  C1:   (2) ->                                            [And
 15                  how.=Just say it bri[efly:
 16  P:    (3) ->                        [That is the: (.) err: this is
 17                  going to be: (.2) er difficulty.=I think a l-lot of
 18                  (.3) err:m (.) misunderstanding about it. .hhh Err:
 19                  generally spe[aking.
 20  C1:   (2') ->               [So (.) pretend I'm [(in) the housing:=
 21  P:                                              [And so I would
 22  C1:             =[what would you say to me Mister Dav[ies.
 23  P:    (3') ->    =[try: and to-                      [Well you can't
 24                   get AI:DS. No matter what I (.8) m-m- did.
```

In (19) and (20) above, there is one 'cycle' of the counsellor's follow-up question and the client's specification of his/her initial
response; and in (21), there are two such cycles. In all extracts the
participants arrive at a more detailed version of the hypothetical
future.

It is noticeable that the more detailed version of the future
achieved through the follow-up questions can also involve more
explicit descriptions of the threatening aspects of the clients' conception of the future. This can be seen in extracts (19) and (20). In
her follow-up question in (19), the counsellor checks with P
whether he is concerned about accepting 'AI:DS or the- (0.2) outcome of AIDS', detailing thereafter these two alternatives in a way
that includes direct reference to 'dying in the en:d' (lines 14–18). In
(20), the follow-up question invites a specification of what about
AIDS 'in particular' bothers the client; and in response, he names
'dying'.

Asymmetries in asking and answering hypothetical questions

Hypothetical questions are powerful means in the conversational production of reality. By proffering answers to these questions, the patients are likely to cooperate in at least two processes: establishing and maintaining the description of a hypothetical future state of affairs as the horizon of the discourse, and dealing with it in terms of the projectables named by the counsellor.

However, the clients' cooperation is not automatic. In this section, I will examine the means that are available for a client *not* to cooperate fully in responding to hypothetical questions. Two types of responses make it possible not to join in building up the future world. First, there are responses that avoid maintaining the hypothetical description as a horizon of the unfolding discourse; and second, there are responses which, while maintaining the hypothetical description, nevertheless avoid dealing with it in terms of the projectables brought forward by the counsellor. Along with the analysis of these means of not cooperating, I will examine the means available for the *counsellors* to pursue answers to hypothetical questions.

Responses that avoid maintaining the hypothetical description

It has been argued above that the very hypothetical quality of the counsellors' questions (which often is particularly marked) makes them difficult to resist. Clients cannot avoid answering by resorting to the improbability of the hypothetical situation: the counsellors are only inviting the clients to 'speak hypothetically'.

However, other kinds of account are available for the clients to give reasons for not answering. Responses which avoid maintaining the counsellor's description of a hypothetical state of affairs operate by offering an account which demonstrates the client's *inability* (or sometimes *unwillingness*) to answer the counsellor's question. In extract (22), the client points out that he does not know and has not thought about the matters raised in the hypothetical question.

(22) (E4-41/3)
```
1   C1:    And if Doctor Jay: if more symptoms developed
2          what would Mr Brown's greatest fear be
3          about that.
```

```
4                (1.4)
5    C1:         er what would be most difficult for him.
6                (1.5)
7    P:  ->      I don't know I haven't thought about that.
```

The availability of accounts like this indicates the participants' orientation to a particular organization of knowledge involved in knowing about the future. This epistemic organization is not unlike the one involved in knowing about other people's minds (see chapter 3). Like another person's mind, the sphere of the future is transcendent. People are not entitled to have knowledge and experience about the future, as they are entitled to know about their past life events, or about their current inner sensations (cf. Sacks 1984).

When asking and answering hypothetical questions, this organization of knowledge is potentially relevant. It does not prevent the conversationalists from constructing the hypothetical future world. But it is available as a resource if for some reason one of them, usually the client, wants to withhold a further production of reality. Propositions like 'I don't know', or 'I haven't thought', and different variations and combinations of them, are ready to hand if needed. Extracts (23) and (24) below provide two further examples.

```
(23)  (E4-41/1)
 1    C2:         Say (.2) say [Mr Brown did die what would=
 2    P:                       [but-
 3    C2:         =be the hardest thing for Helena (0.5) any of
 4                us can die [in ] crashes=
 5    P:                     [yes]
 6    C2:         =or anything but just let's talk it out what
 7                would be the hardest thing for Helena (0.5) .hh
 8                if you did die,
 9                (5.2)
10    P:    ->    I don't think that one- (0.5) is able to a-
11          ->    able to answer that question [before something=
12    C2:                                       [Well I'm just-
13    P:    ->    =happens I REALLY DON'T KNOW I- I-

(24)  (E4-8)
 1    C1:         S[o if:: (1.2) the test came out positive.=I mean=
 2    W:           [(      )
 3    C1:         =what are the thing:s- (1.5) how would you conduct
 4                your life.=What are the thing:s
 5    W:    ->    hhhhhhhh [I don't know hh ].hhh ((teary voice))
 6    C1:                  [IF I WAS TO (SAY IT-)]
```

```
7   C1:        We[ll-
8   W:    ->   [I just don't know. ((teary voice))
```

Also more elaborate accounts are available for the clients to convey their unwillingness to deal with the future in terms of the hypothetical description. Extract (25) provides an example; here the client produces a 'quasi-psychological' reason for not wanting to answer the counsellor's question.[6]

```
(25) (E4-12)
1    C1:        But we are n[ot I think what I heard Doctor
2    P:              [er:
3    C1:        Kaufman saying that answers her question partly .hhh
4               but it doesn't- (1.2) a:nswer the question that
5               (1.6) you raised and I hadn't (.7) WASN'T thinking
6               about it and it made me think in terms of all of us
7               in this room that if any of us should .hh (.5) have
8               some ki:ind of impairment ↑who would we (1.2) want
9               to make those ki:nd of decisions ↑would it be one's
10              parents or would it be (.5) the closest person to
11              one?
12              (1.2)
13   C1:        Just wonder?
14              (2.2)
15   C1:        You don't have to answer to that
16   P:         No[: [I
17   C1:           [to[day
18   ( ):           [(      )
19   P:         think it it's the (.) it's the difficult (.6) decision
20       ->     it's almost li:ke (.4) >there is something< (.6) I
21       ->     think about making a decision like that or: (.7)
22       ->     writing ( ) will: which can feel as if you're
23       ->     almost inviting something to ha:ppen: and I think
24       ->     (it shall wait) for tha- that (.2) that reason (.)
25              er::
```

In sum, due to its transcendent epistemic status, the conversationally created future world is a precarious reality. The clients have available valid accounts for declining the hypothetical questions.

However, the client's claim that he does not know or does not want to think does not determine the next action of the counsellor.

[6] Note how the counsellor's statement in line 15 (You don't have to answer to that), produced after the substantial delay in P's response (lines 12–14), provides P with a marked possibility for withholding his answer.

The unfolding of interaction in (22) and (23) shows different lines of action that the counsellors can take after the client's 'resistance'. Roughly, the counsellors can either *give up* the hypothetical question, or try and find an *alternative route*.

In extract (26) below (which is an extension of extract (22)), the counsellors give up their question and shift to another hypothetical description.

```
(26)   (Extension of (22))
 1     C2:        And if Doctor Jay: if more symptoms developed
 2                what would Mr Brown's greatest fear be
 3                about that.
 4                (1.4)
 5     C2:        er What would be most difficult for him.
 6                (1.5)
 7     P:         I don't know I haven't thought about that.
 8                (1.2)
 9     O: ->      Can I a:sk (.) one final (0.3) I promised to
10                keep quiet but can I ask one question before
11                you move on. .hhhh If: (0.2) Mr Brown
12                (found I mean) (0.2) if you don't want to ask
13                it or he doesn't want to answer it it doesn't
14                matter but I just wondered .hhh=
15     P:         Mm
16     O:         if he found it (0.2) as he says increasingly
17                difficult (0.2) to have a sexual relationship
18                (0.4) in the sense that they used to have:
19                because of this lurking fear .hhh what would
20                that do to their relationship with each other?
21                (1.2)
22     P:         Oh yes:
23                (1.2)
24     O:         Would it have any effect.
25     P:         Ye:s I think it would.
```

In line 9 of (26) above, after the client's account, the observing physician intervenes with another enquiry.[7] The fresh enquiry is also hypothetical, but both the description of a hypothetical state of affairs and the projectable are different. The focus shifts from

---

[7] This is one of the very rare cases where an observer volunteers a turn of talk. In this session, one of the most experienced counsellors was participating, exceptionally, in the session as an observer. Note how she prefaces her intervention with an apology, which seems to request a warrant for her intervention.

'more symptoms' to difficulties in sexual relationships. The construction of the future continues, but the participants, as it were, move to another location on the building site.

In extract (27), the counsellor pursues the client's answer by taking an alternative route.

```
(27)  (Extension of (23))
 1   C2:        Say (.2) say [Mr Brown did die what would=
 2   P:                     [but-
 3   C2:        =be the hardest thing for Helena (0.5) any of
 4              us can die [in  ] crashes=
 5   P:                    [yes]
 6   C2:        =or anything but just let's talk it out what
 7              would be the hardest thing for Helena (0.5) .hh
 8              if you did die,
 9              (5.2)
10   P:         I don't think that one- (0.5) is able to a-
11              able to answer that question [before something=
12   C2:                                     [Well I'm just-
13   P:         =happens I REALLY DONT KNOW I- I-
14   C2:  ->    Look (.2) if you weren't there what would be
15        ->    the hardest thing for her,
16              (3.0)
17   C2:        Just guess?
18              (7.0)
19   W:         ((clears throat))
20              (2.0)
21   C2:        What woul[d be-
22   P:                  [The- (.3) the hard- ha-hardest (.2)
23              thing,=well I mean (0.5) be-bereavement?
24   C2:  ->    Missing you[: o r : ] or managing=
25   P:                    [mi-mis-]  ·
26   C2:  ->    =financially or the house and the children,
27   P:         Ahh (0.5) puts you [on the spot,=
28   W:                            [.hhh
29   W:         =Yes.=
30   P:         =I THINK THE – I THINK MISSING ME
```

In (27), after having faced P's claim that he doesn't know, the counsellor takes an alternative route which finally leads the patient to answer the hypothetical question. First the counsellor rephrases the hypothetical description: 'If *you* weren't there' is substituted for 'if you did die'. Through the new wording, the counsellor retreats from an explicit description of an ultimately sensitive state of affairs into a more ambiguous one. At least nominally, 'if *you* weren't there' allows for various reasons for the person's absence, death being only one of them. Thus the new wording seems to equate death with various other possible reasons for absence.

Through the comparison of death with other forms of absence, the new wording also challenges the patient's initial account. As a response to the first version of the question, trading off the initial description 'if you did die', the patient claimed that he is unable to answer. However, it is questionable whether the patient can justifiably claim that he is unable to say what would be the hardest thing for his wife if he were absent.

After the rephrasing of the hypothetical description, there follows the counsellor's query (lines 14–15). The projectable is spelled out almost exactly in the same words as it was before P's first negative response. Then, as the enquiry has been renewed, there emerges a long (3.0 sec.) pause.

The silence is first broken by the counsellor saying 'Just *guess?*' This *downgrades the knowledge claim* involved in the enquiry. By downgrading the knowledge claim, the counsellor once again challenges P's account: even if he were unable to answer in terms of knowing, nevertheless he could be expected to be able to guess. After another, even longer gap of 7.0 sec. the counsellor initiates a turn, using the question form 'What would be-', which indicates that she has not given up the pursuit. However, the patient also begins a turn; the counsellor relinquishes the floor; and thereafter the delivery of P's response hesitantly begins (line 22).[8]

---

[8] In extract (27), the counsellor's shift of footing is also interesting. At the beginning of the sequence she delivers her question employing the 'live open supervision' format, thus addressing the principal counsellor. However, at line 8 she begins to address the client directly. Notably, C2's shift of footing takes place *after* she has delivered the most threatening part of her utterance ('say Mr Brown *did* die' in line 1): the social distance between questioner and projective answerer (see chapter 5) is maintained until this has been spelled out. Moreover, the footing shift is preceded by P's acknowledgement token in line 5, whereby P has begun to treat himself more or less as the addressee.

It has to be mentioned, however, that this segment is taken from the session where the principal counsellor was inexperienced in operating the 'live open supervision' machinery. Therefore, C2's inclination to shift the footing may have been prompted by the anticipated or actual lack of cooperation on C1's part as well.

To summarize, by offering an account giving reasons for a failure to answer, clients can powerfully influence the unfolding of a conversation involving the use of hypothetical questions. The account may prompt a new enquiry to be asked, or the initial enquiry to be transformed.

Responses that avoid the projectables suggested by the counsellor

Another type of difficulty arises when the client does produce an answer, but this does not fully satisfy the projectable named by the counsellor. Extract (28) is an example of this. The less than fully cooperative answer occurs in response to a follow-up question (employing the live open supervision format) where the counsellors try to elicit a specification of the client's view about what kind of treatments he would not want to have if he were 'very ill'.

```
(28)  (E4-46)
 1   C1:    ((...)) if[:
 2   P:             [Mm
 3          (0.2)
 4   C1:    you were very i:ll
 5          (.)
 6   P:     We[ll uh:m
 7   C1:       [would you want them to do everything (.3)
 8          absolutely possible [to save your li:fe.
 9   P:                         [Hm
10   P:     Well if a machine is sort of keeping me going
11          well then obviously I would (1.0) probably
12          would want- want you to turn it off:.=if it was
13          the machi:ne.
14          (1.7)
15   P:     er:[: i-
16   C1:       [So equally would you want to be put on a
17          machine.
18          (0.2)
19   P:     Not really no I don't thin[k so.
20   C1:                             [So you're- (.) are
21          you saying you wouldn't like anything (1.3)
22          really last ditch. Like a- like a [mach[ine.
23   C2:                                      [But  [let's=
24   P:                                            [Uh::m
25   C2:    = hear what other things then.=
26   C1:    =What other things would you not like.
```

```
27                (1.2)
28    P:    ->    Well I'd like to probably er: (1.2) ( ) try
29          ->    and go with my head up as it were. (1.0) er:
30          ->    (0.3) With a bit of (.) respect still in myself.
```

In (28), the counsellors ask the patient questions about his preferences concerning life-sustaining measures if he were to be critically ill. The projectables in the counsellors' questions involve P's choices concerning his treatment. In the final follow-up question (lines 23–6) the projectable is designed as P's choices regarding 'what other things' he would not like.

In the first part of the sequence, P offers his answers in a manner that cooperates with the counsellor's choice of projectables: he asserts that he would not want to have his life prolonged by 'a machine' (in lines 10–13 and 19). In response to the second follow-up question, however, P is less cooperative. Instead of offering a list of 'things' that he would 'not like' at the end of his treatment (the kind of answer suggested by the question), he produces (in lines 28–30) a metaphorical description of the kind of death he would like to have.[9]

In P's response, therefore, the initial hypothetical description ('if: (...) you were very i:ll') is preserved as the horizon, but the answer does not deal with that in terms of the projectable suggested by the counsellor (the 'other things' that P would not like). The unfolding of the discourse after P's response makes manifest C2's orientation to this misalignment. In her follow-up question (marked with arrows in extract (29) below) the counsellor shifts the focus away from P's metaphorical description of a dignified death; instead, she pursues a line of questioning focusing on P's practical choices in the hypothetical situation:

```
(29) (Extension of (28))
10    P:    Well if a machine is sort of keeping me going well
11          then obviously I would (1.0) probably would want-
12          want you to turn it off:.=if it was the machi:ne.
```

---

[9] P's final answer includes two characteristically *idiomatic* expressions, 'go with my head up' and 'With a bit of (.) respect still in myself'. The work that these idioms do seems to come close to the uses of idioms analysed by Drew and Holt (1988): instead of detailing the issues addressed, idioms *summarize* them; moreover, they seek to elicit *affiliation* from the co-interactants; and they prepare the ground for *topic termination*.

```
13                      (1.7)
14      P:              er:[: i-
15      C1:             [So equally would you want to be put on a
16                      machine.
17                      (0.2)
18      P:              Not really no I don't thin[k so.
19      C1:                                       [So you're- (.) are you
20                      saying you wouldn't like anything (1.3) really last
21                      ditch. Like a- like a [mach[ine.
22      C2:                                   [But [let's=
23      P:                                        [Uh::m
24      C2:             =hear what other things then.=
25      C1:             =What other things would you not like.
26                      (1.2)
27      P:              Well I'd like to probably er: (1.2) ( ) try and go
28                      with my head up as it were. (1.0) er: (0.3) With a
29                      bit of (.) respect still in myself.
30                      (0.2)
31      C2:    ->       .hhh bu- bu- machines are one thing but the other
32             ->       things that one needs is our tablets.
33      P:              Mm
34      C1:             Mm hm=
35      C2:    ->       =So would you want the doctors to try all the
36             ->       tablets.
```

By not attending to P's answer and by returning topically to the 'machines' (the central topical object earlier in the sequence: see lines 10, 12, 16, 21), C2 displays her understanding of P's answer as non-cooperative with the counsellors' line of questioning.

Extracts (30) and (31) provide two other examples of clients' responses which contest the counsellors' choice of projectables.

```
(30)    (E4-46)
        ((Immediately following extract 29))
31      C2:             .hhh bu- bu- Machines are one thing but the
32                      other things that one needs is our tablets.
33      P:              Mm
34      C1:             Mm hm=
35      C2:             =So would you want the doctors to try all the
36                      tablets.
37                      (0.5)
38      C1:             And [b l o o d transfusio::n:[s
39      C2:                 [(            ).        [
40      P:                                          [Well if it
41                      [was uh::m
```

```
42   C1:              [a:nd-
43   ( ):             Mm [( )
44   P:       ->         [if I was probably too ill to even
45            ->      notice any difference well then that wouldn't
46            ->      really make much (.) difference would it. No
47            ->      matter what you pumped into (me)
(31) (E4-12)
                      ((P has expressed his fear of 'contracting some kind of dementia'))
1    C1:              .hh I mean taking things to [ their worst
2    W:                                          [ *(        ) should
3                     happen*
4                     (1.0)
5    C1:              I mean as far as I understand if one- (.7) I'm
6                     not saying this can happen,=but taking it to
7                     its very worst, (.) if .hh you did begin to
8                     fi:nd it difficult to make decisions and all
9                     that,=↑who would you want to make them for you?
10                    (.2)
11   C1:              Who would you want to help you?
12                    (1.4)
13   P:       ->   No one:, I would say, [I'd like to=
14   C1:                                 [No one.
15   P:       ->   =think-(.) No [I don't (think I c-) I=
16   C1:                         [Okay.
17   P:       ->   =could- (1.0) think about it like that.=.hh You
18                    see (it's just) one of those very insidious
19                    things,=because everybody gets days when they
20                    can't r'member anything,=and ((continues with a
21                    description of his worry ))
```

A key feature in the clients' responses in extracts (30) and (31) is that the clients avoid treating the hypothetical future situation in terms of the projectables suggested by the counsellors. In (30) (which occurs immediately after extracts (28) and (29) analysed earlier) the projectables involve P's choices regarding 'tablets' and 'blood trans*fu*sio::n:s'; in his response, P claims that things like that would not make any difference. In (31), the projectable concerns P's choices regarding the persons who could make decisions for him in case he himself would be unable to. In his response, P names no one, and continues by explicitly contesting the question, saying 'I don't (think I c-) I could- (1.0) think about it like that.'

It might be of interest to the reader to see how the contest of projectables, i.e. of the terms of describing the future, begun in the adjacent extracts (28), (29) and (30), finally ended. In this case (as

often happens), the counsellors finally got the upper hand: after a
massive pursuit by the counsellors, the patient yielded in describing
(but less than wholeheartedly) the hypothetical future situation of
his critical illness in terms of his choices regarding the treatment
options. Space does not allow us to analyse the final course of the
interaction, but it will be shown in extract (32) below. The final
turn where the patient nominally cooperates with the counsellors'
choice of projectable is shown with arrows.

```
(32)   (Extension of (30)
32   C2:        .hhh bu- bu- machines are one thing but the
33              other things that one needs is our tablets.
34   P:         Mm
35   C1:        Mm hm=
36   C2:        =So would you want the doctors to try all the
37              tablets.
38              (0.5)
39   C1:        And [b l o o d transfusio::n:[s
40   C2:            [(              ). [
41   P:                                [Well if it
42              [was uh::m
43   C1:        [a:nd-
44   ( ):       Mm [( )
45   P:            [if I was probably too ill to even
46              notice any difference well then that wouldn't
47              really make much (.) difference would it. No
48              matter what you pumped into
49              (0.5)
50   C2:        (Well) (it would)-
51              (0.2)
52   C1:        Well i[t would-
53   C2:              [We never know:.=
54   C1:        =We ne[ver kn(h)ow heh heh=
55   P:               [No.
56   C1:        =whether [t o try: i t
57   C2:                 [That's what I'm trying
58              to [understa:nd.
59   P:             [If I was sort of too ill to realise er what
60              was really going on (.) well obviously you
61              could well virtually do what you like and I
62              wouldn't be that particularly aware of [it.
63   C1:                                               [Well
64              let me try and put it a different way as
65              sometimes people [are very i:ll [when they=
66   P:                          [Mm           [Mm
```

```
67   C1:        =have AI::DS, a[nd we=
68   P:                   [Mm
69   C1:        =ca::n (1.1) in som[e cases the treatment=
70   P:                           [Mm
71   C1:        =wor:ks and they get better but (.) [knowing=
72   P:                                             [Mm
73   C1:        =that (0.5) because they've got AIDS something
74              else may happen.
75   P:         Mm
76   C1:        So (0.4) you know some people may feel they
77              want every heroic measure every ti[:me, and =
78   P:                                           [Mm
79   C1:        =others may say: (0.2) enough is en[ough.
80   P:                                            [Mm
81              (0.2)
82   C1:        It's very difficult for us [to: have an opinion
83   P:                                    [Mm
84   P:         Mm:=
85   C1:        =at a distance,=but supp[osing it was Ha:rry=
86   P:                                [Mm
87   C1:        =and you were asked to make the decision about
88              Harry
89              (0.2)
90   P:         Mm
91              (0.5)
92   C1:        he was too i:ll and you were the next of kin
93              and had to decide whe[ther we should go o:n=
94   P:                              [Mm
95   C1:        =trying or no[t what would your decision be.
96   P:                      [Mm
97   P:         Well I think (0.2) my decision would be based
98              on what he would want.=And I think he probably
99              would want you to keep trying.
100  C1:        Mm
101             (0.3)
102  C1:        So there[fore that's what you'd=
103  P:                 [Mm:
104  C1:        =decide [for him.=If the situation was=
105  P:                 [Yeah.
106  C1:        =reversed what would you want him to decide for
107             you.
108             (1.2)
109  P:    ->   If I- if I was (0.7) really quite ill and ( )
110       ->   there was nothing really much more that you
111       ->   could do: well then that would be it then I
112       ->   suppose I would like to s- to sort of (0.8) be
```

113   ->   left.
114   (0.5)
115   P: ->   As it were. To get on with it.

In summary, then, it appears that through the design of their responses to counsellors' hypothetical questions, clients can avoid dealing with the hypothetical situations in terms of the projectables suggested by the counsellors. This may lead to the future world being constructed in a different way than projected in the counsellors' hypothetical questions. Such moves are, however, regularly challenged with counter-moves by the counsellors, who can try to reinstate the original projectables.

Note on exits from future-oriented talk

Like any other conversational activity, building up the conversationally shared future world cannot go on *ad infinitum*. At some point, the conversationalists leave the reality they have been building.

According to Sacks, as cited by Jefferson (1984a), certain types of topic pose a particular closing problem for conversationalists. 'To get *off* them and to go anywhere else from them, one has specifically to *do* "getting out of them"' (1984a: 191). When exiting from 'embarrassing' or 'controversial' topics, the participants cannot just simply begin to talk about other matters. Thus, in her analysis of 'troubles talk', Jefferson has pointed out that 'overwhelmingly, interactants treat troubles talk as a topic after which there is nothing more to be said' (1988: 345).

In ordinary conversation, most of the topic changes occur in an unmarked fashion, topics flowing one from another (Button and Casey 1984). The movement in and out of 'embarrassing' and 'controversial' topics is, however, typically *boundaried*.

Talking about fear and distress related to the future with HIV-positive patients or people coming for an HIV test is potentially an 'embarrassing' topic. The previous chapter described the methods that participants use in *entering* this topic. *Exiting* requires equally fine conversational manoeuvres.

The topical boundary after the talk about the clients' future is typically marked by a pause, and the nomination of a fresh topic by the counsellor, or elicitation of a new topic from the client(s).[10] In some cases, however, the participants may depart from the future world in a stepwise manner, usually by transforming the future-related themes into generic or present ones, as in extract (36), which I will discuss shortly.

What I will focus on here, however, is not the 'next' moves after the participants have departed from the topic of the future. Instead, I will examine how the conversationalists *prepare* the environment for the exit from future-oriented talk while still in it. Exit from future-oriented talk requires its own *kairos*, the right time (Erickson and Shultz 1982). It appears that the future world is regularly described in a particular way before the participants depart from it. The favourable environment for departure involves the future being portrayed as *manageable*.[11]

Extract (33) below provides an example of a departure from future-oriented talk. The sections of talk constituting the departure from 'future talk' are marked with arrows. Through his questions about the test and about the client's knowledge of it, the counsellor introduces a new topic, thereby focusing away from the topic of future.

(33)   (E4-24)
       ((The participants are talking about P's (non-present) sister's reactions.))
1   C: If she- if (.2) if you <u>did</u> have full-blown AIDS
2   what would she be most <u>wo:</u>rried about (.) do
3   you think?
4   (.8)
5   P: Er::: my health?
6   C: Uh-hum.
7   P: Probably (my morale and)- (.3) probably not me

---

[10] I have not systematically examined shifts between topics that do not involve talk about the future or other sensitive materials. However, Conversation Analytical literature suggests that in institutional talk, boundaried topical movement is usually much more frequently applied than in 'ordinary conversation' (see e.g. Heritage and Sefi 1992). One could expect, then, that the boundaried movement *per se* is not a special feature related to future talk only.

[11] Jefferson (1988: 431–4) has identified three kinds of 'close-implicative elements' for troubles-talk. These include items such as 'optimistic projection', 'invocation of the status quo', and 'making light of the trouble'. The descriptions of the manageability of the future in AIDS counselling seem to operate in a similar fashion as the 'close-implicative elements' of troubles talk.

```
8                passing it on to: (.2) anyone.
9                (.6)
10    C:         [(      )
11    P:         I think- I think she's [more (.8) (aware)=
12    C:                                [uhum
13    P:         =of it than that.
14    C:         Do you think everyone in the family understands
15               how (HIV virus is) passed on
16    P:         Err:::hhhh (.5) I:: (.) really wouldn't know.
17    C:         Would you (.4) know how to talk to them, (.) if
18               there were questions?=.hhh If they said to you
19               (.) Bill if we touch you: are we gonna get
20               AIDS?
21    P:         Er[r::::::::::::::::::::        ] I'd- I would =
22    C:           [(What you wanna say)?]
23    P:         =think that they would- (.3) err:: have enough
24               knowledge of it:, (.2) Maybe not the younger
25               kids but the older ones.
26    C:         Would you know how to (.2) address it if it did
27               come up? (            [            )
28    P:                               [Oh yeah. (.2) I think so.
29               (1.6)
30    (P):       Sure.
31    (C):       All right.
32    C:    ->   .hhhh (1.8) An:d (.) so- (.2) it- you-you come
33          ->   here then to have a test,=today,=is that
34          ->   ri:[ght.
35    P:    ->      [Yeah. I (          ) tested.
36    C:    ->   (All right) what do you know about the te:st.
37    P:    ->   Err:: (.) Really I don't know much::
38               ((continues))
```

In (33) above, the talk immediately preceding the departure from the future world involved descriptions where this world appears manageable. In his responses to the counsellor's questions, the client asserts that he could manage the distribution of necessary information to his family.

In (33), the client's description of a 'manageable hypothetical future' appeared in response to the counsellor's questions. These questions – especially the last one in lines 26–7 – seem to be designed so as to provide for an opportunity for such a description to appear: by employing the yes–no format, the counsellor creates an opportunity for the client to assert that he indeed would know how to 'address it if it did come up'.

Descriptions of a manageable future, however, can also be approached in other ways. In extract (34) below, the description also appears in response to the counsellor's question – but in this case the question is not designed so as to elicit such description. The client takes much more initiative in bringing in the positive tone of voice. Nonetheless, the description of the manageability of the future provides an opportunity for the participants to leave the topic. Again, the moves whereby the participants begin to generate a new topic are marked with arrows.

```
(34)  (N-13)
 1    C:            But say we'd just said that statement your immune
 2                  system is having a struggle now.=What difference
 3                  would it make t[o:-
 4    P:                           [Well no:ne I me- I mean if that was
 5                  the only statement you made, because that th-that it
 6                  (s'rt of) probably is doing anyway.
 7    C:            O:kay,
 8    P:            Err::
 9                  (1.8)
10    P:            But at the same time i-i-it does (.7) most of the
11                  time: (1.0) end up (winning) kicking this ou:t
12                  (.5)
13    C:            Mm[::
14    P:              [eventually.
15    C:            Hm-[mm
16    P:               [Err::
17                  (1.4)
18    P:            S:o
19                  (1.5)
20    C:            Mm
21                  (.8)
22    C:            Mm          (( C is writing
23                  (3.0)       her notes ))
24    C:            Mm
25                  (2.2)
26    C:   ->       Liz is there anything-
27                  (3.8)
28    O:   ->       (No I don't t[hink so.)
```

In (34), the patient, after having been asked about his reactions if his immune system would have a struggle, asserts that his immune system 'most of the time' manages to win its struggles. Therefore he indirectly gives a description of a manageable future. In this case, however, the patient's response is part of an evasive move. In lines 4–6, he contests the relevance of the counsellor's question by asserting that the hypothetical state of affairs is a reality already. By this move he avoids giving a full future-oriented answer to the counsellor's question: the hypothetical future state of affairs would not make any difference, because it is actual now. Nonetheless, even this indirect and evasive description of a manageable future constitutes an occasion for topic closing. By leaving the future talk at this juncture, the counsellor chooses not to challenge the patient's evasive move.

Description of the manageability of the future needs not to be given by the clients only. In extracts (35) and (36), after the clients' responses to future-related questions, the counsellors shift into the statement format, offering concluding future-related descriptions. After the counsellors' statements, which emphasize the manageability of the future, topic shifts occur. These statements are marked with arrows numbered 1, and the topic shifts with arrows numbered 2.

```
(35)  (E4-46/6)
      ((The participants talk about P's preferences concerning a postmor-
      tem examination.))
 1    P:              I don't think I'd be too bothered about that
 2                    because obviously I've had needles shoved in me
 3                    all the time:.
 4    C1:             [Mm:
 5    C2:             [Mm:
 6                    (0.5)
 7    P:              But I don't think I would like to have uh:m
 8                    sort of bits cut out and
 9                    (0.5)
10    C1:   (1) ->    Well perhaps that [something when you've=
11    P:                                [Mm
12    C1:   (1) ->    =thought about it [and if you could talk to Harry=
13    P:                                [Mm
14    C1:   (1) ->    =about [it because if you're going to talk=
15    P:                     [Mm
16    C1:   (1) ->    =about will:s and fune[rals and .hhh af[ter=
17    P:                                    [Mm:            [Well we-
18    C1:   (1) ->    =dea:th [you might as well do it ve(h)ry=
19    P:                      [(sometimes do)
20    C1:   (1) ->    =tho(h)roughly [and put it out of the way and=
21    P:                             [Yeah.
```

```
22    C1:    (1) ->    then it's
23                     (.)
24    P:                Mm:
25    C1:    (1) ->    it's ou:t [and you don't have to talk about it=
26    P:                          [(Yeah)
27    C1:    (1) ->    =again.
28    P:                Mm:
29                     (1.6)
30    C1:    (2) ->    Is there [anything (0.6) that you'd like to=
31    (P):                      [(       )
32    C1:    (2) ->    =[comment on having had this discussion is=
33    P:                [(Mm)
34    C1:    (2) ->    =there anythi:ng you'd like to say right now?
35    P:                Uh:m (0.6) (But) I don't know if you remember:
36                     the time before when I come (0.5) and I said
37                     about the computer and stuff like th[at. Well=
38    C1:                                                 [Mm:
39    P:               =I did get o:ne
40                     (.)
41    (C1):             Mm
42    P:                I've [got er:: an Amstrad PCW,
```

```
(36)  (N-27)
      ((The counsellor is asking the clients how they would respond if
      somebody asked whether he can get AIDS from P.))
1     C1        Miss[is
2     P:            [Yeah.
3     C1:       Davies can you help him to just [finish this off.
4     W:                                        [Yea:h (      )
5     W:        Yes. .hhh You- (.4) oh (.) the only other way is by
6               sexual intercourse.
7     C1:       (A[nd)-
8     W:          [and I'm no(h)t [g(h)oi(h)ng to have [with you so=
9     P:                         [Tha:t's it.          [
10    C1:                                              [O:kay.
11    W:        =it's not [going to worry us.
12    C1:                 [Right.
13    C1:   (1) ->   You could go [e:ven further, (.5) and say (.6) .hh =
14    P:                          [(Good)
15    C1:   (1) ->   =and if I was to have it with you: we would use the
16          (1) ->   condom we['d take-
17    W:                       [Yes
18    W:        Yes.
19    C1:   (2) ->   The reason why Doctor Kaufmann and I're quite keen
20          (2) ->   on asking these questions is because .hhh we feel
21          (2) ->   that you people (.3) are in very: (1.3) in a sense
```

```
22              (2) ->    privileged but difficult position in having having a
23              (2) ->    lot more knowledge: than the general public.
24   W:                   *(Mm-m)*
25   C1:    (2) ->        .hh And t[aking at Mister Davies' thing as that=
26   P:                            [Uh-hum
27   C1:    (2) ->        =there is not a lot of knowledge about it. .hhhh And
28              (2) ->    we feel that if you- (.3) ever
29              (2) ->    had anyone to speak to you could can actually:
30              (2) ->    re[duce
31   (W):                   [hhhh .hh[hh
32   P:                              [Erm:: [(        ) this.
33   C1:    (2) ->                          [fear.
```

In (35), the counsellor advises the patient to talk about postmortems with his brother, and concludes that 'it's ou:t and you don't have to talk about it again' (lines 25 and 27). And finally in (36), the patient's wife and the counsellor consecutively describe how the clients could assure other people about the very limited scope of risk of transmission.

Why, then, does a conversational environment in which the future world is portrayed as manageable appear to be particularly favourable for exiting from talk about future? Trying to answer a question like this takes us outside the scope of strictly sequential analysis of talk. However, two reasons could be suggested: one has to do with the generic dynamics of face-to-face interaction, and the other with the special institutional task of counselling.

(1) The close implicative character of the descriptions of the manageable future can be related to the 'inherent' morality of face-to-face interaction. The concept of 'face', developed by Goffman (1967) and Brown and Levinson (1987), may be useful here. Perhaps it would be a loss of face *par excellence* if a conversationally established future world were to be left in circumstances where the other party, the patient, would have been portrayed only as powerless and suffering. The patient's face is recovered by constructing the future world in such a way where the client is an active, successful agent. After this restoration of the client's 'agency', the participants are free to exit from the world they thus have completed.

(2) The general interactional favourability of the descriptions of manageable aspects of the future (as a close implicative environment for future talk) is probably enhanced by the specific institutional

relevancies of AIDS counselling. If the clients' future involves (and has been described in the session so as to involve) issues like illness and death, any thoroughly 'optimistic' projections are not possible. The counsellors' task is to help the clients to come to terms with their future, whatever this will be like. As soon as the client has described the hypothetical future situation in terms that convey its manageability, a part of the counsellor's task has been fulfilled. The future, which in the beginning of the 'future talk' sequences is in various ways constituted as a sensitive and delicate matter, has now been cast in a new light. The 'dreaded issues' have been locally transformed into 'manageable issues'.

8

Conclusion

Rather than summarizing what has been said in preceding chapters, in the conclusion I wish to bring forward some theoretical and methodological ideas inspired by the data analyses presented in the book. The conclusion is, therefore, fragmentary: a number of themes will be touched upon, all arising from this study, but pointing in various different directions.

Conversation Analysis and Family Systems Theory

The AIDS counselling sessions studied in this book constitute in one respect a new type of data for Conversation Analysis. Unlike the participants in ordinary conversations, and even participants in many forms of institutional talk, the counsellors have a strong theoretical awareness which informs much of their activity. 'Circular questioning', 'live open supervision' and 'future-oriented hypothetical questions' are not spontaneously evolved practices, but the results of conscious theory-building and the development of professional conduct. Therefore, it is important to ask whether Conversation Analysis can say anything about counselling that the professionals have not already said in Family Systems Theory or other theories developed by practitioners.

We can probably distinguish here three types of issue: 'What', 'How', and 'Why' questions (cf. Silverman 1994). The relation of CA with the Family Systems Theory is different with regard to each of these.

'What' questions concern the general regularities in interaction: what is done by the participants. Many of the 'what' questions are answered by texts generated by Family Systems Theory, where

329

techniques like circular questioning, direct open supervision and hypothetical questions are discussed. To find them in the data does not necessarily add anything to what the counsellors already know.[1]

'How' questions concern the techniques of doing what is done in the interaction. This involves, for example, how circular questions and hypothetical questions are asked, received and responded to, and how live open supervision works. Here, it appears, Conversation Analysis operates on an entirely different level of precision from the practitioners' own theory. Usually, Family Systems Theory texts discuss 'how' matters on a very general level, e.g. by giving a paraphrased example of a certain type of question. The implicit assumption seems to be that as members of the common-sense world, the readers of counselling journals and manuals have the knowledge and skills needed for the apprehension and application of the patterns presented. This is, of course, the correct assumption. Therefore, issues like the participants' postural orientation during the delivery of a question, or the appropriate environment for a delicate enquiry need not be addressed in the theoretical texts and manuals primarily targeted at the practitioners.

Conversation Analysis, however, is concerned with exactly these kinds of phenomena. By studying them it seeks to explicate the interactional competencies that counsellors and clients mobilize while operating in a Family Systems Theory framework (or any other theory-based framework of interaction). As this study has indicated, there is a vast array of such skills, most of which are normally activated by the participants in a semi-automatic, non-reflecting manner. Unravelling these can be considered as one of the main contributions of this book.

'Why' questions concern the reasons for, and consequences of, doing the things that are done in counselling. Many answers which Conversation Analysis would consider adequate are given already

---

[1] It is, however, still possible to 'find' these practices from the data. I first encountered 'circular questioning', 'direct open supervision' and 'hypothetical questions' on the tapes and transcripts, and had analysed them for a rather long time before being told by the counsellors about their theories of these practices. The salience of these practices in the data bears witness to the importance of the counsellors' theory in forming interaction with the clients.

in the Family Systems Theory texts. For example, in the classical article on circular questioning (Selvini Palazzoli *et al.* 1980) it was remarked that these types of enquiries are more effective than 'direct' questions in engaging the clients in conversation. Equally, AIDS counsellors have themselves pointed out that 'hypothetical, future-oriented questions' encourage the patients to express their fears and also decrease the pressure upon the counsellor to provide definite answers (Miller and Bor 1988). This study has confirmed that the counsellors have been right in so saying.

What Conversation Analysis can add here to the counselling theory is to explicate the mechanisms which give the counsellors' techniques their effects. For example, I have shown how circular questioning is effective largely because it puts clients in a position where they are 'fishing' for one another's views; and that hypothetical future-oriented questions are so effective because any adequate answer to such a question equally presupposes the hypothesized state of affairs.

However, there are also some other 'why' questions where Family Systems Theory and Conversation Analysis are not complementary. On one hand, for the counsellors, the ultimate reason for doing things in the counselling sessions is the belief that by so doing they will help the clients. For example, circular questioning is practised in order to help clients to perceive the differences between one another's perspectives on AIDS-related issues, and to grasp how their ways of responding to AIDS operate as a 'system'. Research applying Conversation Analysis can say nothing about these kinds of matters, primarily because Conversation Analysis can only deal with phenomena which are observable in the interaction. But on the other hand, Conversation Analysis can try to find unacknowledged uses, or 'latent functions', within the session for the things that occur there. For example, some of the different uses of co-counsellors' questions discussed in chapter 5 were such latent functions. Issues like those are not addressed in the Family Systems Theory textbooks (although there is no a priori reason why they should not be).

In summary, it appears that the concerns of Conversation Analysis and those of the counsellors' own theories are partially overlapping, and partially divergent. There are issues where Conversation Analysis cannot say much more than has already been said in the Family Systems Theory texts. Regarding some other overlapping interests, research based on Conversation Analysis can complement in a constructive way the understanding of counselling based on Family Systems Theory. But there are still other matters where Conversation Analysis invests a great deal of interest (related to the explication of the participants' taken-for-granted competencies and skills), which may appear as irrelevant from the point of view of Family Systems Theory or a practising counsellor. Investigating them is not primarily motivated by a belief that it will help to develop counselling (although it may one day turn out to be so), but by an interest in advancing the sociological understanding of talk-in-interaction.

Implications for counselling practice

The most fundamental implication of this study for counselling practice is to have shown that the techniques based on Family Systems Theory can be adopted successfully in counselling with HIV-positive patients. Throughout the various chapters we have seen that AIDS counselling based on Family Systems Theory 'works': the counsellors and their clients produce unique interaction scenes and episodes which are unlike ordinary conversation and probably also unlike any other type of counselling or therapy. Conversation Analytical study cannot make any claims regarding the therapeutic effectiveness of these interactions – but what we have demonstrated is that Family Systems Theory is most effective in shaping, in a controlled and conscious fashion, the way that people interact with one another in the counselling setting.

With regard to the three specific questioning practices studied in this book, a general remark needs to be made: all these techniques are most powerful devices for *engaging the clients in talking*. These practices do have their tasks in demonstrating for the clients the 'systemic' nature of their problems and in helping the clients to cope. But an even more fundamental task is engagement in talking. It is more fundamental because without the clients' engagement, a counselling session would not be possible at all. 'Circular questioning', the questions that employ the 'live open supervision' format, and 'hypothetical future-oriented questions' are all techniques of amazing interactional power, especially for eliciting clients' talk about matters that they initially may feel reluctant to discuss. It is important that the counsellors continuously bear in mind what kind of forceful machinery they control.

Interactional difficulties were observed, too. In particular, these were related to questions employing the 'live open supervision' format. As we have seen, the format was occasionally abandoned by the counsellors themselves, sometimes apparently due to lack of experience, and sometimes when the co-counsellor engaged in a series of questions. Therefore, out of the three questioning techniques analysed in this book, the one applying the 'live open supervision' format seems to be least routinized and in need of some further development.

On the other hand, we have also been able to demonstrate the usefulness of this questioning technique beyond the objectives discussed in Family Systems Theory. Questions employing the 'live open supervision' format allow for the possibility of the local differentiation of the interactional profiles of the two professionals: one of them can take a more 'demanding' footing, whereas the other may remain more aligned with the client(s). This aspect of live open supervision could in future be more consciously utilized and controlled.

Regarding talk about the clients' future, our analysis has emphasized the importance of *preparatory work* before 'hypothetical questions' are asked. The counsellors' own theoretical statements concerning talk about the future focus almost exclusively on the 'hypothetical questions'. Here the counsellors' own practice is even more sophisticated than their theory: in a most systematic way, they prepare their clients for the hypothetical questions concerning the future, by means of careful topic elicitation and topic development. The importance of this preparatory work could possibly be given specific attention in the teaching of counselling skills.

Implications for Conversation Analysis

Two overarching technical concepts of Conversation Analysis have been frequently used in this book: turn-taking and participation framework. Regarding the former, our data analyses have demonstrated the complexities of the organization of the 'quasi-conversational' (Heritage and Greatbatch 1991) turn-taking. We have demonstrated the clients' amazing compliance with an asymmetric and uniform pattern of interaction; compliance that was not motivated by an orientation to norms related to turn-taking *per se*, but by their orientation to the local interactional activities and to the vagueness of the general frame of the encounter.

One of the possibly generalizable observations in this study concerns the use of *sanctions, accounts* and *requests for permission* in the management of turn-taking. The occasional use of these devices in AIDS counselling sessions might suggest a similarity between AIDS counselling and more institutional turn-taking systems. However, as we have shown, in AIDS counselling these devices operate exclusively within the framework of conversational rules of turn-taking. Therefore, we might suggest that sanctions, accounts and requests for permission *per se* cannot be considered as an indication of the formal, institutional character of turn-taking. The devices can be used for multiple purposes; their function has to be determined individually, case by case.

The management of the participation frameworks in institutional talk has thus far been a much less investigated area than turn-taking. Therefore, a primary contribution of this study is to have demonstrated that the concept of the participation framework contains huge potential for the investigation of institutional talk. Levinson's (1988: 197) suggestion that in various institutional contexts production and reception roles may be 'surgically dissected for institutional purposes' has been shown to be very much to the point. It has to be emphasized that what has been presented in this study by no means covers all such 'surgical dissection' even in AIDS counselling sessions. There is much unexamined territory to be covered.

One of the new themes that our analysis of participation frameworks has brought forward is the link between *epistemic structure* and participation structure. The participants' knowledge and their epistemic positions (i.e. what they expect one another to know) create great relevance for their interaction. Possessing knowledge and being able to know are practical and socially organized matters.

In chapters 3 and 4 we saw how the epistemic structure was closely involved in the management of participation frameworks. The speakers and hearers were allocated participation statuses which corresponded to their epistemic statuses. In chapter 3, we saw how the 'owner' of the experience was allocated a specific reception role when his or her inner experience is described by someone else; and in chapter 4, we analysed how the client got treated as the 'target' of a co-counsellor's question addressed to the main counsellor, by virtue of the 'content' of the question concerning matters that the client is expected to know best.

Our observations confirm the general thesis put forward by Goffman: 'At the very center of interaction life is the cognitive relation we have with those present before us' (1983: 4; cf. also Goodwin 1981: 149–66). In future studies developing the notion of the participation framework in institutional or non-institutional contexts, the involvement of the epistemic structures with the management of the participation framework could be one of the themes to be looked at more closely.

Management of delicacy through indirectness is a single analytical theme that binds together much of the data analyses presented in this study. We have observed how different questioning techniques can be used in the careful and cautious elicitation of the clients' talk about potentially sensitive issues. Care and caution operate through different forms of indirectness. In 'circular questioning', the sensitive descriptions of experience are not elicited directly from the experiencing person, but are first asked from his or her close associate. With questions employing the 'live open supervision' format, the sensitive questions are not posed directly to the client, but are first addressed to one of the professionals. Finally, in 'hypothetical questions', the client's fears concerning the future are not formulated as features of a real world, but as happening in a markedly hypothetical reality.

The use of different forms of indirectness in the management of delicacy has been recently discussed in various papers (cf. Brown and Levinson 1987; Silverman and Peräkylä 1990; Bergmann 1992). The questioning practices studied in this book are of particular interest because forms of indirectness that would occur relatively rarely in ordinary conversation have been conventionalized as central elements of a therapeutic technique. Indirectness has become a part of the routinized professional practice. In AIDS counselling based on Family Systems Theory, the structure of these 'indirect' questioning patterns is recurrent and relatively stable; and, most importantly, awareness of these practices is a part of the counsellors' theoretical knowledge of their own work.[2]

Following Bergmann (1992), we can suggest that these forms of indirectness have a double, reflexive function in the management of delicacy. On the one hand, by using indirect questioning patterns the counsellors approach the client's predicament in a courteous and polite manner: they do not demand that the client speak in a blunt and straightforward way. In this respect, indirect questions are 'softer' questions. But on the other hand, through the very indirectness the counsellors also *constitute* as sensitive and delicate the issues that the questions concern. By employing indirect patterns of questioning, counsellors suggest to the clients that these are matters that *have to be* approached carefully. Therefore, apart from deference to the clients' predicament, indirect questioning patterns also embody an expectation that the clients, in the first place, are in this predicament.

It is also very important to bear in mind that 'softer' questions need not be less powerful. The data analyses in this book have demonstrated how the AIDS counsellors' questioning practices are structured so as to forestall the clients' resistance. In circular questioning, clients in effect end up fishing for descriptions of one another's experience. In live open supervision, two counsellors, rather than one, collaboratively operate in the delivery of a question. In hypothetical questions, the clients are nominally talking about only a fantasy world, not about their real lives. To avoid answering direct questions may, therefore, be much easier than to avoid answering these kinds of indirect ones.

On a more general level, this study has suggested a new area of research for Conversation Analysis: the examination of *theory-based interaction*. As has been emphasized again and again throughout the book, the questioning practices studied here are based on a particular therapeutic theory. Conversation Analysis

---

[2] This does not mean to say, however, that the counsellors' theoretical knowledge would regard these questioning techniques *primarily as devices for the management of delicacy*. The different questioning patterns are differently attended to: the function of 'hypothetical questions' as a means for management of delicacy is quite explicitly discussed in the counsellors' theory, whereas the primary task of the other two questioning practices is understood by the counsellors to be other than management of delicacy.

made it possible to examine in detail how these techniques operate. It also helped us to see how the operation of a unique theory-based questioning technique rests upon the participants' general interactional competences, which have their home-base in mundane conversation.

Research on theory-based interaction offers a future challenge for Conversation Analysis. AIDS counselling is by no means the only setting where professionals are engaged in theory-building, with the intention to understand and develop their interaction with the clients. In counselling and psychotherapy, there are various theories and traditions operating; any specific bearing that these theories may have on the actual interaction between the clients and professionals is a matter that can be examined through Conversation Analysis. Growing awareness about the importance of face-to-face interaction is also becoming characteristic of medical work, education and even business.

To put it briefly and simply, the challenge for Conversation Analysis in research on theory-based interaction is to show in detail how the theoretical ideas are worked through in the practice of interaction. The pioneering studies of Gale (1991) and Buttny (1990, 1994) on family therapy interaction demonstrate the promise of this kind of approach. Like Gale's and Buttny's studies, the research reported in this book concerned the application of *one* counselling theory in *one* clinic. In future studies, a more *comparative* approach should be introduced. It would be of great interest, both theoretically and practically, to study in detail how the alternative theoretical frameworks are worked through in the actual interaction between professionals and clients.

For example, in primary health care, there are competing theoretical ideas operating at the moment: unlike the traditional 'biomedical' thinking, new ideas emphasize a more holistic ('biopsychosocial' or 'patient-centred') approach (Engel 1977 and 1980; McWhinney 1989). If the doctor's theoretical commitment to either of the competing models has any bearing on the ways in which she or he interacts with the patient, the difference can be studied using Conversation Analysis. (For developments in this direction, see e.g. Silverman 1987; Frankel and Beckman 1989.)

Or to give another example, in psychotherapy research there has been a longstanding dispute over whether or not the therapist's theoretical orientation matters at all. Reports of outcome-oriented quantitative research have recurrently pointed out that the theoretical orientation of the therapist has very little bearing on the outcome of the therapy, measured by standard assessment interviews and self-report inventories (Stiles, Shapiro and Elliot 1986; Leiman and Stiles 1993). On the other hand, it has been pointed out that quite a different kind of process-oriented research is needed in order to find out the actual interactive structures and practices of psychotherapy (see e.g. Rice and Greenberg 1984; Moon *et al.* 1990; Wahlström 1992). Conversation Analytic research will make it possible to examine, in a new level of precision, how therapies operating within different theoretical frameworks are different in actual interaction. It will also be possible to identify those interactive features that are *common* to different schools of therapy. (As examples of qualitative developments towards this direction, outside the realm of Conversation Analysis, see Agnus and Rennie 1988 and 1989; Gubrium 1992).

For the conversation analyst, a prerequisite for working in these fields is to familiarize him- or herself with the theories that the professionals are using. This may require a considerable amount of time and energy; but it is impossible to fully appreciate professional forms of interaction without understanding the theories that inform their production.

There are, however, definite limits in the applicability of the practitioners' theory in data analysis. The most important part of the actual data analysis – i.e. the detailed case-by-case examination of data extracts – has to remain just as inductive as any other Conversation Analytical work is. This means that the conversation analyst has to be able to 'bracket' his or her knowledge of the professionals' theory, in order to find out what is happening in the actual, incorporate interaction. Only after the inductive data analysis should the conversation analyst mobilize his or her knowledge about the professionals' theory, in order to be able to identify all the implications of the findings.

Implications for medical sociology

This book has been about face-to-face interaction. Apart from the reference to counsellors' theories and their tasks, I have consciously avoided linking the results of the data analysis with any larger-scale cultural or social structures and processes. In other words, I have treated the world of interaction as an *autonomous* realm of social reality (cf. Goffman 1981). The linkages between interaction and the larger-scale cultural or social phenomena are, however, potentially to be found – even though revealing their exact nature would require much more analytical work than is possible here. But I would like to close this book by indicating one such linkage.

Almost all the practices examined in this book have had a common denominator: in one way or another, they can all be used to *encourage the clients to speak*. It has been argued that by recurrently setting up the question–answer sequence, by asking circular and hypothetical questions, and even by applying live open supervision, counsellors create contexts where it is possible for clients to speak about their concerns.

The clinic where clients are helped to talk is a relatively recent phenomenon. Two well-known American historians of medicine working in a Foucauldian framework, W.R. Arney and B.J. Bergen (1984; see also Armstrong 1983), have argued that 'a new medical revolution' began in the Western world in the 1950s. Before that, modern medicine concentrated on the patient's body only: the body, and only the body, was the site of illnesses and cures. In the 'new medical revolution', the *experience* of the patient was discovered. Since then, Arney and Bergen argue, medicine has increasingly sought to include the mind and the social relations of the patient in its scope. A central feature in this new medicine is *incitement to speak*:

Medicine has been undergoing a transition in the structure of its discourse that not only allows the patient to speak as an experiencing person, but *needs*, *demands*, and *incites* him to speak.   (Arney and Bergen 1984: 46)

According to Arney and Bergen, the beginning and the end of human life – birth and death – are so far the biographical environments most thoroughly influenced by the new medicine that concentrates on the experiencing subject.

Present-day medicine increasingly constructs the patient, through various discursive practices, as an experiencing, communicating subject (Silverman 1987). Therefore, the clinic needs the patients' disclosures of their experience as much as the patients need the clinicians to listen to them.

The observations presented in this book have shown how AIDS counsellors are working in the forefront of this new medicine. Bearing in mind the centrality of counselling in the medical response to AIDS, it seems that HIV/AIDS is a new illness, not only in a bio-medical sense, but also socially. A new kind of talking – profession-ally guided talk about experience, feelings and social relations – accompanies HIV/AIDS probably more than any other serious illness.

Appendix: the data base

The data used in this study are video recordings from AIDS counselling sessions at two clinics in the Royal Free Hospital, London. The bulk of the data is from the Haemophilia Centre of that hospital, and some additional data has been collected from the HIV/AIDS clinic of the same hospital.

Due to my appointment as a Glaxo Research Fellow in the research project 'Counselling with people who may be HIV positive' (based at Goldsmiths' College and led by Professor David Silverman) I was granted access to the video archives of the Haemophilia Centre and the HIV/AIDS clinic of the Royal Free Hospital. The counselling sessions at the Haemophilia Centre are routinely video recorded for the purpose of using them for the preparation of subsequent sessions with the same patients, and for teaching and research. Recordings are made only if the patients give their consent. By the time of the beginning of the research project, the counsellors at the HIV/AIDS clinic had also begun to video record their sessions; but due to an increasing workload, they gave up this practice after about six months. The video archives of the two clinics currently consist of approximately 450 hours of counselling sessions.

Only a small fraction of the existing recordings could be used in this research. Some 40 sessions were initially examined. These were more or less randomly sampled, although interviews involving more than one client (a patient with his close associates) were preferred at some stages of the selection. Out of the sessions initially watched, 32 were used as data in the research. (The remaining recordings were examined at the earliest part of the research, and the transcripts and analyses from them were discarded as the standard of work got better.)

Most of the patients involved in the 32 sessions used as data were HIV-positive haemophilic males. There were nineteen patients and their ages varied from the early teens to the fifties. Of these nineteen patients, three were counselled in two sessions used as data, and another two in three sessions. Five sessions used as data were from pre-test counselling in the HIV/AIDS clinic; and one session was from counselling in that clinic with a patient newly diagnosed as HIV positive. Of the HIV/AIDS clinic material, one of the patients was female (in other words, she was the only female patient in the whole data set); of the male patients, most identified themselves as gay.

Two sessions (one pre-test and one with an HIV-positive haemophiliac) out of the 32 were transcribed from beginning to end. From the rest of the sessions, only extracts were transcribed. The length of the extracts varies from about 30 seconds to 25 minutes. They were collected to cover talk about the patients' future, about safe sex practices, and to cover instances where one client is asked to describe the experience of another. Most of the data used in this study were from extracts related to the first and the last themes. Together the data transcribed comprises more than 10 hours of talk.

About two-thirds of the transcripts were initially prepared by Dr David Greatbatch and the rest by myself, apart from a few extracts transcribed by Ms Outi Paloposki. However, during the course of the analysis of the data, I reworked most of the segments that were examined in detail. The notation that we used was the one developed by Gail Jefferson, which is currently followed in almost all Conversation Analytical studies.

In the data analysis, Conversation Analytical methods were used (for general accounts about Conversation Analytical methods, see Heritage 1988 and Wootton 1989). In practical terms, this involved in the first place careful listening to the talk and meticulous examination, word by word and turn by turn, of the transcripts.

In choosing the segments of data which were to be examined in detail, the point of departure was a rough classification of interactional phenomena that appeared to be interesting in analytical terms. It included categories such as 'departures from question–

answer pattern', 'management of the different versions of the same (family) events', 'interaction between the counsellors' and 'talking about delicate issues'. These categories arose from the initial contacts with the data. Events belonging to these kinds of category were collected from the transcribed data and examined in detail. Single case analyses, comparisons of different patterns that were found in them, meticulous examination of deviant cases (cf. Silverman 1989), memo-writing, and discussions with the other people involved in the project gradually led to the uncovering of the structures and practices described in the text.

References

Agnus, L. & Rennie, D. (1988) Therapist participation in metaphor generation: collaborative and non-collaborative styles. *Psychotherapy* 25: 552–60.

(1989) Envisioning the representational world: the client's experience of metaphoric expression in psychotherapy. *Psychotherapy* 26: 372–9.

Alexander, J. (1988) *Action and Its Environments. Towards a New Synthesis.* New York: Columbia University Press.

Armstrong, D. (1983) *The Political Anatomy of the Body.* Cambridge University Press

Arney, W. and Bergen, B. (1984) *Medicine and the Management of Living.* Chicago University Press.

Atkinson, J.M. (1982) Understanding formality: the categorization and production of 'formal' interaction. *The British Journal of Sociology* 33(1): 86–117.

Atkinson, J.M. and Drew, P. (1979) *Order in Court. The Organisation of Verbal Interaction in Judicial Settings.* London: Macmillan.

Atkinson, J.M. and Heritage, J. (1984) (eds.) *Structures of Social Action. Studies of Conversation Analysis.* Cambridge University Press.

Austin, J.L. (1962) *How to Do Things with Words.* Oxford: Clarendon Press.

Baldock, J. and Prior, D. (1981) Social workers talking to clients: a study of verbal behaviour. *British Journal of Social Work* 11: 19–38.

Bergmann, J.R. (1992) Veiled morality: notes on discretion in psychiatry. In Drew, P. and Heritage, J. (eds.): *Talk at Work. Interaction in Institutional Settings.* Cambridge University Press, pp. 137–62.

Boden, D. and Zimmerman, D.H. (eds.) (1991) *Talk and Social Structure.* Cambridge: Polity Press.

Bor, R. and Miller, R. (1988) Addressing 'dreaded issues': a description of a unique counselling intervention with patients with AIDS/HIV. *Counselling Psychology Quarterly* 1: 397–405.

Bor, R., Perry, L., Miller, R. (1989) A systems approach to AIDS counselling. *Journal of Family Therapy* 11: 77–86.

Boscolo, L., Cecchin, G., Hoffman, L., Penn, P. (1986) *Milan Systemic Family Therapy. Conversations in Theory and Practice.* New York: Basic Books.

Brown, G. and Yule, G. (1983) *Discourse Analysis.* Cambridge University Press.

Brown, P. and Levinson, S. (1987) *Politeness: Some Universals in Language Usage.* Cambridge University Press.

Burnard, P. (1992) *Perceptions of AIDS Counselling.* Aldershot: Avebury.

Burnham J. and Harris, Q. (1985) Therapy, supervision, consultation: different levels of a system. In Campbell, D. and Draper, R. (eds.) *Applications of Systemic Family Therapy. The Milan Approach.* London: Grune & Stratton, pp. 59–67.

Buttny, R. (1990) Blame-account sequences in therapy: the negotiation of relational meanings. *Semiotica,* 78: 219–48.

(1994) Problem reformulation in therapy: clients and therapist joint construction of the clients' problems. Paper presented at the American Association of Applied Linguistics Conference, Baltimore.

Button, G. and Casey, N. (1984), 'Generating topic: the use of topic initial elicitors', in Atkinson, J.M. and Heritage, J. (eds.), *Structures of Social Action: Studies in Conversation Analysis,* Cambridge University Press, pp. 167–90.

(1985) Topic nomination and topic pursuit. *Human Studies* 8: 3–55.

Byrne, P.S. and Long, B.E.L. (1976) *Doctors Talking to Patients: A Study of the Verbal Behaviours of Doctors in the Consultation.* London: HMSO.

Cade, B. and Cornwell, M. (1985) New realities for old: some uses of teams and one-way screens in therapy. In Campbell, D. and Draper, R. (eds.) *Applications of Systemic Family Therapy. The Milan Approach.* London: Grune & Stratton, pp. 47–57.

Campbell, D. and Draper, R. (eds.) (1985) *Applications of Systemic Family Therapy. The Milan Approach.* London: Grune & Stratton.

Carballo, M. and Miller, D. (1989) HIV counselling: problems and opportunities in defining new agenda for the 1990s. *AIDS Care,* 1: 117–23.

Chester, R. (1987) *Advice, Support and Counselling for the HIV Positive.* A report for DHSS, University of Hull.

Clayman, S.E. (1992) Footing in the achievement of neutrality: the case of news interview discourse. In Drew P. and Heritage J. (eds.): *Talk at Work. Interaction in Institutional Settings.* Cambridge University Press, pp. 163–98.

Dijk, T. A. van (1985) Introduction: discourse analysis as a new cross-discipline. In Dijk, T. A. van (ed.) *Handbook of Discourse Analysis.* London: Academic Press.

Dingwall, R. (1980) Orchestrated encounters: an essay in the comparative analysis of speech-exchange systems. *Sociology of Health and Illness* 2 (2): 151–73.

Dingwall, R. and Robinson, K.M. (1990) Policing the family: health visiting and the public surveillance of private behaviour. In Gubrium, J. and Sankar, A. (eds.) *The Home Care Experience*. Newbury Park: Sage.

Drew, P. (1990) Conversation Analysis – who needs it. *Text* 10 (1/2): 27–35.

(1992) Contested evidence in courtroom cross-examination: the case of a trial for rape. In Drew, P. and Heritage, J. (eds.) *Talk at Work. Interaction in Institutional Settings*. Cambridge University Press, pp. 470–520.

Drew, P. and Heritage, J. (eds.) (1992) *Talk at Work. Interaction in Institutional Settings*. Cambridge University Press.

Drew, P. and Holt, E. (1988) Complainable matters: the use of idiomatic expressions in making complaints. *Social Problems* 35 (4): 398–417.

Drew, P. and Wootton, A., (eds.) (1988) *Erving Goffman: Exploring the Interaction Order*. Cambridge: Polity Press.

Duranti, A. (1988) Ethnography of speaking: toward a linguistics of the human praxis. In Newmeyer, F.J. (ed.) *Linguistics: The Cambridge Survey*. Vol. IV: *The Socio-Cultural Context*. Cambridge University Press, pp. 210–28.

Duranti, A. and Goodwin, C. (eds.) (1992) *Rethinking Context. Language as an Interactive Phenomenon*. Cambridge University Press.

Durkheim, E. (1964) *The Rules of Sociological Method*. New York: Free Press.

Engel, G.L. (1977) The need for a new medical model: a challenge for biomedicine. *Science* 196: 129–36.

(1980) The clinical application of the biopsychosocial model. *American Journal of Psychiatry* 137 (5): 535–44.

Erickson, F. and Shultz, J. (1982) *The Counselor as Gatekeeper. Social Interaction in Interviews*. New York: Academic Press.

Feinberg, P.H. (1990) Circular questions: establishing the relational context. *Family Systems Medicine* 8(3): 273–7.

Fleuridas, C., Nelson, T.S., Rosenthal, D.M. (1986) The evolution of circular questions: training family therapists. *Journal of Marital and Family Therapy* 12 (2): 113–27.

Frankel, R. (1990) Talking in interviews: a dispreference for patient-initiated questions in physician–patient encounters. In G. Psathas (ed.) *Interactional Competence*. University Press of America, pp. 231–62.

Frankel, R. and Beckman, H. (1989) Evaluating the patient's primary problem(s). In Stewart, M. and Roter, D. (eds.) *Communicating with Medical Patients*. Newbury Park: Sage, pp. 86–98.

Gale, J.E. (1991) *Conversation Analysis of Therapeutic Discourse: The Pursuit of a Therapeutic Agenda*. Volume XLI in the series 'Advances in Discourse Processes'. Norwood, New Jersey: Ablex Publishing Corporation.

Garcia, A. (1991) Dispute resolution without disputing: how the interactional organization of mediation hearings minimizes argumentative talk. *American Sociological Review* 56: 818–35.

Garfinkel, H. (1967) *Studies in Ethnomethodology*, Englewood Cliffs, NJ: Prentice-Hall.

George, H. (1989) Counselling people with AIDS, their lovers, friends and relations. In Green, J. and McCreaner, A. (eds.), *Counselling with HIV-Infection and AIDS*. Oxford: Blackwell Scientific Publications, pp. 69-87.

Goffman, E. (1967) *Interaction Ritual: Essays on Face-to-Face Behavior*. New York: Doubleday Anchor.

(1974) *Frame Analysis: An Essay on the Organization of Experience*. New York: Harper and Row.

(1979) Footing. *Semiotica* 25: 1–29. (Reprinted in Goffman 1981)

(1981) *Forms of Talk*. Oxford: Basil Blackwell.

(1983) The interaction order. *American Sociological Review* 48(1): 1–17.

Goodwin, C. (1979) The interactional construction of a sentence in natural conversation. In Psathas, G. (ed.) *Everyday Language: Studies in Ethnomethodology*. New York: Erlbaum, pp. 97–121.

(1981) *Conversational Organization: Interaction Between Speakers and Hearers*. New York: Academic Press.

(1984) Notes on story structure and the organization of participation. In Atkinson, J.M. and Heritage, J.C. (eds.) *Structures of Social Action: Studies in Conversation Analysis*. Cambridge University Press, pp. 225–46.

(1992) Transparent vision. Unpublished manuscript, Department of Anthropology, University of South Carolina.

(1993) Perception, technology and interaction on a scientific research vessel. Unpublished manuscript, Department of Anthropology, University of South Carolina.

Goodwin, C. and Duranti, A. (1992) Rethinking context: an introduction. In Duranti, A. and Goodwin, C. (eds.) *Rethinking Context: Language as an Interactive Phenomenon*. Cambridge University Press.

Goodwin, C. and Harness Goodwin, M. (1992) Professional vision. Plenary lecture at the Conference of Discourse and the Professions, Uppsala, Sweden, August 1992.

Greatbatch, D. (1988) A turn-taking system for British news interviews. *Language in Society* 17: 401–30.

(1992) The management of disagreement between news interviewees. In Drew, P. and Heritage, J. (eds.) *Talk at Work. Interaction in Institutional Settings*. Cambridge University Press, pp. 268–301.

Grice, H.P. (1975) Logic and conversation. In Cole, P. and Morgan, J.L. (eds.) *Syntax and Semantics 3: Speech Acts*. New York: Academic Press, pp. 41–58.

Gubrium, J. (1992) *Out of Control: Family Therapy and Domestic Disorder*. London: Sage.

Gumperz, J.J. (1982) *Discourse Strategies*. Cambridge University Press.

(1992a) Interviewing in intercultural situations. In Drew, P. and Heritage, J. (eds.) *Talk at Work. Interaction in Institutional Settings*. Cambridge University Press, pp. 302–27.

(1992b) Contextualization and understanding. In Duranti, A. and Goodwin, C. (eds.) *Rethinking Context: Language as an Interactive Phenomenon*. Cambridge University Press, pp. 229–52.

Hanks, W.F. (1990) *Referential Practice. Language and Lived Space among the Maya*. University of Chicago Press.

Have, P. ten (1989) The consultation as a genre. In Torode, B. (ed.) *Text and Talk as Social Practice*. Dordrecht: Foris, pp. 115–35.

Heath, C. (1986) *Body Movement and Speech in Medical Interaction*. Cambridge University Press.

(1989) Pain talk: the expression of suffering in the medical consultation. *Social Psychology Quarterly* 52 (2): 113–25.

Heritage, J. (1984) *Garfinkel and Ethnomethodology*. Cambridge: Polity Press.

(1985) Analyzing news interviews: aspects of the production of talk for an overhearing audience. In van Dijk, T.A. (ed.), *Handbook of Discourse Analysis Vol 3.*, London: Academic Press, 299–345.

(1988) Explanations as accounts: a conversation analytic perspective. In Antaki, C. (ed.) *Analysing Everyday Explanation: A Case Book of Methods*. London: Sage, pp. 127–44.

(1989) Current developments in conversation analysis. In Roger, D. and Bull, P. (eds.), *Conversation: an Interdisciplinary Perspective*. Clevedon: Multilingual Matters, pp. 21–47.

Heritage, J. and Greatbatch, D. (1991) On the institutional character of institutional talk: the case of news interviews. In Boden, D. and Zimmerman, D.H. (eds.) *Talk and Social Structure. Studies in Ethnomethodology and Conversation Analysis*. Cambridge: Polity Press, pp. 93–137.

Heritage, J. and Sefi, S. (1992) 'Just a chat': dilemmas of advice giving in interactions between health visitors and first time mothers. In Drew, P. and Heritage, J. (eds.) *Talk at Work*. Cambridge University Press, pp. 359–417.

Hoffman, L. (1981) *Foundations of Family Therapy. A Conceptual Framework for Systems Change*. New York: Basic Books.

(1988) A constructivist position for family therapy. *The Irish Journal of Psychology* 9: 110–29.

Hughes, D. (1982) Control of the medical consultation. *Sociology* 16 (3): 359–76.

Hymes, D. (1974) *Foundations of Sociolinguistics: An Ethnographic Approach*. Philadelphia: University of Pennsylvania Press.

Jefferson, G. (1974) Error correction as an interactional resource. *Language and Society* 2: 181–99.

(1980) Final report to the SSRC on the analysis of conversations in which 'troubles' and 'anxieties' are expressed (no. HR 4805). Mimeo.

(1981) 'Caveat speaker': a preliminary exploration of shift implicative recipiency in the articulation of topic. End of Grant Report. London: Social Science Research Council. Mimeo.

(1984a) On stepwise transition from talk about a trouble to inappropriately next-positioned matters. In Atkinson, J.M. and Heritage, J.C. (eds.) *Structures of Social Action: Studies in Conversation Analysis.* Cambridge University Press, pp. 194–222.

(1984b) On the organisation of laughter in talk about troubles. In Atkinson, J.M. and Heritage, J. (eds.) *Structures of Social Action: Studies in Conversation Analysis.* Cambridge University Press, pp. 347–369.

(1984c) Notes on a systematic deployment of the acknowledgement tokens 'Yeah' and 'Mm hm'. *Papers in Linguistics* 17: 197–216.

(1985a) On the interactional unpacking of a gloss. *Language in Society* 14: 435–66.

(1985b) An exercise in the transcription and analysis of laughter. In Dijk, T.A. van (ed.), *Handbook of Discourse Analysis, Vol. 3.* London: Academic Press, pp. 25–34.

(1988) On the sequential organisation of troubles talk in ordinary conversation. *Social Problems* 35 (4): 418–41.

Jefferson, G. and Lee, J.R.E. (1981) The rejection of advice: managing the problematic convergence of a 'troubles telling' and a 'service encounter'. *Journal of Pragmatics* 5: 339–422.

Kendon, A. (1990) *Conducting Interaction. Patterns of Behavior in Focussed Encounters.* Cambridge University Press.

Labov, W. and Fanshel, D. (1977) *Therapeutic Discourse: Psychotherapy as Conversation.* New York: Academic Press.

Lee, J.R.E. (1987) Prologue: talking organization. In Button, G. and Lee, J.R.E. (eds.) *Talk and Social Organization.* Clevedon: Multilingual Matters, pp. 19–53.

Leiman, M. and Stiles, W.B. (1993) Semiosis in psychotherapy. Research symposium on semiotic processes in psychotherapy, Heinävesi, Finland, 6–9.6.1993. Unpublished paper.

Levinson, S.C. (1983) *Pragmatics.* Cambridge University Press.

(1988) Putting linguistics on a proper footing: explorations in Goffman's concepts of participation. In Drew, P. and Wootton, A. (eds.) *Erving Goffman: Exploring the Interaction Order.* Cambridge: Polity Press, pp. 161–227.

Linell, P., Gustavsson, L., Juvonen, P. (1988) Interactional dominance in dyadic communication: a presentation of initiative–response analysis. *Linguistics,* 26: 415–42.

McCreaner, A. (1989) Pre-test counselling. In Green, J. and McCreaner, A. (eds.), *Counselling with HIV-Infection and AIDS*. Oxford: Blackwell Scientific Publications, pp. 21–7.

McHoul, A. (1978) The organization of turns at formal talk in the classroom. *Language in Society* 7: 183–213.

McIntosh, J. (1986) *A Consumer Perspective on the Health Visiting Service*. University of Glasgow: Social Paediatric and Obstetric Research Unit.

McWhinney, I. (1989) The need for a transformed clinical method. In Stewart, M. and Roter, D. (eds.) *Communicating with Medical Patients*. Newbury Park: Sage, pp. 25–40.

Manning, P. (1989) Ritual talk. *Sociology* 23 (3): 365–85.

Mauksch, L.B. and Roesler, T. (1990) Expanding the context of the patient's explanatory model using circular questioning. *Family Systems Medicine* 8 (1): 3–13.

Maynard, D.W. (1988) Language, interaction and social problems. *Social Problems* 35 (4): 311–34.

(1991a) Interaction and asymmetry in clinical discourse. *American Journal of Sociology* 97 (2): 448–95.

(1991b) The perspective-display series and the delivery and receipt of diagnostic news. In Boden, D. and Zimmerman, D.H. (eds.) *Talk and Social Structure. Studies in Ethnomethodology and Conversation Analysis*. Cambridge: Polity Press.

(1992) On clinicians co-implicating recipients' perspective in the delivery of diagnostic news. In Drew P. and Heritage, J. (eds.) *Talk at Work. Interaction in Institutional Settings*. Cambridge University Press, pp. 331–58.

Mehan, H. (1979) *Learning Lessons: Social Organisation in the Classroom*. Cambridge, Mass: Harvard University Press.

(1985) The structure of classroom discourse. In Dijk, T.A. van (ed.) *Handbook of Discourse Analysis, Vol. 3*. London: Academic Press, 120–32.

Merritt, M. (1976) On questions following questions (in service encounters). *Language in Society* 5: 315–57.

Merton, R.K. (1957) *Social Theory and Social Structure*. Revised and enlarged edition. New York: Free Press

Miller, D. (1987a) HIV counselling: some practical problems and issues. *Journal of the Royal Society of Medicine* 80: 287.

(1987b) Counselling. *British Medical Journal* 294: 1671–4.

Miller, R. and Bor, R. (1988) *AIDS: A Guide to Clinical Counselling*, London: Science Press.

Moerman, M. (1988) *Talking Culture: Ethnography and Conversation Analysis*. Philadelphia: University of Pennsylvania Press.

Moon, S.M., Dillo, D.R., Sprenkle, D.H. (1990) Family therapy and qualitative research. *Journal of Marital and Family Therapy* 16 (4): 357–73.

Nelson-Jones, R. (1982) *The Theory and Practice of Counselling Psychology.* London: Cassel.

(1988) Practical counselling and helping skills. Second Edition. London: Cassell.

Olson, U.-F. and Pegg, P.F. (1979) Direct open supervision: a team approach. *Family Process* 18: 463–9.

Parsons, T. (1937) *The Structure of Social Action.* New York: McGraw-Hill.

(1951) *The Social System.* New York: Free Press.

Penn, P. (1982) Circular questioning. *Family Process* 21 (3): 267–80.

(1985) Feed-forward: future questions, future maps. *Family Process* 24(3): 299–310.

Peräkylä, A. (1989) Appealing to the 'experience' of the patient in the care of the dying. *Sociology of Health and Illness* 11 (2): 117–34.

(1991) Hope work in the care of seriously ill patients. *Qualitative Health Research* 1(4): 407–33.

Peräkylä, A., Silverman, D. Rethinking speech-exchange systems: communication formats in AIDS counselling. *Sociology* 25 (4): 627–51.

Pike, K.L. (1967) *Language in Relation to a Unified Theory of the Structure of Human Behaviour.* Second revised edition. The Hague: Mouton.

Pollner, M. (1987) *Mundane Reason. Reality in Everyday and Sociological Discourse.* Cambridge University Press.

Pomerantz, A. (1980) Telling my side: 'Limited Access' as a 'Fishing Device'. *Sociological Inquiry* 50: 186–98.

(1984) Agreeing and disagreeing with assessments: some features of preferred/dispreferred turn shapes. In Atkinson, J.M. and Heritage, J.C. (eds.) *Structures of Social Action: Studies in Conversation Analysis.* Cambridge University Press, 57–101.

Rice, L.N. and Greenberg, L.S. (1984) *Patterns of Change. Intensive Analysis of Psychotherapy Process.* New York: Guildford.

Sacks, H. (1971) Lecture, 10 May.

(1972) An initial investigation of the usability of conversation data for doing sociology. In D. Sudnow (ed.) *Studies In Social Interaction.* New York: Free Press, pp. 31–74.

(1974) On the analyzability of stories of children. In Turner, R. (ed) *Ethnomethodology. Selected Readings.* Harmondsworth: Penguin, pp. 216–32.

(1984) On doing 'being ordinary'. In Atkinson, J.M. and Heritage, J. (eds.) *Structures of Social Action: Studies in Conversation Analysis.* Cambridge University Press, pp. 413–29.

(1987) On the preference for agreement and contiguity in sequences in conversation. In Button, G. and Lee, J.R.E. (eds.) *Talk and Social Organization.* Clevedon: Multilingual Matters, pp. 54–69.

(1992a) *Lectures on Conversation. Volume 1.* Edited by G. Jefferson; with an introduction by E.A. Schegloff. Oxford: Blackwell.

(1992b) *Lectures on Conversation. Volume 2.* Edited by G. Jefferson; with an introduction by E.A. Schegloff. Oxford: Blackwell.

Sacks, H., Schegloff, E.A., Jefferson, G. (1974) A simplest systematics of turn-taking for conversation. *Language* 50, 696–735.

Scheflen, A. E. (1973) *Communicational Structure: Analysis of a Psychotherapy Transaction.* Bloomington: Indiana University Press.

Schegloff, E. A. (1968) Sequencing in conversational openings. *American Anthropologist* 70: 1075–95.

(1972) Notes on conversational practice: formulating place. In Sudnow, D. (ed.) *Studies in Social Interaction.* New York: Free Press, pp. 75–111.

(1979) The relevance of repair to syntax-for-conversation. *Syntax and Semantics* 12: 261–86.

(1980) Preliminaries to preliminaries: 'Can I ask You a Question'. *Sociological Inquiry* 50: 104–52.

(1981) Discourse as an interactional achievement: Some uses of 'uh huh' and other things that come between sentences. In *Georgetown University Round Table on Languages and Linguistics* 1981. Ed. Deborah Tannen. Washington, DC: Georgetown University Press, pp. 71–93.

(1986) The routine as achievement. *Human Studies* 9: 111–51.

(1987) Between macro and micro: contexts and other connections. In Alexander, J., Giesen, B., Munch, R., Smelser, N. (eds.) *The Micro-Macro Link.* Berkeley and Los Angeles: University of California Press, pp. 207–34.

(1988) Goffman and the analysis of conversation. In Drew, P. and Wootton, A. (eds.) *Erving Goffman: Exploring the Interaction Order.* Cambridge: Polity Press, pp. 89–135.

(1991) Reflections on talk and social structure. In Boden, D. and Zimmerman, D. (eds.) *Talk and Social Structure.* Cambridge: Polity Press, pp. 44–70.

(1992a) Repair after next turn: the last structurally provided defense of intersubjectivity in conversation. *American Journal of Sociology* 98: 1295–345.

(1992b) On talk and its institutional occasion. In Drew, P. and Heritage, J. (eds.) *Talk at Work. Interaction in Institutional Settings.* Cambridge University Press, pp. 101–34.

(1992c) Introduction. In Sacks, H. *Lectures on Conversation. Volume 1.* Ed. G. Jefferson. Oxford: Blackwell, pp. ix–lxii.

Schegloff, E.A. and Sacks, H. (1973) Opening up closings. *Semiotica* 7: 289–327.

Schutz, A. and Luckmann, T. (1974) *The Structures of Life World.* London: Heinemann.

Searle, J.R. (1969) *Speech Acts.* Cambridge University Press.

(1976) The classification of illocutionary acts. *Language in Society* 5: 1–24

Selvini Palazzoli, M., Boscolo, L., Cecchin, G., Prata, G. (1978) *Paradox and Counterparadox. A New Mode in the Therapy of the Family in Schizophrenic Transaction.* New York: Jason Aronson.

(1980) Hypothesizing–circularity–neutrality: three guidelines for the conductor of the session. *Family Process* 19 (1): 3–12.

Selvini, M. and Selvini Palazzoli, M. (1991) Team consultation: an indispensable tool for the progress of knowledge. Ways of fostering and promoting its creative potential. *Journal of Family Therapy* 13: 31–52.

Sharrock, W. (1974) On owning knowledge. In Turner, R. (ed.) *Ethnomethodology.* Harmondsworth: Penguin, pp. 45–53.

Sharrock, W. and Anderson, B. (1987) Work flow in a paediatric clinic. In Button, G. and Lee, J.R.E. (eds.) *Talk and Social Organization.* Clevedon: Multilingual Matters, pp. 244–60.

Silverman, D. (1973) Interview talk: bringing off a research instrument. *Sociology* 7(1): 31–48.

(1985) *Qualitative Methodology and Sociology.* Aldershot: Gower.

(1987) *Communication and Medical Practice. Social Relations in the Clinic.* London: Sage.

(1989) Telling convincing stories: a plea for cautious positivism in case-studies. In Glassner, B. and Moreno, J. (eds.) *The Qualitative–Quantitative Distinction in Social Sciences.* Dordrecht: Kluwer, pp. 57–77.

(1990) The social organization of HIV counselling. In Aggleton, P., Davies, P., Hart, G. (eds.) *AIDS: Individual, Cultural and Policy Dimensions.* Lewes: Falmer Press.

(1993) *Interpreting Qualitative Data. Methods for Analysing Talk, Text and Interaction.* London: Sage.

(1994) Ethnography and conversation analysis in the study of professional–client interaction: a question of 'How' and 'Why'. Paper delivered at the World Congress of Sociology, Bielefeld, Germany.

Silverman, D., Bor, R., Miller, R., Goldman, E. (1992) Advice-giving and advice-reception in AIDS counselling. In Aggleton, P., Davies, P., Hart, G. (eds.) *AIDS: Rights, Risk and Reason.* Lewes: Falmer Press.

Silverman, D. and Peräkylä, A. (1990) AIDS counselling: the interactional organization of talk about delicate issues. *Sociology of Health and Illness* 12 (3): 293–318.

Sinclair, J.M. and Coulthard, R.M. (1975) *Towards an Analysis of Discourse: the English Used by Teachers and Pupils.* Oxford University Press.

Sluzki, C. (1983) Process, structure and world-view: an integrated view on systemic models in family therapy. *Family Process* 22: 469–76.

Smith, D. and Kingston, P. (1980) Live supervision without a one-way screen. *Journal of Family Therapy* 2: 379–87.

Sorjonen, M.-L. and Heritage, J. (1991) And-prefacing as a feature of question design. In Laitinen, L., Nuolijärvi, P., Saari, M. (eds.)

Leikkauspiste. Kirjoituksia kielestä ja ihmisestä. Helsinki: SKS, pp. 59–74.

Speed, B., Seligman, P., Kingston, P., Cade, B. (1982) A team approach to therapy. *Journal of Family Therapy* 4: 271–84.

Stiles, W.B., Shapiro, D.A., Elliot, R. (1986) 'Are all psychotherapies equivalent?'. *American Psychologist* 41: 165–80.

Strong, P.M. (1979) *The Ceremonial Order of the Clinic: Parents, Doctors and Medical Bureaucracies.* London: Routledge and Kegan Paul.

Stubbs, M. (1983) *Discourse Analysis.* Oxford: Basil Blackwell.

Sudnow, D. (1967) *Passing On. The Social Organization of Dying.* Englewood Cliffs, NJ: Prentice-Hall.

Tannen, D. (1990) *Talking Voices.* Cambridge University Press.

Taylor, T.J. and Cameron, D. (1987) *Analysing Conversation: Rules and Units in the Structure of Talk.* Oxford: Pergamon Press.

Tomm, K. (1985) Circular interviewing: a multifaceted clinical tool. In Campbell, D. and Draper, R. (eds.) *Applications of Systemic Family Therapy: The Milan Approach.* London: Grune & Stratton.

Wahlström, J. (1992) *Merkitysten muodostuminen ja muuttuminen perheterapeuttisessa keskustelussa* [Semantic change in family therapy]. Jyväskylä: Jyväskylä Studies in Education, Psychology and Social Research 94.

West, C. (1983) 'Ask Me No Questions . . . '. An analysis of queries and replies in physician–patient dialogues. In Fisher S. and Todd, A.D. (eds.) *The Social Organization of Doctor–Patient Communication.* Washington DC: Centre for Applied Linguistics, pp. 75–106.

Wootton, A.J. (1989) Remarks on the methodology of conversation analysis. In Roger, D. and Bull, P. (eds.) *Conversation: An Interdiscplinary Perspective.* Clevedon: Multilingual Matters, pp. 238–58.

Wowk, M.T. (1989) Emotion talk. In Torode, B. (ed.) *Text and Talk as Social Practice.* Dordrecht: Foris, pp. 51–71.

Zimmerman, D.H. (1988) On conversation: the conversation analytic perspective. *Communication Yearbook 11*, pp. 406–32.

Index

For EU product safety concerns, contact us at Calle de José Abascal, 56–1°,
28003 Madrid, Spain or eugpsr@cambridge.org.

www.ingramcontent.com/pod-product-compliance
Ingram Content Group UK Ltd.
Pitfield, Milton Keynes, MK11 3LW, UK
UKHW010852090126
466816UK00011B/177